# Essential Child Psychiatry

*To Barbara, Zara, Jessica and George*

*For Churchill Livingstone*

*Publisher:* Lucy Gardner
*Copy Editor:* Susan Hunter
*Production Controller:* Mark Sanderson
*Sales Promotion Executive:* Douglas McNaughton

# Essential Child Psychiatry

**Peter Hoare** DM MRCPsych
Senior Lecturer in Child Psychiatry, Edinburgh University; Honorary Consultant,
Royal Hospital for Sick Children, Edinburgh, UK

Foreword by
**Neil McIntosh** MB BS BSc FRCP FRCPE
Edward Clark Professor of Child Life and Health, University of Edinburgh, UK

CHURCHILL LIVINGSTONE
EDINBURGH LONDON MADRID MELBOURNE NEW YORK AND TOKYO 1993

CHURCHILL LIVINGSTONE
Medical Division of Longman Group UK Limited

Distributed in the United States of America by Churchill
Livingstone Inc., 650 Avenue of the Americas, New York,
N.Y. 10011, and by associated companies, branches and
representatives throughout the world.

First published 1993

ISBN 0-443-04464-3

British Library Cataloguing in Publication Data
A catalogue record for this book is available from the British
Library.

Library of Congress Cataloging in Publication Data
A catalog record for this book is available from the library of
congress.

Produced by Longman Singapore Publishers (Pte) Ltd
Printed in Singapore

# Contents

# Contents

# Foreword

One of the greatest strengths of *Essential Child Psychiatry* is the ability of Peter Hoare to write a book which is both erudite and simple — a rare gift amongst medical practitioners. The book is free of jargon and on the occasions when specialist terminology is used there is an excellent glossary.

Psychiatric disturbance is seen in about 7–15% of children at any given age, and 50% of such disturbed children remain disturbed from childhood to adolescence and on to adult life. Such disturbance greatly affects the child's balance of health and development often leaving the child isolated, not only within the community but also within the family.

The frequency of psychiatric disturbance in children and the resulting unhappiness in the child and the family, mean that a basic understanding of the principles of child psychiatry is important for all students whether they intend to be general practitioners or paediatricians.

Most books on general paediatrics, affordable by undergraduates, are too sketchy to be informative even about the normal psychological development of children — an element fundamental for the appreciation of abnormal development. Although some large reference textbooks in general paediatrics may deal with well recognised conditions, they can allocate only one or two Chapters to the subject and their approach is often dogmatic. The openness and lack of dogmatism in *Essential Child Psychiatry* is refreshingly different. The breadth of its material means that although primarily aimed at undergraduates, it is extremely useful for general practitioners, paediatricians and any postgraduate dealing with parents and children.

The material is well organised. Its sequence is logical and the text is illustrated by examples and tables allowing the student to appreciate the subject and understand the theories of child development in their historical and philosophical context. The first Chapter on normal and abnormal psychological development briefly revues the theories of child development in a clear, interesting and stimulating way, revealing the complexity of the subject, the wide diversity of theories and the many unanswered questions. A clear disposition follows on how to recognise childhood psychopathology and the general features of disturbance. Before beginning the more traditional description of psychiatric problems and management, a most useful Chapter describes how children should be referred when there is a problem and how they should be assessed with their parents. The basic data that is needed and the specialised interview techniques and psychological tests that are used are simply explained.

The core of the work consists of ten Chapters, the first and last describing disturbances which occur in pre-school children and in adolescence. The other eight Chapters revue the disturbances of mood, conduct, emotion and elimination etc. seen in the preadolescent schoolchild. Each Chapter makes excellent use of Tables to draw out the critical elements of diagnosis and action. The final Chapters consider the particular emotional strains placed on children by chronic organic disease or handicap and explain important aspects of the law on childcare and common medicolegal and forensic problems.

As a general paediatrician with an undergraduate and postgraduate teaching commitment I have been aware for a long time of the turgid style of most works on child psychiatry. *Essential Child Psychiatry* is an enjoyable and informative book. It should have widespread appeal for those who would like further insights into child behaviour both normal and deviant, whether they are working for undergraduate or postgraduate examinations or simply wanting to broaden their understanding of child life and health.

1993 Neil Mcintosh

# Preface

Child psychiatrists are often asked to provide an overview of their subject, preferably in one hour, to a diverse group of medical personnel at the undergraduate and postgraduate levels of training. Medical students, psychiatrists and paediatricians in training as well as family doctors all require some working knowledge of the subject. Similar requests are also received from tutors in psychology, social work, occupational therapy and speech therapy. As I have often had to respond to such requests, I have devised over the years a series of lectures to cover the topic in a didactic but nevertheless wide-ranging manner. While hoping to convey the richness of the subject matter, I recognise that simple, clear presentation is essential to retain the interest of the reader and also to help him or her to acquire the necessary knowledge. This is the main aim of this short book.

Two other points have influenced the format of the book. First, I have made extensive use of tables and figures to summarise the key points of the text, so that the reader can use them as an aide-memoire and as a reference source. Second, I have quoted references liberally throughout the text in order to justify the statements made and also to provide the more interested reader with the opportunity to pursue the topic further.

The book has three sections: the first part reviews normal and abnormal development, the general features of childhood disturbance and the principles of diagnosis and assessment; the middle section describes the features of the main clinical syndromes; and the final section discusses a miscellaneous group of topics including mental handicap, the psychiatric aspects of chronic illness and treatment methods. I have given more emphasis to chronic illness and to treatment methods as I think these subjects are not well covered in the available comparable textbooks. I have also written a short chapter on adolescence to round off the subject in a more complete manner. The chapter on legal and forensic aspects is included because this topic is of increasing importance in contemporary child psychiatric practice. The last chapter on multiple choice questions is included for two reasons: this form of assessment is used increasingly in examinations; and secondly but more importantly, it gives the student a simple and reliable method of self-assessment. Hopefully, the inclusion of the explanatory section with the answers will assist the student further. A brief glossary is also provided for the reader with a non-medical background in order to help with the more specialised terms. My final point is about style. I have used the male gender throughout the book whenever this could refer to either sex as the alternative is cumbersome and wordy.

I would like to end by thanking Georgina Bentliff and Lucy Gardner from Churchill Livingstone for their unstinting support and encouragement in the preparation of the book. Similar heartfelt thanks are also extended to my secretary Sheila Clunas for her forbearance and patience in the completion of the book.

Edinburgh 1993                                                                          P.H.

# 1. Introduction

Child psychiatry is concerned with the assessment and treatment of children's emotional and behavioural problems. These problems are very common, with prevalence rates of 10–20% in several community studies (Rutter et al 1970b, Shepherd et al 1971, Richman et al 1982). The Isle of Wight study (Rutter et al 1970b) showed that less than one in ten disturbed children was seen by specialist psychiatric services with the majority looked after by general practitioners, paediatricians, community health doctors and other professionals working with children, such as teachers or residential care staff. Clearly, familiarity with the range and management of children's emotional and behavioural problems is essential for all doctors involved in the care of children.

Psychological disturbance in childhood is most usefully defined as an abnormality in at least one of three areas, emotions, behaviour or relationships. However, unlike most other branches of medicine, it is not helpful to regard these abnormalities as strictly defined disease entities with a precise aetiology, treatment or prognosis. Rather, it is preferable to regard them as deviations or departures from the norm which are distressing to the child or to those involved with his upbringing. Although child psychiatric disorders do not conform to the strict medical model of illness, this does not mean that the disorders are trivial or unimportant. Some disorders such as childhood autism or conduct disorder have major implications for the child's development and adjustment in adult life.

In childhood, the distinction between disturbance and normality is often imprecise or arbitrary. Isolated symptoms are common and not pathological. For example, many children will occasionally feel sad, unhappy or have temper tantrums. This does not mean however that the child is disturbed, as disturbance is determined by the number, frequency, severity and duration of symptoms rather than by the form of the symptomatology. In addition, disturbed children rarely have unequivocally pathological symptoms such as hallucinations or delusions. In clinical practice, it is often more important to establish why the child is the focus for concern rather than adopt the more narrow perspective of whether the child is disturbed or not.

Another distinctive feature of childhood psychiatric disturbance is that several factors rather than one contribute to the development of disturbance.

1

This makes their assessment and treatment more difficult, so that an essential prerequisite for successful treatment is the correct evaluation of the relative contribution of the different aetiological factors. Aetiological factors are usually categorised into two groups, constitutional and environmental. The former include hereditary factors, intelligence and temperament. The three major environmental influences are the family, schooling and the community. Another factor, physical illness or disability, if present, can have a profound effect on the child's development and on his vulnerability to disturbance.

Three other considerations are of general importance in understanding children's behaviour: the situation-specific nature of behaviour; the impact of current stressful life circumstances; and the role of the family. Several studies (Rutter et al 1970b, Shepherd et al 1971) have shown that children's behaviour varies markedly in different situations. For instance, a child may be a major problem at school, but not at home, or vice versa. Consequently, there may well be an apparent discrepancy between the account of the child's behaviour provided by the parents and that provided by the teachers. The most likely explanation for this discrepancy is that the child does indeed behave differently, as the demands and expectations on the child vary in the two situations. It is therefore essential to obtain several independent accounts about the child's behaviour wherever possible in order to obtain an accurate and realistic assessment of the problem. The situation-specific nature of the behaviour also has implications for treatment. It is important as well to explain to the parents and the teachers the reasons for the discrepancy, thereby reducing the chances of misunderstanding.

Children are immature and developing individuals. Childhood is also a period of life characterised by change and the necessity for adaptation. Consequently, it is not surprising that symptoms of disturbance may arise at times of stress when the demands upon the child are too great. Recent research (Goodyer et al 1985, Goodyer 1990) has shown that stressful life events are associated with an increased psychiatric morbidity among children, findings similar to those reported for adults (Brown & Harris 1978). Some stresses, such as the birth of a sibling or starting school, are of course normal and usually uneventful, whereas others, such as marital break-up or life-threatening illness, are serious with long-term implications for the child's well-being.

The child may cope successfully with these stresses, which as a result enhance the child's self-esteem and confidence. Alternatively, the child may be overwhelmed, responding with the development of symptomatic behaviour. The latter may involve regressive behaviour (behaving in a more immature, dependent fashion), or be more clearly maladaptive, for instance aggression, excessive anxiety or withdrawal. A crucial feature of the assessment procedure is the identification of the stressful factors that may be contributing to the problem, as this will influence treatment strategies and also the prognosis.

The family is a most powerful force for the promotion of health as well as for the production of disturbance in the child's life. Assessment of parenting qualities, the marital relationship and the quality of family interaction are essential components of child psychiatric practice. It is a frequent observation that it is the parents who are disturbed and not the child. One consequence of this observation is that in many cases the focus of treatment is likely to be the parents or the whole family rather than the referred child. Indeed in many instances, the main emphasis of treatment may be the promotion of normal healthy family interaction as much as in the specific treatment of the child's disturbed behaviour.

Finally, many disturbed children do not complain openly about their distress nor admit to problems. It is usually their parents or other adults involved with their care who bring the child to the attention of professionals. Disturbed children also frequently manifest their distress or unhappiness indirectly through the development of symptoms such as abdominal pain, aggression or withdrawal. Direct questioning of the child on first acquaintance is unlikely to reveal the true extent of the child's feelings and his degree of distress. Sensitive observation during the interview and the use of indirect approaches such as play therapy techniques are necessary to elicit a more accurate view of the child's feelings. This is only likely to be successful once a relationship of trust has been established between the child and the therapist.

# 2. Normal and abnormal psychological development

## INTRODUCTION

Children are not small adults, but developing individuals. A child aged 2 years is very different from a teenager, whereas a 25-year-old may not differ that much from someone 10 years older. During childhood, the child undergoes a remarkable transformation from a helpless, dependent infant to an independent, self-sufficient individual with his own views and outlook, capable of embarking on a career and living separately from his family. Knowledge of the mechanisms, processes and the sequences underlying these events is necessary in order to understand the nature of psychological disturbance in childhood. This knowledge also helps to define more clearly age-appropriate behaviour and to distinguish the pathological from the normal. This chapter has three sections: developmental theories, developmental psychopathology and personality development.

## DEVELOPMENTAL THEORIES

### Terminology

It is useful to define some key terms at the outset as they are often used interchangeably. *Growth* is usually defined as the incremental increase of a character, feature or attribute, whereas *maturation* is that aspect(s) of development mainly due to innate or endogenous factors. *Development* describes the changes in the organism's structure and behaviour that are systematically related to age. Many behaviours, for example walking or talking, have a substantial maturational component, whereas others, for instance emotional or social development, are strongly influenced by environmental factors. The continuous interaction between maturational and environmental factors throughout childhood helps to mould the personality development of the child.

Developmental theories tend to focus on at least one of three areas: cognitive, emotional or social. The various theories differ widely in their theoretical orientation, supporting empirical evidence and in the relative importance attributed to experience as an influence on development. No single theory is satisfactory, so that most clinicians use some parts of the various theories to explain different aspects of development.

Another important aspect of development is the acquisition of motor and visuo-spatial skills. These have a predominantly maturational component and are of more immediate interest to paediatricians than to child psychiatrists. Nevertheless, knowledge about motor development is useful for those involved with the care of disturbed children. Consequently, this aspect of development is summarised briefly later in the chapter.

## Stage and non-stage theories of development

There are two broad categories of developmental theory: stage theories and non-stage theories. Examples of the former are the theories of Piaget and Freud, whereas learning theory is an example of the latter. Stage theories have the following characteristics:

- Each stage represents a distinctive, coherent and structured mode of thinking, feeling etc
- Stages are hierarchically organised, so that later stages incorporate remnants from earlier stages
- Sequence of stages is invariable and no stage can be skipped or missed
- Stages are universal, though environmental factors can modify the form but not the structure of the stage
- Successive stages are more complex and integrated than earlier phases.

By contrast, non-stage theories regard development as continuous rather than discontinuous, so that they do not emphasise the distinction between periods of relative stability and times of change. In addition, they do not stipulate an invariable sequence to development, though they acknowledge that there is a hierarchical organisation of behaviour as development proceeds.

## COGNITIVE DEVELOPMENT

Jean Piaget, a Swiss psychologist, has elaborated the most comprehensive theory of cognitive development (Piaget 1929). Many of his conclusions were based on experiments conducted on his own children over a number of years. He has had a tremendous impact on educational concepts and teaching, particularly in primary schools over the last 30 years. More recently, the theoretical basis and correctness of Piaget's conclusions have been questioned by further empirical studies (see later this section). Despite these criticisms, Piaget's views remain the most useful account of cognitive development.

Piaget's theory is a well elaborated stage theory of development set within a biological framework. Survival of the fittest and most adaptable is the driving force underlying development. Accordingly, in order to survive, the individual must have the capacity to adapt to the demands of the environment. Cognitive development is the result of interaction between the individual and the environment. Four factors influence cognitive development:

- Progressive neurological development enables the child to appreciate new aspects of experience and to apply more complex reasoning
- The child has the opportunity to practise newly acquired skills
- The child has the opportunity for social interaction and to benefit from schooling
- Internal psychological mechanisms or structures emerge that allow the child to construct successively more complex cognitive models based on maturation and experience.

## Piaget's major concepts (Table 2.1)

Piaget believed that the genetic endowment provided the individual with an invariant pattern or structure to development. He proposed two types of cognitive structure, *schemas* and *operations*, to explain the process of development. Schemas are relatively simple mental structures present from birth onwards. They are the internal representations of some specific action or behaviour. Typical examples would include the sucking or grasping reflexes. By contrast, operations only arise much later in cognitive development and they are considerably more complex. They represent internal structures of a high order which have the distinctive feature that they are reversible. For example, multiplication is reversible by division.

The child adapts his cognitive structure to the demands of the environment through two main processes, *assimilation* and *accommodation*. The former refers to the incorporation of new objects, thoughts and behaviour into existing structures, whereas the latter describes the change of existing structures in response to novel experiences. A third structure, *equilibration*, is the means by which the individual balances the competing forces of assimilation and accommodation. In general, the child attends and learns to adapt to his environment most easily when there is a degree of novelty in the environment which challenges his curiosity, but which is not so strange that it becomes too confusing.

The following example illustrates the dynamic interaction between these processes. An 8-month-old child will be able to grasp certain objects, say a finger, but not something very small or very large. The gradual acquisition of the ability to grasp other-sized objects can be seen as an example of accommodation. However before the accommodation can take place, the objects must be in some sense 'graspable', that is the schema must to some degree assimilate the object before accommodation occurs. The schema has therefore been accommodated and equilibrium returns with the new type of grasping assimilated. The child is now able to proceed on to another task.

**Table 2.1**   Piaget's major concepts

| Concept | Description | Examples |
|---------|-------------|----------|
| Adaptation | Basic process of all human activity, including assimilation and accommodation | Pupils alter size according to brightness |
| | | Language changes according to whether the person is friend or stranger |
| Assimilation | Adaptation of experiences or objects in accordance with existing strategies or concepts | A baby assimilates when he/she reaches for a toy |
| | | Inclusion of new object into existing category |
| Accommodation | Modification of strategy as a result of new experience or information | Baby alters grasp to get hold of differently shaped object |
| | | Concept of justice changed after experience of war |
| Equilibration | The process of balancing assimilation and accommodation | Change of strategy to solve problem, e.g. from trial and error to systematic search |
| Schema | Internal representation of some specific action, present from birth | In the infant, sucking and grasping responses |
| Operations | Internal cognitive rules that arise during later childhood | Multiplication and division |
| | | Acquisition of conservation concepts for number, volume and weight |

## Piaget's stages of cognitive development (Table 2.2)

Piaget describes four main phases: sensorimotor, pre-operational, concrete operational and formal operational. The age range given for each stage is the average, though this can vary considerably depending upon intelligence, cultural background and socioeconomic factors. However, the order is assumed to be the same for all children. Schemas predominate in the sensorimotor and preoperational stages, operations in the concrete operational and formal operational stages.

### Sensorimotor (birth–2 years)

Initially, behaviour is dominated by innate reflexes such as feeding, sucking and following, hence the name for this stage. Gradually, the infant realises the distinction between *self* and *non-self*, namely where his body ends and the world outside begins. The infant also realises that his behaviour can influence the environment, so that intentional and purposeful behaviour begins. Finally, the infant achieves *object permanence*, whereby he recognises that an object still exists even though it is no longer visible. This is the beginning of the internal representations of objects, the forerunner of memory.

**Table 2.2**   Piaget's stages of cognitive development

| Stage | Age | Key features |
| --- | --- | --- |
| Sensorimotor | 0–2 years | Recognises self as distinct from other objects in the world |
| | | Able to initiate actions, e.g. to reach out to grasp object |
| | | Achieves object permanence (objects exist even when no longer visible) |
| Preoperational | 2–7 years | Uses language and is able to represent objects by images and words |
| | | Thinking is egocentric (difficulty in recognising another point of view) |
| | | Thinking is animistic (every object has feelings and thoughts) |
| | | Objects classified solely on basis of single feature, for instance colour or shape |
| Concrete operational | 7–12 years | Thinks logically about objects and events |
| | | Achieves conservation of number (age 6), volume (age 7) and mass (age 9) |
| | | Objects classified on several dimensions as well as in a rank series e.g. size |
| Formal operational | 12 years and upwards | Thinks logically about abstract propositions and is able to test hypotheses |
| | | Becomes concerned about the hypothetical, the future and ideological problems |

- The ages given are averages
- Rate of progression is dependent on intelligence, cultural background and socioeconomic factors
- Sequence is assumed to be the same for all children
- Schemas predominate in the sensorimotor and preoperational stages
- Operations predominate in the concrete operational and formal operational stages

*Pre-operational period (2–7 years)*

Language development greatly facilitates cognition, so that the individual begins to represent objects by symbols and words. Thinking is, however, *egocentric* and *animistic*. The former refers to the child's tendency to regard the world solely from his own position with the inability to see a situation from another viewpoint. Animistic thinking describes the child's tendency to regard everything in the world as endowed with feelings, thoughts and wishes. For instance, the moon is watching over you when you sleep, or again, the child says 'naughty door' when the door bangs behind him.

The child has problems with the principles of conservation for number, volume and mass. The essential principle underlying conservation is that the number, volume and mass of objects are not changed by any visual alteration in their display or appearance. For instance, the child readily believes that the more widely spaced of two rows of counters has more counters than the more densely packed row, or that there is more water in a tall beaker when it is poured from a shorter, more squat beaker.

The child also believes that every event has a preceding cause, rejecting the concept of chance or coincidence. Again, the child's moral sense is rigid and inflexible, so that punishment is invariable, irrespective of the circumstances. The child's concept of illness is radically different from that of the adult, with illness a consequence for misdeeds or a punishment for a misdemeanour.

### Concrete operational (7–12 years)

Thinking becomes more logical and less dominated by immediate perceptual experience or events such as changes of appearance or arrangement. Conservation of number, volume and mass is successively achieved during this period. The child becomes less egocentric, capable of seeing events from another person's standpoint. The child is able to appreciate and utilise reversibility, for example if 2 and 2 equals 4, then 4 minus 2 must equal 2.

### Formal operational (12 years and upwards)

This stage represents the most complex mode of thinking. Its main characteristics are the ability to think in an abstract fashion, to formulate general laws and principles and to devise and test hypotheses, an approach similar to that used in mathematics or in scientific investigation. An example of such reasoning is the following: Joan is fairer than Susan; Joan is darker than Anne. Who is the darkest? (Answer: Susan). Prior to the formal operational stage, the child would require the aid of dolls to solve this problem. (It should be pointed out that not everyone achieves this stage of thinking, even as an adult!) The content of thinking also alters markedly, with an emphasis on the hypothetical, the future and ideological problems.

### Critical comment on Piaget

Though most developmental psychologists accept the Piagetian idea of an orderly sequence to cognitive development, more recent experimental research has failed to demonstrate the existence of specific cognitive structures proposed by Piaget for the concrete and formal operational stages. This problem is highlighted by experiments showing that children are often consistently inconsistent in their approach to problem solving despite using the same cognitive structures. Additionally, the Piagetian explanation for the younger child's inability to solve conservation problems, for example the absence of the necessary cognitive structures, has been questioned by more recent studies (Bryant 1974, Donaldson 1978, Bee 1989) showing that the critical factor in the child's failure to solve such problems may be inadequate memory capacity rather than inadequate cognitive ability per se. These criticisms of Piaget are substantial, but they should not detract from the major conceptual contribution that he has made to the knowledge of cognitive development in children.

## Other aspects of cognitive development

Psychologists and psychiatrists have become increasingly interested in the development and application of cognitive theory to the understanding and treatment of psychiatric disorders (Beck et al 1979, McAdam & Gilbert 1985, Hawton et al 1989). The use of cognitive therapy in the treatment of psychiatric disorders is discussed in Chapter 17.

Cognitive therapy proposes that the individual's beliefs or cognitions determine his mood, outlook and behaviour. This idea of cognitive set is similar in some ways to the Piagetian notion of schema. Three key aspects of this cognitive appraisal are the individual's views about a) himself, b) the world and c) the future. Cognitive therapy explains depression in the following manner: when a person is depressed, his thoughts are self-defeating and he commits certain cognitive errors. Three examples of these are given below:

- *minimalisation*: distorting evidence so that a positive achievement is not fully recognised. Example: 'So I got very good marks in my exams – anyone could if they worked as hard as I did!'
- *personalisation*: blaming oneself for someone else's behaviour when there is no justification for this. Example: 'The reason my parents separated is because of me.'
- *dichotomous* or *absolute thinking*: all experiences are placed in one of two opposing categories, 'black' or 'white', and the extremely negative view is taken. Example: 'I'm no good at tennis, so I'm bound to be useless at any other sport.'

Treatment with cognitive therapy involves the exploration into the style and content of the distorted thinking in order to enable the person to think in a more realistic manner and to function more adaptively.

### Self-concept and self-esteem (Harter 1983)

The first phase in the development of the self-concept is a sense of separateness or separate self, that is *self* versus *non-self*. This is one of the most important achievements of the sensorimotor period in Piaget's model. Along with the attainment of object permanence and intentional behaviour, this development enables the infant to explore and to investigate his environment with considerably more confidence. The newly acquired notion of selfness is shown clearly by the infant's ability for self-recognition. This is usually acquired around 18 months, though some rudiments of self-recognition may come earlier. The child's first categories or dimensions are usually age, gender and sex, so that a 3–5-year-old begins to label himself and other people as 'big', 'little', 'young' or 'old'. School-age children expand their self definition to include their likes and dislikes as well as more explicit comparisons with other children. During adolescence, there is an extended period of re-assessment and re-evaluation of one's self, corresponding to Erikson's 'identity crisis/identity diffusion' phase (see below).

An important facet of the self-concept is the evaluative, that is the individual's favourable or unfavourable assessment of himself. This aspect of the self-concept is usually referred to as *self-esteem*. James (1890) provided a useful way to conceptualise self-esteem. He believed that self-esteem was a ratio of successes to pretensions or of attainments to aspirations with a value around unity indicating high self-esteem.

Self-esteem has also attracted increasing interest from developmental psychologists and child psychiatrists in recent years. This is probably linked with the increasing application of cognitive theory to the understanding and treatment of psychiatric disorders. Bee (1989), reviewing recent studies of self-esteem in children and adolescents, concluded that children with high self-esteem seemed to do better academically at school, saw themselves as in control of their own destiny, had more friends and got along better with their families. Children with high self-esteem tend also to come from families where independent achievements are valued and praised and in which there is a warm, affectionate relationship between children and parents with clear limits set upon the children's behaviour. These findings echo those of Baumrind (1972), who found that children with high self-esteem had parents whose parental style was characterised as *authoritative* (clear limits, responsive and interested) in contrast to either *authoritarian* (detached, controlling and less warm) or *permissive* (non-controlling and non-demanding but quite warm and affectionate).

Interestingly, Bee (1989) noted that previous studies had showed that there were gender differences in the association between popularity and maturity. More mature girls tended to be popular and also leaders of their group, whereas the most popular boys tended to be less mature, with interests centred mainly around their friends and their acceptance by the peer group. By contrast, the more mature boys tended to be rather introspective, with an emphasis on the achievement of future goals.

Recently, psychologists have attempted to devise satisfactory instruments to measure self-esteem in childhood. Harter (1985) reported on the development of a new questionnaire to assess self-esteem in children. The questionnaire is a 36-item self-completed questionnaire which measures global self-worth as well as five separate subscales:

- scholastic performance
- social acceptance
- athletic competence
- physical appearance
- behavioural conduct.

The psychometric properties of the questionnaire, including internal reliability and factor analysis, have been thoroughly tested on a population basis (Harter 1985). Hoare and colleagues (Hoare et al 1992) have now completed a British standardisation, so that it should be possible to use the newly modified questionnaire on British populations with some degree of confidence. This modified questionnaire could be useful in several situations: to measure the continuity or discontinuity of self-esteem throughout childhood; to assess the impact of stressful events on the child, for instance the onset of illness; and to compare groups of children with different illnesses or handicaps.

## THEORIES OF EMOTIONAL AND SOCIAL DEVELOPMENT

This section discusses four theories devoted to social and emotional development in childhood. The theories differ markedly in their theoretical basis, the scope of their explanatory theories and the amount of independent supporting evidence. Three of the theorists, Freud, Erikson and Bowlby, have a common background in psychoanalytic thinking, whereas the fourth, the social learning theory, is based upon the application of learning theory principles to various aspects of the child's development. While social and emotional development is discussed separately, this aspect of development is closely affected by cognitive development and in turn affects cognitive development.

### Freudian or psychoanalytic theory (Table 2.3)

Freud (1953) elaborated the most comprehensive theory of emotional development, mainly derived from clinical work with adult patients. Others, including his daughter Anna, Melanie Klein and Winnicott, have extended and developed psychoanalytic concepts as a result of their own work with child patients. The contribution of these writers will be mentioned briefly at the end of this section.

Freudian theory emphasises the biological and maturational compo- nents of development with an invariant sequence to development for everyone. Like Piaget's, this is a stage or phase theory with the individual progressing successively through each phase. A major criticism of Freudian theory is that its concepts do not lend themselves readily to empirical or scientific investigation, so that it is difficult to prove or more importantly, disprove the validity of the theory. Freud proposed

**Table 2.3**   Freud's stages of psychosexual development

| Stage | Age | Major developmental task | Adult characteristics arising from incomplete resolution of the stage |
| --- | --- | --- | --- |
| Oral | 0–1 | Weaning | Addictive behaviour such as smoking, drinking and overeating; also passivity and gullibility |
| Anal | 2–3 | Toilet training | Obsessional, obstinacy or the opposite (extreme untidiness, for example) |
| Phallic | 4–5 | Oedipus complex: identification with parent of same sex | Vanity, recklessness (and the opposite) |
| Latency | 6–12 | Development of ego defence mechanisms | None |
| Genital | 13–18 | Mature sexual intimacy in adulthood | Adults who have successfully integrated earlier stages should emerge from this stage with a clear sense of their own identity and interests |

that the individual goes through five stages prior to adulthood, a) oral, b) anal, c) phallic, d) latency and e) genital. These terms refer to the major developmental task or potential conflict that the individual has to achieve or resolve during this period.

*Oral stage (0–1 year)*

The oral region (mouth, lips and tongue) is the main source of satisfaction or pleasure. Adequate and regular feeding is of prime importance to the infant. There should however be a balance between too much and too little. Otherwise, the infant becomes over-involved or 'fixated' at that stage, and is unable to make the transition to the next developmental stage. One consequence of the unsatisfactory resolution of a particular stage is that the individual is said to manifest some of the traits or characteristics of this phase in later adult life. For instance, incomplete resolution of the oral stage is said to provide the basis for the psychopathology of addictive behaviour such as overeating, smoking or drinking.

*Anal stage (2–3 years)*

The main feature of this stage is the child's acquisition of voluntary bowel and bladder control. The child becomes increasingly aware of his ability to regulate and modify his excretory and digestive functions. The increased control of these functions is matched by similar gains in locomotor and cognitive skills. The child derives enjoyment and pleasure from increasing control over bodily functions as well as from his developing autonomy.

Toilet training is seen as the first and also as the prototype of co-operative activity between the child and the parent. The parent–child interaction must be a balance between independence and compliance, oppositionality and co-operation. Ensuring the successful completion of toilet training requires adaptability and sensitivity by the parent because of the child's immaturity and also because of the child's enjoyment of oppositional behaviour. Too rigid and/or too flexible an approach is said to influence the child's emerging personality with an undue emphasis on over-control or alternatively its opposite, under-control. The adult personality characteristics of tidiness and obsessionality are regarded as the remnants of an incomplete resolution of the anal phase.

*Phallic stage (3–5 years)*

The child becomes increasingly aware of his/her genitals, the enjoyment to be derived from them and the differences between the sexes. Freud developed these ideas most clearly for boys and coined the term *Oedipus complex* to describe the conflictual situation arising between the boy and his parents during this phase. He proposed the following sequence of events to explain the development of the Oedipus complex: the boy becomes attached to his mother, leading to rivalry with the father for the affection of the mother; the boy also recognises that his father is powerful and would be likely to punish him severely if he pursues the rivalry too far (the basis for the castration complex). The resolution of the crisis is for the boy to 'identify' with his father and use him as a role model, so that he can hopefully not only reduce the risk of retaliation but also increase his own power by emulating his father. Similar explanations are applied for the girls' sexual conflict, for which the term *Electra complex* is used.

The conflictual situation is also thought to explain the emergence of another mental structure, the *superego* or conscience. The child's realisation that he may do wrongful things, particularly involving his parents, induces a sense of guilt or shame. This notion of guilt is gradually extended and developed to include most situations where an ethical or moral conflict can arise. The other prominent feature of this stage is the emergence of jealous and competitive feelings towards peers and siblings. The child's developing social skills ensure that peer group activity is an important feature of play and daily activity.

The unsatisfactory resolution of the Oedipus conflict manifests itself in later life as sexual conflicts concerning sexual role and identity and also the inability to form intimate sexual relationships.

*Latency stage (5–12 years)*

This period is so called because of its relative tranquillity compared with the emotionally stormy periods of the phallic and genital periods. Freud believed that sexual feelings subside after the resolution of the oedipal crisis. The child focuses his attention on the same-sex parent, leading to increased identification with and role-modelling on this parent. Similarly, peer group relationships are predominantly with the same sex. Though overt interest in sexual matters does decrease during this period, Freud certainly oversimplified his description when he maintained that they were absent.

A major feature of this period is the establishment of the ego mechanisms of defence. Anxiety and its management have always been a pivotal part in the psychoanalytic theory of neurosis. Anna Freud (1936), partly through her observations of child patients, postulated that an important function of the developing *ego* (the reality-testing function of the child's mental processes) was to manage the excessive anxiety that arises from the inevitable stressful nature of some childhood experiences. Anna Freud believed that these mechanisms are protective and adaptive for the child, providing that they are not used excessively and thereby preventing the child from experiencing manageable amounts of stress. The exposure to stress and anxiety is essential for the child's well-being, as it provides the child with the opportunity to learn to cope with unpleasant or distressing feelings. Successful management of the anxiety also improves the child's self-esteem, as the child has an enlarged repertoire of coping skills.

Table 2.4 defines and gives examples of the main defence mechanisms. The most common defence mechanisms used in children are as follows:

- *denial* – the reluctance to accept the impact of a potentially stressful event or situation
- *rationalisation* – the attempt to excuse or minimise the psychological consequences of an event
- *regression* – the occurrence of developmentally immature behaviour, often at times of stress
- *displacement* – the transfer of hostile or aggressive feelings from their original source to another person, usually less powerful or important.

Other mechanisms such as *sublimation* or *intellectualisation* are not as frequently developed in children, though they may become apparent in adolescence and in early adult life. Defence mechanisms become incorporated into the individual's repertoire of responses to anxiety-inducing situations. Individual variation in the range and strength of the defence mechanisms is the norm, with the individual pattern becoming established during adolescence.

Finally, another variation of the defence mechanism in childhood is the phenomenon of *somatisation*. Here, instead of the anxiety being transformed into a psychological symptom as with a defence mechanism, the anxiety is transposed into physical symptoms. Common examples include abdominal pain, headaches and limb pains of unexplained origin.

**Table 2.4** Ego mechanisms of defence

| Name | Definition | Example |
| --- | --- | --- |
| Denial | Denial is the inability or reluctance to accept the psychological impact of a potentially stressful event or situation | The child denies stealing even though it is obvious that he is responsible. This is because the open admission of the theft would induce such a loss of self esteem and sense of guilt that it becomes impossible, hence the use of denial |
| Rationalisation | Rationalisation is a strategy to excuse or minimise the psychological consequences of an event | The child who fails to gain selection to the school football team may say to his friend 'I don't like football anyway, so I am not bothered about playing for the team' |
| Regression | Regression is the occurrence of developmentally immature behaviour, often at times of stress | Many children have a recurrence of enuresis at the start of primary school |
| Displacement | Displacement is the transfer of hostile or aggressive feelings from their original source to another person usually less important | A school child may be aggressive in the playground with other pupils rather than be aggressive towards the teacher in the classroom |
| Reaction formation | Transfer of hostile or aggressive impulses into their opposite, more socially desirable form | The over-solicitous concern for the welfare of his sibling may indicate that the child has underlying feelings of jealousy and rivalry |
| Sublimation | Transfer of unacceptable impulses into a socially accepted form | Aggressive and competitive impulses are utilised in the promotion of athletic and sporting prowess |
| Intellectualisation | Discussion of emotionally significant event in an abstract or logical manner without acknowledgement of the emotional component | Improved prognosis for childhood leukaemia means that the emotional distress caused by the condition is now much less |

*Genital stage (12–18 years)*

The endocrinological and physiological changes occurring at puberty rekindle the individual's interest in sexual matters and heterosexual relationships. Freud regarded heterosexual relationships as the norm. A good outcome of this stage is dependent on how well or otherwise the individual has dealt with earlier stages. Two stages, the oral and the phallic, are particularly crucial. Poor resolution of the oral phase may preclude the foundation of close, trusting relationships with the opposite sex, whilst unresolved phallic conflicts may lead to confusion over sexual role and behaviour. In addition to the successful establishment of the sexual role, the older adolescent has other tasks such as separation from parents, career choice and the acquisition of own ethical and moral values.

## Erikson

Erikson (1965), a trained psychoanalyst, was particularly interested in and influenced by anthropology, so that his major contribution has been to give developmental theory a social and cultural dimension, hence his term *psychosocial* rather than *psychosexual*. He elaborated a phase or stage theory covering the whole lifespan from birth to death. Each stage had a development task with success or failure polarised as two extremes or opposites. Like Freud, he believed that the unsuccessful or unresolved residues of earlier phases had a continued impact on later adjustment and on the successful resolution of subsequent phases. For example, an unsatisfactory first phase leading to a basic sense of mistrust rather than trust is likely to cause major problems with personal relationships in later life.

There are five important stages of the theory as applied to childhood (Table 2.5).

*Phase I – Trust versus mistrust (age 0–1).* This phase occupies the first year and is mainly concerned with the establishment of secure and stable relationships, primarily between mother and child. This idea is clearly similar to that of Freud and Bowlby (see below). The successful outcome, the establishment of basic trust, is that the child believes that the world is predictable, safe and secure and that he is able to exert an influence over the outcome of events. By contrast, a basic sense of mistrust implies that the world is cruel, erratic and unable to meet the child's needs. The role of the care-giver, usually the mother, is crucial to the achievement of a successful outcome.

*Phase II – Autonomy versus shame, doubt (age 2–3).* This phase is characterised by the child's increasing powers of mobility and locomotor skills, providing the basis for the development of some independence and autonomy. The new skills are initially very vulnerable and only precariously developed, so that the child's self-confidence is easily undermined leading to the negative outcome of shame and doubt. The role of the parent(s) is crucial in fostering the sense of achievement rather than failure.

*Phase III – Initiative versus guilt (age 3–5).* The child's rapidly ex-panding skills, particularly in language, enable the child to initiate and sustain activities, so that exploration and activity are the order of the day. If the child's exuberance and enthusiasm are too restricted or thwarted by parents or others, then despondency and defeatism predominate, leaving the child with a sense of guilt.

*Phase IV – Industry versus inferiority (age 6–12 years).* Schooling and peer relationships dominate this period, so that the successful child becomes literate, numerate and socially integrated with his peers. Failure to

**Table 2.5** Erikson's life cycle theory of development

| Age | Phase | Task |
|---|---|---|
| 0–1 | Trust versus mistrust | Establishment of social relationships<br>*Good outcome* – secure, stable relationships<br>*Bad outcome* – insecure, unsatisfactory relationships |
| 2–3 | Autonomy versus shame, doubt | Beginning of independence and of skill acquisition<br>*Good outcome* – capable and competent<br>*Bad outcome* – dependent and unsure |
| 4–5 | Initiative versus guilt | Successful pursuit of certain goals or aims<br>*Good outcome* – confident about skills<br>*Bad outcome* – hesitant, uncertain |
| 6–12 | Industry versus inferiority | Acquisition of scholastic and social skills<br>*Good outcome* – literate, numerate and socially integrated<br>*Bad outcome* – failure to acquire scholastic skills, socially isolated |
| 13–18 | Identity versus role confusion | Clear sense of own individuality and of aims in life<br>*Good outcome* – suitable career choice, satisfactory heterosexual relationships<br>*Bad outcome* – uncertain of career, poor peer relationships |
| 19–25 | Intimacy versus isolation | Establishment of satisfactory long-term intimate relationships<br>*Good outcome* – stable relationships and good career<br>*Bad outcome* – poor intimate relationships and career choice |
| 26–40 | Generativity versus stagnation | Rear children in stable union<br>*Good outcome* – successful career, family stability<br>*Bad outcome* – poor career attainment, unstable relationships |
| 41+ | Ego integrity versus despair | Acknowledgement of life's successes and failures<br>*Good outcome* – acceptance of life's limitations and vagaries<br>*Bad outcome* – despondency and despair |

achieve these goals leads to a sense of inferiority and inadequacy with a low self-esteem.

*Phase V – Identity versus identity diffusion.* Two tasks, 'sexual identity' and 'career identity', are the major focus of interest for the individual. Independence from the family and developing one's own value system become important during late adolescence. The successful accomplishment of these tasks provides the individual with a strong sense of identity and self confidence, enabling the adolescent to make the transition to adulthood relatively easily. By contrast, poor peer relationships and uncertain career choice are prominent features of an unsatisfactory adjustment, resulting in role diffusion and an aimless lack of direction.

Erikson's writings are a compelling and coherent account of development with their emphasis on the active interaction between the individual and his environment shaping the final outcome. A major weakness is the lack of empirical evidence to support his conclusions. It should be said, however, that Erikson's ideas on identity and self-esteem have many similarities to the contemporary ideas of modelling and cognitive appraisal proposed by cognitive and behavioural theories.

## Attachment theory

### Development of attachment

A characteristic of human beings is their predilection for and interest in social relationships. Although Freud and Erikson refer to social relationships, it is only recently with the elaboration of attachment theory by Bowlby (1969) and Ainsworth (1982) that a plausible theory for this phenomenon has been described. Attachment theory proposes that social relationships develop in response to the mutual biological and psychological needs of the mother and the infant. The mother–infant interaction promotes social relationships. Each member of the diad has a repertoire of behaviours that facilitates interaction: the infant by crying, smiling and vocalisation and the mother by facial expression, vocalisation and gaze. A mother can also regulate the infant's state of alertness – for instance, soothing the child by rocking and stroking and stimulating the child by talking and facial expression.

*Attachment* describes the infant's predisposition to seek proximity to certain people and to be more secure in their presence. Bowlby maintains that there is a biological basis for this behaviour, as it has been found extensively in other primates (Harlow & Harlow 1969, Hinde & Spencer-Booth 1970) as well as in most human societies. The behaviour has considerable survival and adaptive value for the species, as it enables the dependent infant to explore the environment from a secure base and also to use the base as a place of safety at times of distress.

Before 7 months, the infant is not selective or discriminating in its social relationships. The main qualities facilitating social interaction are novelty and reciprocity, that is, the infant is attracted to objects that are visually interesting as well as responsive, qualities ideally shown by the human face. From 7 months onwards, the infant begins to develop selective attachments, initially usually to the mother but not exclusively to her. The infant gradually extends the number of attachment figures, so that a hierarchy of attachments based upon their strength emerges, with the child showing clear preferences for different individuals. Though Bowlby refers to a *critical period*, that is, a time when attachments develop most readily, there is no convincing evidence that this is so important in the development of human relationships.

Ainsworth (1982) emphasises the importance of the quality of the attachment behaviour between the infant and parent(s). She distinguishes between secure and insecure attachments, with the former seen as preferable to the latter. Ainsworth also devised a technique, the so called *stranger situation*, to measure the security of attachment. The technique involves observing the child in the following situations:

- with the mother
- with the mother and a stranger
- alone with a stranger
- completely alone
- reunited with the stranger
- reunited with mother.

The child's responses to these situations are used to classify the child into *securely attached* or *insecurely attached*, the latter being further categorised into *detached/avoidant* and *resistant/ambivalent*. Table 2.6 shows the main characteristics of the three types of response.

**Table 2.6**  Behaviour of securely and insecurely attached infants in the stranger situation

| Group | Behaviour |
| --- | --- |
| Securely attached: | Baby seeks and maintains contact with or proximity to mother |
| | Infant clearly prefers mother to stranger |
| | Infant greets mother with smile or cry after separation |
| Insecurely attached: detached/avoidant | Child avoids or ignores mother at reunion |
| | Little tendency to seek contact with mother |
| | Child does not hold on if picked up |
| | Child treats stranger about the same as mother |
| Insecurely attached: resistant/ambivalent | Infant actively seeks contact with mother |
| | Infant seems ambivalent as if wanting contact but resisting |
| | Infant distressed when separated from mother |

Bowlby, based upon his work with children who had suffered severe deprivation and also from observing the effects of hospitalisation on children, described the sequence of reactions following a period of separation, the so-called *separation anxiety response*. He maintained that there was a recognisable sequence to this experience which he categorised into protest, despair and detachment:

- *Protest* is the initial response, in which the child is overtly distressed at the absence of the familiar person
- The continued absence of this person subsequently leads to the period of *despair*, which is categorised as one of grief and mourning for the absent figure
- Finally, if unresolved, the child enters the phase of *detachment*, in which the child has abandoned hope of the return of the attachment figure and appears uninterested and indifferent, even when the person returns.

The separation response is regarded by Bowlby and colleagues as the prototype for the experience of loss in later life. He maintains that the quality of the first attachment response is crucial in determining the success or otherwise of subsequent interpersonal relationships. Additionally, the separation response is seen as similar in many ways to the depressive reaction following the experience of loss. Despite their attractiveness, independent evidence in support of these ideas is not well substantiated.

The term *bonding* has been used to describe the persistence of relationships over time, that is, the child's capacity to retain the relationship despite the absence of the other individual. Much of the infant's behaviour promotes the development of attachments by ensuring close proximity and interaction with the mother. These ideas have many implications for obstetric and paediatric practice, and for the reduction in the stress associated with hospitalisation, as well as providing some insight into the possible origins of non-accidental injury in childhood.

## Other contributions to psychoanalytic thinking on child development

Two other people, Klein and Winnicott, have made important contributions to the theory of child development and to the practice of child psychotherapy. Melanie Klein (1932, 1948) believed that the infant's fantasy life in the first year was crucial for subsequent personality development. Primitive defence mechanisms such as *projection, projective identification* and *splitting* arise at that time, and are seen as the forerunners of later 'psychotic' mechanisms. The first stage in development is the *paranoid/schizoid* position, where the infant attempts to deal with the frightening and hostile world. Subsequently, the infant realises that the source of the conflict resides within himself, leading to the *depressive* position around the age of 1 year. The major developmental task for the child is to work through these feelings and to make 'reparation' for the fantasised attacks on the mother. Adult analysts treating patients with schizophrenia or borderline personality disorder have found Kleinian concepts particularly helpful.

Winnicott (1957, 1958), who had a paediatric training, developed important ideas about maternal role, for instance *good-enough mothering*, and other ideas such as the *true self*, the *false self* and the use of *transitional objects* by the child to reduce and allay anxiety. His therapeutic contributions also included the development of the *squiggle game* between the child and the therapist, whereby the therapist interprets the child's ambiguous drawings in terms of underlying anxieties.

## Social learning theories (Table 2.7)

This umbrella term has been used to describe those theories that derive from the application of findings from experimental psychology to the study of child development. Social learning theories differ from the other theories discussed in this section in the following ways:

- they are not stage theories
- they are not solely concerned with childhood but can be applied to all age groups
- they are based on learning theory principles
- they are ahistorical in their approach to understanding behaviour, that is, they concentrate on contemporary circumstances for explaining behaviour rather than emphasising the role of previous events or experiences.

Several important consequences arise from this approach. The theories do not regard child development as an invariant, unalterable or rigid sequence of development but maintain rather that cognition, language and experience shape and modify the child's behaviour. Cognition and language are crucial ingredients as they are the prerequisites for the child to understand and make sense of his world. These abilities enable the parents to communicate with the child about the world, and also enable the child to communicate with the parent. Experience is vital, not only because it provides the opportunity for various behaviours to emerge, but also because it influences the outcomes or contingencies of behaviour, thereby providing the basis for the modification of behaviour.

The main principle underlying the social learning theory approach is the application of learning theory to the understanding of children's behaviour. Psychologists commonly define learning as: 'a permanent change in behaviour as a result of experience'. Consequently, understanding the major influences of behaviour is an important aspect of experimental and clinical psychology. Psychologists distinguish many types of learning, with a comparable number of theories to explain the phenomena. The three most relevant to child development will be mentioned here: these are a) learning

**Table 2.7**    Key terms in learning theory

| Term | Definition |
|---|---|
| Classical conditioning | A major type of learning in which an automatic unconditioned response (UR) such as a reflex becomes triggered to a new cue, called the conditioned stimulus (CS), after the CS has been paired several times with the original unconditioned stimulus (US) |
| Conditioned stimulus | In classical conditioning this is the stimulus that, after being paired a number of times with an unconditioned stimulus, comes to trigger the unconditioned response |
| Extinction | A term used in operant conditioning to describe the weakening or disappearance of a response due to the absence of the previously reinforcing event |
| Modelling or observational learning | Learning of behaviour through observing someone else perform the behaviour |
| Negative reinforcement | The strengthening of a behaviour by the removal or cessation of an unpleasant stimulus |
| Operant conditioning | A type of learning in which behaviours are increased or decreased as a function of the events that follow them (the reinforcers) |
| Positive reinforcement | The strengthening of a behaviour by the presentation of some pleasurable or positive stimulus |
| Punishment | The unpleasant consequences administered after some undesired behaviour in order to extinguish the behaviour |
| Unconditioned response | In classical conditioning this is the basic unlearned response that is triggered by the unconditioned stimulus |
| Unconditioned stimulus | In classical conditioning this is the cue or signal that automatically triggers the unconditioned response |

by direct reinforcement, b) learning by imitation and 3) learning by induction.

These theories highlight the importance of the *social context* in which learning occurs. The antecedents and consequences of behaviour determine whether the behaviour increases or decreases in frequency. The present dictates the outcome and the past is only important in that previous experience may influence the response bias or preference in the present circumstances.

### Learning by direct reinforcement

Reinforcement, that is, the presentation or removal of a stimulus after a response which alters the subsequent frequency of that response, is the central idea underlying this approach to the acquisition or modification of behaviour. There are two major paradigms or examples with this type of learning, *stimulus-contingent* or *classical conditioning* and *response-contingent* or *operant conditioning*.

*Stimulus-contingent reinforcement,* originally studied by Pavlov, is as follows: an unconditioned stimulus (UCS) is presented, thereby eliciting a reflex unconditioned response (UCR), e.g. the presentation of food elicits salivation from the animal. Subsequently, another neutral stimulus (CS), e.g. a bell, is presented simultaneously with the UCS. Repeated presentation of the two stimuli leads over time to the establishment of a conditioned response or CR, in this case salivation, occurring in response to the sole presentation of the condition stimulus, in this case the bell. The response has become conditioned to the new stimulus.

*Response-contingent reinforcement* was extensively studied by Skinner. Here, the paradigm is that the individual's behaviour is modified or shaped according to the contingencies or reinforcers associated with that behaviour. For instance, pigeons can be trained to peck one shape or colour on a disc rather than another by rewarding one behaviour with some food and not the other. The strength and persistence of the behaviour is influenced by the schedule or pattern of reinforcement.

It is evident that these two types of learning can easily result in adaptive or maladaptive patterns of behaviour depending upon the circumstances. For instance, classical conditioning can result in the child developing adaptive avoidance of dangerous situations or equally a maladaptive response, for instance becoming phobic about school or social situations. Similarly, operant conditioning can lead to the establishment of adaptive or 'socialised' patterns of behaviour or alternatively produce maladaptive behaviour, for example a mother inadvertently reinforcing temper tantrums by appeasing the child with sweets.

The principles of learning theory have been applied extensively in the treatment of children's behaviour problems (see Ch. 17).

*Learning by imitation*

Everyday observation shows clearly that 'observable' learning or imitation is a common method for altering behaviour. Bandura (1969) showed that observation or modelling of behaviour occurred readily among children in many situations. Two factors influence the acquisition of such behaviour, the direct or inherent consequences of the behaviour and the indirect consequences. For example, a child may observe that a person who greets someone in a friendly situation is usually happy themselves (*direct effect*) and in turn this behaviour is usually followed by a warm response from another person (*indirect effect*). The two consequences are seen as desirable by most children, so that pro-social behaviour is therefore promoted. Many people believe that the alleged adverse effects of television violence on children arise from the child witnessing a deviant role-model who is apparently successful in many situations.

*Learning by induction*

Though conditioning and modelling may explain the acquisition of more simple behaviours, it is more difficult to explain the contingencies for more complex and mature social behaviour. The *cognitive–behavioural model* or *learning by induction* maintains that in order for the individual to acquire more complex and sophisticated behaviour, he needs to be able to extract the general principles underlying the behaviour, that is, to induce from the particular to the general. As children mature, their increased cognitive capacity enables them to establish some general principles governing pro-social behaviour, for example 'they can see the wood for the trees'. Parents have a crucial role through the parent–child relationship in the facilitation of this development in the child. These cognitive ideas of learning are similar to Piaget's notion of abstract or formal operational thinking.

## SPECIAL TOPICS

### Language development

Language acquisition plays a central role in the child's development. It facilitates the emergence of complex cognitive skills such as reasoning and abstract thinking as well as enabling the child to communicate with other people. The processes and factors influencing language development are complex and not fully understood. Instead of attempting to discuss these issues in detail, a brief summary is provided.

Language is commonly defined as a system of symbols with recognised meanings that enable an individual to send and to receive an infinite variety of messages. The two key elements of the definition, the symbols and the infinite variety of messages, emphasise that language is distinct from other sounds by its ability to communicate meaning. The development of language follows a consistent pattern in most children and in most cultures, though some variation does occur. Several phases are delineated: a) the prelinguistic stage, b) the word stage, c) the sentence stage and d) the acquisition of rules stage.

*The pre-linguistic stage (birth–1 year)*

This proceeds through crying, cooing, babbling and echolalia, the repetition of the last heard phrase or sound.

*Crying* is the first means by which the infant uses sound to communicate. The infant has a repertoire of crying sounds to indicate various types of distress or problem. Mothers soon learn to discriminate between the different varieties, and many are able to distinguish the crying of their own infant from that of others. In some cases, the quality of the infant's crying is indicative of an underlying abnormality.

*Cooing* (beginning around one month) is the production of vowel sounds, particularly *ooh, ooh, ooh*, hence the name. It is usually a sign of pleasure or contentment, so that it is the source of mutual satisfaction for mother and infant.

*Babbling* (around 6 months onwards) is the addition of a consonant to a vowel to produce a syllable such as *ba, gi* and *da*. Interestingly, the babbling sounds produced are common to all cultures and often includes sounds that the infant has not heard. Babbling sounds are subsequently elaborated into more complex structures using *echolalia* to produce sounds such as *da, da, da, da* and *gi, gi, gi, gi.*

### The word stage

Words, defined as symbols that consistently refer to the same object(s), appear from 9 months onwards. Initially, the words are only intelligible to someone who knows the child, and are frequently used to convey a whole sentence of meaning, the so-called *holophrase*. The acquisition of new words is also slow at the beginning, so that an 18-month-old will typically have a vocabulary of 40–50 words, mostly nouns referring to a class of object or persons. The child's ability to understand language (*receptive language skills*) is more advanced than the production of words (*expressive language skills*). New word categories are acquired in an orderly sequence: nouns first, followed by verbs. Prepositions, adjectives and adverbs do not appear until the end of the second year, followed by pronouns and conjunctions.

### The sentence stage

Around 18 months, the child begins to combine two words to form a sentence, an important landmark for the child and parent. Typically, the first sentences are noun–verb action statements such as 'daddy gone'. Such sentences are often described as *telegraphic*, as only essential words are included.

### Acquisition of rules stage

From 18 months onwards, rapid progress is made in the length, complexity and precision of sentences. Children begin to use rules in a consistent fashion to generate more complex sentences. Important rules are inflections (adding -*ing* to make 'running', 'jumping' etc.), prepositions ('in' and 'on'), plurals -*s* ('cats'), irregular past ('was' and 'saw') and possessive *s* 'mummy's', 'daddy's') and the article ('a' and 'the'). A notable feature during this phase is the rapid increase in vocabulary (from 200 words at the age of 2 to over 2000 words at the age of 5).

*Transformational rules.* This phrase refers to the ability to re-order or re-arrange the meaning of sentences. This occurs much later in language development. Example: 'I can ride a bicycle' can be negatively transformed into 'I cannot ride a bicycle' or interrogatively into 'Can you ride a bicycle?'

### Theories of language development

Chomsky's (1965) influential notions of the *surface* and *deep structure* of language and that of the hypothetical 'language acquisition device' are examples of theories emphasising the maturational and innate components to language development. Contemporary theories, while acknowledging the role of maturation, favour an integrative approach with maturation, cognition and socialisation each making a contribution.

## Gender and sex role concepts (Kohlberg 1966)

While acknowledging the historical importance of Freudian theory in the development of ideas about sexual behaviour and sex roles, current views on these topics emphasise individual plasticity or variability in the acquisition of these roles. Increasing cognitive skills, social interaction and differential social reinforcement of sex roles are seen as the major influences on the acquisition of these concepts.

*Gender identity*, the awareness of one's own sex and that of the difference between the sexes, is regarded primarily as a cognitive achievement. Most children acquire this concept around the age of 2 years, whereas *gender stability*, i.e. the individual remains the same sex throughout life, and *gender constancy*, i.e. the individual remains the same sex despite appearing differently or changing clothes, is not attained until around 6 years. This progression is seen as another example of the concept of *conservation*, that change in appearance does not necessarily mean change of form.

Once children have acquired gender stability, they seem to go through a phase of applying this idea too rigidly, so that 'sex-role stereotyping' occurs. This is shown by the predominance of same-sex friendships during middle childhood (6–10 years) and the acquisition of fixed attitudes and beliefs about the two sexes. For example, boys will maintain that 'girls are weak, whereas boys are strong' or 'boys are good at sports, whereas girls are not'. This attitude is another example of the way in which children overextend concepts when they are initially acquired. Later on, the child's greater cognitive skills enable him to apply the ideas in a more flexible manner. Sex-role behaviour, that is, the behaviour that matches the child's expectation for his or her own sex role, can be seen in children's play and behaviour from the toddler period onwards. It becomes a prominent feature during middle childhood.

## Moral and ethical behaviour

Kohlberg's (1964) adaptation of Piagetian views about preoperational thinking and operational thinking is a useful way to conceptualise this topic. Kohlberg described a stage theory extending from the preschool period into adult life. He recognised three main divisions, preconventional, conventional and postconventional morality, with further subdivisions of these categories.

### Preconventional morality (3–10 years)

This starts from the premise that bad is punished and good is not, similar to Piaget's idea of authoritarian morality, that is every bad deed is punished without exception and that if you are punished, you must have done something wrong. The child gradually extends this concept, so that what feels right for the child and brings pleasurable results must be right. Ideas about fairness and keeping a bargain become important.

### Conventional morality (10 onwards)

The child shifts his focus from himself to his immediate family group with their values superseding his own as the ultimate source of authority. Mutual trust and respect for other family members engenders in return a sense of trust, loyalty and appreciation from other family members towards him. In adolescence, the focus of attention may shift from the family to society at large. Respect for and compliance with society's values are seen as worthwhile, as they contribute to the good of society, an objective that the child endorses.

### Postconventional morality (adolescence onwards)

The adolescent now begins to distinguish between the relative value of different principles. For example, the laws should be observed as they promote stability and cohesion within society, though there may be some extreme circumstances when the person may disregard these rules. The philosophy of utilitarianism or 'the greatest good for the greatest number' is an underlying principle. Some principles are, however, seen as inalienable or unalterable, for instance the right to life and to liberty. It should be noted that many adolescents and adults do not reach the sophistication of postconventional morality and operate at the conventional level.

## Motor, visual and auditory development

Though these aspects of development are clearly of more relevance to the paediatrician than to the child psychiatrist, they are nevertheless important for all professionals working with disturbed children for two reasons:

**Table 2.8**   Summary of developmental milestones (average of achievements)

| Posture and movement | Vision and manipulation | Hearing and speech | Social behaviour |
|---|---|---|---|
| **3 months** | | | |
| *Prone*: rests on forearms, lifts up head and chest<br>*Held standing*: sags at knees | *Vision*: alert, watches movement<br>Follows toys dangling in front of face<br>*Hands*: loosely open | Quietens to interesting sounds<br>Chuckles and coos when pleased | Shows pleasure appropriately |
| **6 months** | | | |
| *Prone*: lifts self up on extended legs<br>*Held standing*: sags at knees | Watches ball rolling 2 m away<br>Reaches out for toys and takes in palmar grasp, puts to mouth | Localises sounds at 0.5 m at either side<br>Makes tuneful noises | Alert, interested<br>Still friendly with strangers |
| **9 months** | | | |
| *Prone*: wriggles or crawls<br>*Held standing*: bounces or stamps | Looks for toys when dropped<br>Scissors grasp and transfers objects to other hand before placing object in mouth | Quick localisation of quiet sound at 1 m at either side | Distinguishes strangers and shows apprehension<br>Chews solids |
| **1 year** | | | |
| Crawls on all fours Walks around furniture<br>Stands for a second or two | Drops toys deliberately and watches where they go<br>Index finger approach to tiny objects, then pincer grasp | Understands simple commands<br>Babbles incessantly | Co-operates with dressing<br>Waves 'bye bye' |
| **18 months** | | | |
| Walks alone and can pick up a toy from the floor without falling | Builds tower of 3 cubes<br>Scribbles | Uses several words | Drinks from cup with two hands<br>Demands constant mothering |
| **2 years** | | | |
| Runs<br>Walks up and down stairs two feet at a time | Builds tower of 6 cubes | Joins words together in simple phrases | Uses spoon<br>Indicates toilet needs, dry by day |
| **3 years** | | | |
| Walks upstairs one foot per step, and down two feet per step | Builds tower of 9 cubes<br>Copies an O | Speaks in sentences<br>Gives full name | Eats with spoon and fork<br>Can undress with help<br>Dry by night |
| **4 years** | | | |
| Walks up and down stairs one foot per step<br>Stands on one foot for a few seconds | Builds 3 steps from 6 cubes after demonstration<br>Copies an O and an X | Talks a lot<br>Speech contains many infantile substitutions | Dresses and undresses alone<br>Washes and dries face and hands |
| **5 years** | | | |
| Skips<br>Hops | Draws a man<br>Copies an O, X and a ▢ | Fluent speech with few infantile substitutions | |

- Significant motor, visual or hearing impairment may have an adverse effect on cognitive, emotional or social development
- Children with physical handicap or disability are significantly more likely to be psychiatrically disturbed than healthy children (Rutter et al 1970b).

Rather than describe the stages in detail, Table 2.8 summarises the major developmental milestones.

## SUMMARY

This brief review of child development has revealed the complexity of the subject, the wide diversity of theories and the many unanswered questions. Hopefully, the reader has not become too overawed or confused, but rather has been stimulated by the richness of the topic. The best approach to child development in the present state of knowledge is to be eclectic. Choose models or parts of them that make most sense for you. Despite the uncertainty, it is important to have a framework of child development, so that the understanding and interpretation of abnormal or deviant behaviour become easier.

## DEVELOPMENTAL PSYCHOPATHOLOGY

The previous section discussed the various theories of cognitive, social and emotional development. The next questions are: how do we recognise disturbed behaviour and how does it arise? The term *developmental psychopathology* has been introduced to describe the two important dimensions necessary to make an adequate assessment of children's behaviour: the *developmental* (or, is the behaviour age appropriate?); and the *psychopathological* (or, is the behaviour abnormal?). The developmental aspect is illustrated with reference to separation anxiety. The latter is a normal reaction in children between the ages of 9 months and 4 years. However, the same response in a 6-year-old would be abnormal. Similarly, the occurrence of temper tantrums in a 3-year-old would not in itself be pathological. The determining factor would be the frequency, severity and persistence of this behaviour.

Childhood psychopathology is most usefully considered under three main headings: a) abnormality of emotions, b) abnormality of behaviour and c) abnormality of social relationships. Both psychoanalytic and social learning theories provide mechanisms to explain the onset of symptoms. As these theories have been discussed earlier, they will only be mentioned briefly. Moreover, detailed discussion of the psychopathology of clinical syndromes will be found in the relevant chapter.

Anxiety and depressive symptoms are important features in emotional disturbance. Anxiety has physical manifestations such as palpitations or dry mouth as well as psychological components such as fear or apprehension. Exposure to anxiety is a normal, indeed essential, part of a child's experience. It arises in many situations: in response to external threat; in new or strange situations; and in response to the operation of conscience or guilt. Anna Freud's concept of defence mechanisms (see earlier section on psychoanalytic theories of development) explains, at least in psychoanalytic terms, the means by which the developmentally immature child learns to cope with excessive anxiety. The mechanisms are seen as adaptive unless they are used excessively, thereby preventing the child from learning to cope with a normal degree of anxiety. Social learning theories explain anxiety in terms of exposure to situations which become associated with anxiety through classical conditional or modelling mechanisms.

Psychoanalytic theories believe that depression arises in response to separation and loss. Bowlby's attachment theory is central to these ideas. Separation anxiety and the separation response are seen as the prototype for the development of depressive responses in later childhood and adult life. Cognitive-behavioural and social learning theories similarly regard loss or perceived loss as the trigger for depressive cognitions or thoughts, with the subsequent elaboration of depressive symptomatology. Harris (1989) has shown that young children are able to discriminate between different degrees of sadness and have expectations that the sadness will lessen over time. These findings would also imply that children may be able to recognise that their sadness is excessive or inappropriate.

Behavioural deviance is most readily conceptualised in terms of social learning theories. The operant conditioning paradigm explains behavioural problems as a deficit or excess of the particular skill or behaviour. For instance, a child with encopresis or enuresis can be regarded as showing a deficit in toileting skills. Similarly, the aggressive child can be seen as displaying excessive belligerent or oppositional behaviour at an inappropriate time. This conceptualisation also has implications for treatment strategies, as the latter often use behavioural techniques in order to increase or decrease the frequency of certain behaviours. Modelling theories, similarly, regard many behavioural problems as arising from the lack of exposure to normal behavioural patterns and/or exposure to deviant models. Treatment approaches accordingly focus on exposure and reinforcement of socially approved behaviour.

Social relationships are often impaired in disturbed children. This may be the primary failure in some instances, such as pervasive developmental disorders, but is more commonly a secondary phenomenon. Children with emotional or behavioural problems are usually socially isolated and unpopular with their peer group as they exclude themselves or are themselves excluded as a result of their deviant behaviour. In addition, the behaviour usually brings them into conflict with parents or other adults such as teachers.

**Table 2.9**   Determinants of personality in childhood

**Constitutional**
- Intelligence
- Temperament
- Gender

**Environmental**
- Family
- Community
  - Schooling
  - Neighbourhood

**Physical illness/handicap**
- Especially neurological disease

# PERSONALITY DEVELOPMENT

Childhood is the time when personality is formed. Wordsworth's aphorism 'the child is father to the man' is substantially true. Personality is a broad concept, encompassing the enduring and uniquely individual constellation of attributes that distinguish one person from another. It consists of the cognitive, emotional, motivational and temperamental attributes which shape the individual's view of himself, his world and the future. Throughout childhood, the various elements interact with each other to mould the child's personality. Moreover, this process occurs in the context of the child's life experiences, particularly within the family but also subsequently in the world outside the family. Healthy personality functioning is an important prerequisite for satisfactory adjustment during childhood and also during adult life.

Personality formation is influenced by two main groups of factors, constitutional and environmental (Table 2.9).

## Constitutional factors

These comprise

- genetic factors
- intelligence
- temperament
- gender differences.

The evidence for a *genetic component* in some child psychiatric disorders – for instance childhood autism and Gilles de la Tourette syndrome – is clear though, even in these instances, it is likely to be polygenic rather than a single gene effect (Rutter et al 1990). A major problem with the application of

**Table 2.10**    Temperamental dimensions (Thomas & Chess)

| Temperamental dimension | Description |
| --- | --- |
| Activity level | Position on the overactivity–underactivity dimension |
| Rhythmicity | Degree of irregularity with various functions, e.g. sleeping, eating |
| Approach/withdrawal | Initial response to new situation, e.g. food, person, toy |
| Adaptability | Ability to manage new situations effectively |
| Threshold of responsiveness | The intensity level of stimulation necessary to evoke a response |
| Intensity of response | Strength of response irrespective of its quality |
| Quality of mood | Predominant balance of contentedness versus discontentedness in behaviour |
| Distractibility | Ease with which stimuli can distract from current task |
| Attention span and persistence | Ability to persist with task |

modern genetic techniques to childhood psychiatric disorders, however, is the inadequate definition of the phenotype (the agreed criteria for what constitutes abnormality) in many psychiatric syndromes in childhood (McGuffin 1987).

*Intelligence*, often defined as the individual's ability to think rationally about himself, clearly affects the child's ability to understand the world and also to adapt successfully.

*Gender differences*, for instance differences in exploratory activity, aggression and activity levels between boys and girls, are also likely to shape the child's emerging personality.

*Temperament* is that facet of personality that refers to the individual's style of interacting with the environment (how they react) as opposed to the motivational (why they react) or the developmental (what they can do). Temperamental characteristics are seen as genetically determined predispositions to react or respond to the environment in certain characteristic ways or style. This 'biological' approach to personality development has become increasingly popular and influential through the studies of Thomas & Chess (1982). They undertook a longitudinal study of children from infancy through to adulthood. They categorised the infant's behaviour along nine dimensions: activity level; rhythmicity; approach/withdrawal; adaptability; threshold of responsiveness; intensity of response; quality of mood; distractibility; and attention and persistence (Table 2.10). Each child has their own position on the nine dimensions, so that a distinct and individual profile or pattern is found for each child. For example, some children are highly active, irregular in their habits and easily distressed, whereas others are placid, regular and unperturbed.

**Table 2.11** Clusters of temperamental characteristics

| Cluster | Description |
| --- | --- |
| Easy temperament | Typically comprises combination of regularity, approach tendencies in new situations, quick adaptability and predominantly positive mood |
| Difficult temperament | Irregularity, withdrawal tendencies, poor adaptation and predominantly negative mood (opposite of easy temperament) |
| Slow to warm up | Withdrawal tendencies in new situations and slow adaptability and frequent negative reactions Often labelled as 'shy' |

Thomas & Chess (1982) found that certain characteristics or styles were more likely to be associated with the subsequent development of behaviour problems. Table 2.11 describes the three broad groups that they found: the easy, the 'slow to warm up' and the difficult. The latter two groups were more at risk for behaviour problems. More recently, Buss & Plomin (1975) have proposed another system based upon four dimensions: active versus lethargic; emotional versus impassive; gregarious versus detached; impulsive versus deliberate. Though this system is intuitively attractive, it has not been used extensively on clinical populations, so that its usefulness has not been determined.

Temperament is seen as important in shaping the child's development of personality in several different and interacting ways:

- Different temperaments elicit different responses from other people, particularly in early childhood. There may be a 'good fit' or a 'bad fit' between the child and his parents with important consequences for the child's development
- Temperament may influence the type and range of environment that the child experiences. For instance, an active, exploratory child is likely to have more new experiences and social experiences than his inactive and passive sibling
- Different temperamental characteristics may be important in different situations. For instance, parents may find one sort of child more easy to handle than another
- Adaptable children are less likely to be affected by the adverse experiences they inevitably encounter during the course of childhood.

### Environmental factors

The main influences on children are:

- the family
- schooling
- the community (Table 2.12).

**Table 2.12**    Role of the family and schooling

**Family**
- Satisfaction of physical needs such as food and shelter
- Provision of love and security
- Development of social relationships with adults/peers
- Promotion of cognitive and language skills
- Exposure to appropriate role models and socialisation
- Acquisition of ethical and moral values

**Schooling**
- Acquisition of scholastic skills
- Promotion of peer relationships
- Acceptance of adult authority outside the family

*The family* fulfils many functions for the child. These include

- the satisfaction of physical needs such as food and shelter
- the provision of love and security
- the development of social relationships with adults and peers
- the promotion of cognitive and language skills
- the exposure to appropriate role models and socialisation
- the acquisition of ethical and moral values.

If the family achieves its objectives, it should provide the child with an extremely healthy environment. If it fails, this is likely to have wide-ranging and long-standing deleterious effects on the child. Parental psychiatric disorder and marital disharmony, often unfortunately present together, are the two most important ways in which a child's life within the family is seriously adversely affected. Many studies, reviewed by Rutter (1985a), have shown that children reared in such families are exposed to frequent quarrelling, criticism, lack of warmth and inconsistent discipline. This is often coupled with the 'pig in the middle' experience, that is the child has to take sides or choose one parent rather than the other.

*Schools* have three main roles for children (Table 2.12):

- the acquisition of scholastic skills
- the promotion of peer relationships
- the acceptance of adult authority outside the family.

Some research (Rutter et al 1979) among secondary school age children has shown that some schools have better 'results' than others with respect to attendance rates, academic success, delinquency rates and subsequent employment prospects, despite similar intakes of pupils at the start of secondary school. Though the results have been criticised, Rutter and his colleagues maintain that schools have a common and distinct 'ethos' which is responsible for the good outcome in some schools.

*The community*, through its neighbourhood resources such as housing or leisure facilities, can clearly have a major influence on the quality of the child's life. Richman et al (1982) showed that unsatisfactory housing increases the risk of behaviour problems among preschool children, whilst Rutter et al (1975b) found that children living in urban areas were twice as likely to be disturbed as children in rural areas. They argued that this difference was not due to the operation of different causative factors in the two areas, but rather that the causative factors were more frequent in cities than in rural areas.

Finally, *physical illness or handicap*, if present, can exert an important influence on personality development. This arises not only from the direct restrictions or limitations that it may impose upon the child's activities and abilities, but more importantly through its indirect effects. The latter include an adverse effect on the child's self-esteem, over-protectiveness of parents and poor social relationships with peers and siblings.

# 3. General features of disturbance

This chapter discusses three aspects of disturbance: causes, classification and prevalence.

## CAUSES OF PSYCHIATRIC DISTURBANCE

A single cause is rarely responsible for the development of disturbance in childhood. The usual pattern is for several factors to be involved, usually in an interactive manner. Not surprisingly, the factors influencing personality development in childhood are also likely to affect the risk of disturbance. Consequently, three main factors are identified (Table 3.1).

**Table 3.1** Causes of psychiatric disturbance

**Constitutional**
- Genetic
- Temperamental
- Intra-uterine disease or damage
- Birth trauma

**Environmental**
- Family
- School
- Community

**Physical damage or illness**
- Especially neurological disease

## Constitutional factors

These are present at birth. So far, specific *genetic factors* have not been identified for many child psychiatric disorders. There is however good evidence from twin studies and adoption studies that genetic factors, probably polygenic, are important determinants of intelligence and temperament, so that it would not be surprising if they also influenced other aspects of behaviour, including deviant behaviour. Pervasive developmental disorders, hyperkinetic syndrome and enuresis are examples of childhood psychiatric syndromes where a genetic component has been established in many studies. The clearest example of the relationship between genetic factors and behaviour is seen in several syndromes associated with mental retardation, for example Down's syndrome, where a chromosome abnormality (trisomy 21) is associated with a definite phenotype, that is, a characteristic physical appearance and intellectual retardation.

*Intra-uterine infection and damage* can adversely affect the fetus in many ways during pregnancy. Infections such as rubella or toxoplasmosis, and more recently the AIDS virus, can impair fetal development with long-term consequences. The *fetal alcohol syndrome*, caused by severe alcohol abuse on the part of the mother during pregnancy, produces a child with a characteristic facial appearance, growth impairment and mental retardation. *Birth trauma*, usually associated with asphyxia or impaired oxygen supply to the fetus during labour, has been shown to affect subsequent intellectual development, thereby placing the child at risk for behavioural problems.

## Environmental factors

As discussed in Chapter 2, the family, schooling and the community are powerful influences, for good or ill, on the child's development. They are the major determinants of the child's adjustment as well as the focus for treatment strategies for many disturbed children.

## Physical handicap or disability

This can be a direct or indirect cause of disturbed behaviour. Brain damage, for example from trauma or infections, has been shown to increase the risk of behavioural disturbance (Rutter et al 1970a). This can arise because of the consequent neurological or intellectual impairment as well as from the adverse effects on the child's self-esteem and family relationships. Other chronic illnesses not affecting the brain also make the child more vulnerable to disturbance, probably due to the indirect effects on the child and family functioning (Rutter et al 1970b).

## CLASSIFICATION (TABLE 3.2)

A single cause is rarely responsible for the development of disturbance in children. The usual pattern is for several factors to be involved with a broad distinction into constitutional and environmental factors. One consequence of this multiple causation is that it is inappropriate to devise a diagnostic classification on the basis of aetiology, as the relative contribution of each factor is often unclear. Diagnostic practice is therefore descriptive or phenomenological, with three main categories of abnormality:

**Table 3.2**  DSM-III-R and ICD-10 classification systems (modified for child psychiatry)

| DSM-III-R | ICD-10 |
|---|---|
| **Axis 1**<br>Clinical syndrome | **Axis 1**<br>Clinical syndrome |
| **Axis 2**<br>Mental retardation<br>Pervasive developmental disorders<br>Specific developmental disorders | **Axis 2**<br>Disorders of psychological development |
| **Axis 3**<br>Physical disorders/illnesses | **Axis 3**<br>Mental retardation |
| **Axis 4**<br>Severity of current psychosocial stressors | **Axis 4**<br>Medical illness |
| **Axis 5**<br>Highest level of adaptive functioning in<br>past year | **Axis 5**<br>Abnormal psychosocial conditions |
| **Axis 6** | **Axis 6**<br>Psychosocial disability |

- emotions
- behaviour
- relationships.

### Definition of disturbance

A commonly used definition of disturbance is as follows:

'an abnormality of emotions, behaviour or relationships which is sufficiently
severe and persistent to handicap the child in his social or personal functioning
and/or to cause distress to the child, his parents or to people in the community'.

Another feature of contemporary diagnostic practice in child psychiatry
is the adoption of a multiaxial framework to describe the various
abnormalities or disabilities that are frequently present together in one child.
This is also a further recognition of the multifactorial nature of disturbance
in childhood. The two common systems are the ICD (WHO 1992) and the
DSM-III-R (American Psychiatric Association 1987). Both systems have
similar underlying principles with an emphasis on a clinical–descriptive
approach to diagnosis and the categorisation of disorder along five separate
dimensions with the child having a position on each dimension, even when
there is no abnormality. The newly available ICD-10 uses a glossary and
DSM-III-R operationally defined criteria to provide the basis for diagnosis
(Table 3.3). An important difference between ICD-10 and DSM-III-R is
that the latter allows for more than one diagnosis on the clinical syndrome
axis, whereas ICD-10 prefers a single diagnosis, an approach more widely
used.

**Table 3.3**   Clinical syndromes of DSM-III-R and ICD-10

| DSM-III-R | ICD-10 |
|---|---|
| **Axis 1** | **Axis 1** |
| Disruptive behaviour disorders | Conduct disorders |
| • Attention-deficit hyperactivity disorder (ADHD) | Emotional disorders |
| • Conduct disorder | Mixed disorders of conduct and emotions |
| • Oppositional defiant disorder | |
| Anxiety disorders of childhood or adolescence | Hyperkinetic disorders |
| • Separation anxiety disorder | Disorders of social functioning |
| • Avoidant disorder of childhood and adolescence | Tic disorders |
| • Over-anxious disorder | Pervasive developmental disorders |
| Eating disorders | Other behavioural and emotional disorders |
| • Anorexia nervosa | |
| • Bulimia nervosa | |
| • Pica | |
| • Rumination disorder of infancy | |
| Gender disorders | |
| Tic disorders | |
| Elimination disorders | |
| • Functional encopresis | |
| • Functional enuresis | |
| Miscellaneous disorders | |
| **Axis 2** | |
| Pervasive developmental disorders | |

The two systems have very many similarities, but have a few important differences. Both have axes for the clinical syndrome, any associated medical illness and current stress; ICD calls the latter *abnormal psychosocial conditions* and DSM *current psychosocial stressors*. ICD has separate axes for mental retardation and developmental disorders, whereas DSM combines the two categories into one axis. Axis 5 of DSM-III-R, the highest level of adaptive functioning in the past year, is not represented in ICD. It is intended to show the contrast between the individual's most adjusted level of function and that shown by his current disturbed behaviour. The newly created axis 6 of ICD, the psychosocial disability, is designed to provide an estimate of the impairment or restriction that the disorder imposes on the child and his development.

DSM and ICD have different principles underlying the diagnostic process. ICD uses a detailed glossary which consists of a description of the clinical features of the syndrome along with the differential diagnosis and the diagnostic guidelines for inclusion or exclusion criteria. This approach mirrors in many ways the clinical practice of clinicians. By contrast, DSM has operationally-defined criteria to define a disorder with few guidelines about exclusion criteria or hierarchical rules to rank the importance or otherwise of individual symptoms. This difference in approach has an important consequence for the diagnostic practice: DSM allows, and to some extent favours, several diagnoses on the clinical axis, whereas ICD prefers and expects a single diagnosis. At present, there is no clear evidence about whether it is better to be an ICD 'lumper' or a DSM 'splitter'.

ICD and DSM have renamed and reclassified infantile autism as childhood autism in a new diagnostic category called *pervasive developmental disorders*. Other disorders in this new group include Rett's syndrome and Asperger's syndrome (see Ch. 6). Earlier versions of ICD and DSM classified infantile autism in the category of *childhood psychosis*. The term 'psychosis' is probably not strictly correct when applied to infantile autism, as psychosis implies a period of normal development which is not usually characteristic of autism. 'Pervasive developmental disorder' is probably a more satisfactory term, as it emphasises the developmental aspect. The choice of 'pervasive' is more problematic as, although autistic behaviour occurs in most situations, the disorder does not affect all aspects of development. For example, some cognitive attainments such as memory may be normal or even superior.

Unfortunately, pervasive developmental disorders are placed on different axes in the latest versions of DSM and ICD, Axis 1 or the clinical syndrome axis on ICD and Axis 2 or disorders of psychological development on DSM. The DSM-III-R Axis 2 also includes mental retardation and specific developmental disorders. The two systems also categorise pervasive developmental disorders in different ways. DSM has only two categories, pervasive developmental disorder and pervasive developmental disorder not otherwise specified, whereas ICD has eight categories including childhood autism, Rett's syndrome, childhood disintegrative disorder and Asperger's syndrome.

Table 3.3 compares the classification of the clinical syndromes in the two systems. DSM-III-R has re-organised attention-deficit and conduct disorder along with oppositional disorder into a new category, *disruptive behaviour disorders*. ICD-10's solution for the classification of this behaviour is to have two categories, *conduct disorder* and *mixed disorder*. Important differences still exist in the way the two systems treat symptoms of hyperactivity, impulsivity and inattention. British child psychiatrists (Taylor 1985) have long maintained that overactivity, hyperactivity and hyperkinesis are common symptoms in many psychiatric disorders, particularly conduct disorders, so that it is more sensible to use the term 'hyperactive' when the behaviour is *pervasive*, i.e. present in all situations, and not just in some situations, i.e. *situational*. Similarly, the terms 'impulsivity' and 'inattention' are extremely difficult to define accurately, so that it may be more sensible to leave them out of the diagnostic criteria. Consequently, ICD restricts the term *hyperactivity disorder* to those children whose major symptom is pervasive hyperactivity.

Another problem for the two systems is how to categorise those disorders which also occur in adult life. This applies particularly to emotional disorders such as anxiety. Theoretically, the two systems propose that those disorders that have the same quality and persistence as adult disorders should be classified in that category. In practice however, it is likely to prove difficult to differentiate the severity of the condition sufficiently accurately to make the correct diagnosis. Again unfortunately, DSM and ICD have different categories of emotional disorder: DSM has three, separation anxiety disorder, avoidant disorder and over-anxious disorder; and ICD four, separation disorder, phobic disorder, social anxiety and sibling rivalry. There is, however, no clear evidence as to which system has the better approach.

## PREVALENCE OF CHILD PSYCHIATRIC DISORDER (TABLES 3.4, 3.5)

Epidemiological research has been an important research interest in the UK for the past 30 years. Professor Michael Rutter and his colleagues have

---

**Table 3.4**   Epidemiological research findings on childhood disturbance

**Isle of Wight study on 10-year-olds**

- Prevalence – approximately 7%
- Emotional, conduct and mixed disorders account for over 80% of psychiatric disorder
- Emotional disorders more common in girls, anxiety being the commonest type
- Conduct disorders more common in boys, frequently associated with specific reading retardation

**Isle of Wight findings on adolescents (14-15 years old)**

- Prevalence – approximately 8%
- Depressive disorders more frequent
- 40% of disorders persisted from the age of 10
- Persistent disorders were more common in boys and were associated with family discord and educational problems
- New disorders were more similar to adult disorders and had an equal sex incidence

**Waltham Forrest study on 3-year-olds**

- 7% had severe problems, 15% mild problems
- Strong association between disturbance and language delay
- Persistence of problems was associated with:
  - marital discord
  - maternal psychiatric ill health
  - large family size
  - poor housing conditions
- Follow up at age 8 showed 60% of problems persisted, most commonly among overactive boys of low ability

---

pioneered the use of epidemiological research to provide basic information about the frequency and distribution of disturbance in childhood. Their findings were immensely successful because they were meticulous in ensuring that they successfully screened and subsequently interviewed the population under investigation and also devised questionnaires and interview schedules with good reliability and validity. Consequently, the findings have become accepted as the 'gold standard' against which to judge other findings. Another important spin off from these studies has been that the questionnaires that they devised have been used in many subsequent research studies, sometimes inappropriately!

The Isle of Wight (IOW) studies provided accurate information about the frequency and distribution of disturbance throughout childhood and adolescence (Rutter et al 1970b), the differences between urban and rural areas (Rutter et al 1975a) and the effects of illness and handicap on vulnerability to disturbance (Rutter et al 1970a), as well as providing clues about the relative importance of various aetiological factors (Rutter et al 1975b).

Most epidemiological studies have shown prevalence rates of between 10% and 20% depending upon the criteria for disturbance. The original Isle of Wight study, using strict definitions of disorder, found rates of disturbance of approximately 7% among 10–11-year-old children. Follow-up of these children into adolescence indicated a prevalence rate of around 7%, with more than 40% of the children with conduct disorder continuing to have major problems. Disorders arising for the first time during adolescence were more adult-like in presentation, with a preponderance of females. Over 80% of the disorders were in the emotional, conduct or mixed categories. Emotional disorders were more common among girls, anxiety

**Table 3.5**  Causative factors in childhood disturbance (epidemiological research findings)

**Family discord**
- Marital discord
- Children in care
- Children not living with both natural parents

**Parental deviance**
- Psychiatric disorder in the mother
- Criminal record in the father

**Social disadvantage**
- Large family size
- Overcrowding
- Father in unskilled occupation

**Schooling**
- High pupil/staff ratio
- High turnover of teachers

being the commonest type. By contrast, conduct disorders, and to an important extent mixed disorders, were more common among boys, with an association with specific reading retardation.

A comparative study of 10-year-olds living in London (Rutter et al 1975a) showed a rate of disturbance over twice that on the Isle of Wight. This study also showed that the difference in prevalence rate was entirely accounted for by the increased frequency of predisposing factors among children and their families in London compared with those on the Isle of Wight. These factors were family discord, parental psychiatric disorder, social disadvantage and inferior quality of schooling.

The IOW study (Rutter et al 1970b) also showed that children with chronic illness or handicap had much higher rates of disturbance than healthy children. For instance, children with central nervous diseases such as epilepsy or cerebral palsy had a rate over five times that of the general population, while children with other illnesses such as asthma or diabetes were twice as likely to be disturbed as healthy children.

Studies of preschool children, most notably Richman et al 1975, have found that about 20% of children have significant behaviour problems, with 7% classified as severe. Follow-up studies (Richman et al 1982) indicated that about 60% of the problems persisted, most commonly among overactive boys of low ability. An important association was found between language delay and disturbed behaviour. Finally, problems were more likely to continue when there was marital discord, maternal psychiatric ill-health and psychosocial disadvantage such as poor housing or large family size.

# 4. Assessment procedures

Assessment is more time-consuming in child psychiatry than in other branches of psychiatry or medicine. It has three components:

- the diagnostic assessment interview
- psychological assessment
- information about the child and parents from other professionals.

## THE DIAGNOSTIC ASSESSMENT INTERVIEW

This has many similarities with traditional methods, though with important modifications. Interview skills are essential in the elucidation, understanding and treatment of emotional and behavioural problems in children. Training in interview skills should be an important part of medical undergraduate and postgraduate training. Recent research (Maguire & Rutter 1976) has shown the lack of skills among doctors in training and also how these skills can be improved. It is of general importance that the interviewing doctor manages to:

- clarify the nature of the problem and the reason for referral
- obtain adequate factual information
- elicit emotional responses and attitudes to past and current events
- observe behaviour during the interview
- establish the trust and confidence of the child and family
- provide the parents with a summary of problems and a provisional plan of treatment at the end of the initial assessment interview.

*Appointment letter (Fig. 4.1)*

There are no absolute rules about the arrangements for the initial interview, so that it is simplest to make some general comments. Most clinicians would normally write an initial appointment letter similar to that shown in Figure 4.1. The letter invites the whole family to attend the initial interview for three reasons:

- to find out from each family member their views about the nature of the problem and also their explanation for the problem

47

---

*SPECIMEN FORMAT FOR LETTER*

DEPT OF CHILD AND FAMILY PSYCHIATRY
ROYAL HOSPITAL FOR SICK CHILDREN
EDINBURGH

Dear ..................................... (Parents and referred child)

.....................................(Referrer) has recently written to us about your concerns for
..................................... (Referred child). We would like to offer you an appointment on
..................................... (Day, date and time of interview).

We find it very helpful if everyone who lives at home attends for the first interview. This
will enable us to find out what everyone at home thinks about the problem.

We would be grateful if you could confirm that the appointment time is convenient by
telephoning or writing to the Department beforehand. We enclose a small map to show
you where the Department is situated. We look forward to seeing you at the clinic.

Yours sincerely


..................................... (Name of therapist)


*REAL LETTER*

DEPT OF CHILD AND FAMILY PSYCHIATRY
ROYAL HOSPITAL FOR SICK CHILDREN
EDINBURGH

Dear Mr and Mrs Jones and Brian

Dr Abraham has recently written to us about your concerns for Brian. We would like to
offer you an appointment on Wednesday 25 November at 2 pm.

We find it very helpful if everyone who lives at home attends for the first interview. This
will enable us to find out what everyone at home thinks about the problem.

We would be grateful if you could confirm that the appointment time is convenient by
telephoning or writing to the Department beforehand. We enclose a small map to show
you where the Department is situated. We look forward to seeing you at the clinic.

Yours sincerely


Dr P. Hoare

---

**Fig. 4.1**   Format of appointment letters

- to allow the therapist to observe family interaction during the interview
- to enable the therapist to enlist the support of other family members to help resolve the problem.

*Diagnostic interview schedule*

A flexible approach is essential in order to ensure that the interview fulfils its two main objectives: firstly, to obtain an accurate account of the problem(s) and their associated features; and secondly, to establish a good relationship with the child and the family. In many circumstances, it may be sensible to conduct the interview with all family members present, particularly with young children who may be upset by separation from the parents. One section of the interview may involve a separate interview with the child and/or the parents. Older children and adolescents often appreciate the opportunity to talk separately about their own views of the problem. Similarly, parents may want to talk with the clinician by themselves in order to discuss more intimate or personal aspects of the problem or again to let the clinician know about their own problems, for instance the marital relationship. Often the separate interviews may be more suitably left until the second interview. Finally, it is good practice to encourage as much eye-to-eye contact and interaction with the family as possible rather than spend the interview writing copious notes – keep note-taking to a minimum.

## 1. Arrangement/layout of the interview room

*General points*

- The interview room should be large enough to seat the family comfortably and also allow the children to use the play material in a relaxed manner
- Arrange the seating so that everyone can see each other easily without barriers — for instance, a desk between the clinician and the family
- Have a variety of play materials available suitable for a wide age range of children. Common items are crayons and paper, dolls' house, play telephones, miniature domestic and zoo animals, jigsaws, simple games and books (for a rough estimate of reading ability).

## 2. The initial phase of the interview

*General points*

- Meet the family in waiting room in a friendly, welcoming manner
- Introduce yourself and get the family to introduce themselves
- Take the family to the interview room (don't go too fast or you will lose them!)
- Show the children the available toys and suggest seating arrangements

- Make introductions again to ensure everyone knows everyone else
- Outline the purpose of the interview and the proposed duration (never normally longer than 1 hour)
- It is often helpful to begin by checking factual details (e.g. ages, names and schools), as this allows the introduction of topics such as schooling, neighbourhood etc
- Ask someone to tell you about the problem.

Before beginning detailed questioning, it is crucial to put the family at ease and begin to develop their trust and confidence, and to show them that you understand them and their problem. The clinician must develop a repertoire of verbal and communication skills based on his own style, personality and experience to facilitate this process. Though it is not possible to be too prescriptive about these skills, certain types of question are invaluable. For example:

- open-ended questions ('How did that make you feel?') rather than closed questions ('Did that make you feel depressed?')
- facilitatory and empathic questions ('You must have been upset. Could you say a bit more about that?')
- clarification of the problem ('Have I got this right?')

The hardest therapeutic task is to win the support and co-operation of both the parents and the child, a difficult balancing act. Unless constant vigilance is maintained throughout the interview, it is likely that one group, the parents or the child, will feel understood and the other misunderstood.

### 3. Detailed history taking and examination

Once the child and family are sufficiently at ease, it is possible to begin to obtain information on the topics mentioned below. It must be emphasised that the list is exhaustive. It is neither feasible, nor indeed desirable, to obtain all this information at the initial interview. The list is meant to be used as an aide-memoire. The bold type highlights the important aspects of assessment and provide a framework to enable a formulation to be made for the individual case.

*Basic data*

Name, address, date of birth, date seen
1. **Presenting problem(s): frequency; severity; onset; course; exacerbating/ameliorating factors; effect on family; help given so far**
2. Other problems or complaints:
   - general health: eating, sleeping, elimination, physical complaints, fits or faints
   - interests, activities and hobbies

- **relationship with parents and sibs**
- relationship with other children: special friends
- mood: happy, sad, anxious
- level of activity, attention span, concentration
- antisocial behaviour
- **schooling: attainments, attendance, friendships, relationship with teachers**
- sexual knowledge, interests and behaviour (when relevant)

3. **Any other problems not previously mentioned**
4. Family structure:
   - **parents: ages; occupations; current physical and psychiatric state**; previous physical and psychiatric history
   - sibs: ages; problems
   - home circumstances
5. Family function:
   - **quality of parenting: mutual support and help; level of communication and ability to resolve problems**
   - **parent–child relationship; warmth, affection and acceptance; level of criticism, hostility and rejection**
   - sibs' relationship
   - pattern of family relationships
6. Personal history:
   - pregnancy and delivery
   - early mother–child relationship: postpartum depression; early feeding patterns
   - temperamental characteristics: easy or difficult, irregular, restless baby and toddler
   - developmental milestones
   - **past illnesses and injuries: hospitalisation**
   - separations greater than one week
   - previous schooling
7. **Observation of child's behaviour and emotional state**
   In younger children, it is not possible to formally examine the child's mental state, though this may be the case with older children. Every opportunity should be taken to observe the child's behaviour which should be noted down systematically and objectively. **Avoid global statements about the child's behaviour. Do not forget to obtain the child's view of the situation, including his likes, dislikes and hopes for the future.**
   - **appearance: nutritional state; signs of neglect or injury**
   - activity level: involuntary movements; concentration
   - mood: expressions or signs of sadness, misery, anxiety
   - reaction to and relationship with the doctor: eye contact; spontaneous talk; inhibition and disinhibition
   - relationship with parents: affection/resentment; ease of separation

- habits and mannerisms
- presence of delusions, hallucinations, thought disorder
8. Observation of family relationships:
   - patterns of interaction
   - clarity of boundaries between parents and child
   - communication
   - emotional atmosphere of family: mutual warmth/tension; criticisms
9. Physical examination:
   a. Screening neurological examination
      - note any facial asymmetry
      - eye movements: ask child to follow a moving finger and observe eye movement for jerkiness, lack of co-ordination
      - finger–thumb apposition: ask child to press the tip of each finger against the thumb in rapid succession; observe clumsiness, weakness
      - copying pattern; drawing a man
      - observe grip and dexterity in drawing
      - observe visual competence when drawing
      - jumping up and down on the spot
      - hopping
      - hearing: capacity of child to repeat numbers whispered 2 m behind him.
   b. Further medical examination (if relevant)

## 4. Conclusion of interview

At the end of the interview, the clinician has the following tasks to perform with the family:

- to summarise his own assessment of the problems based upon their opinions and his observations
- to indicate whether further assessment interviews and/or special investigations are required
- to outline provisional treatment plan where indicated
- to indicate that he will be writing to the referrer to inform him of his findings
- to ensure that the family has understood what has been said.

## 5. Formulation: (see Appendix)

At the completion of the assessment, the clinician should be able to make a *formulation*. This is a succinct summary of the important features of the individual case and is set out in Table 4.1. The formulation should be included in the case-notes, thereby providing the clinician with a record of his views at referral.

**Table 4.1** Principles of formulation

- Succinct summary of main problems
- Diagnosis and differential diagnosis
- Aetiology, with relative contribution of constitutional and environmental factors
- Further information required (including special investigations)
- Probable short-term and long-term outcome
- Initial treatment plan

## Specialised interview techniques

### Individual assessment of child

The individual interview with the child follows the same principles of interviewing with important modifications. The establishment of trust and confidence between the child and clinician is essential. General points are as follows:

- Put the child at his ease through use of an informal and relaxed manner
- Explain the purpose of the interview ('a chance to get to know you')
- Set limits on behaviour ('The toys are here for you to play with or not. It's your choice')
- Avoid direct and intrusive questions about feelings and ideas
- Show concern and interest for the child as a person and value the child's point of view.

Clearly, it is only with older children and adolescents that it is possible to rely upon verbal exchanges to complete the assessment. Other verbal techniques for eliciting the child's feelings are:

- the child's response when asked 'Do you have good dreams or bad dreams? Tell me one of your dreams.'
- the child's response when asked 'If you could have three wishes, what would you wish for?'
- the 'squiggle game'. Winnicott (1970) devised this game as a way of getting into contact with the child. The clinician explains briefly to the child that he will make a squiggle with a pencil or crayon on a sheet of paper and the child will then make it into something and then it will be the clinician's turn. As they take turns, a theme may emerge from the series of the squiggles drawn. The clinician uses the drawings, the child's approach to the game and the child's description of the squiggles as a way to help him and the child gain some understanding into the child's concerns and feelings.

With younger children, indirect methods using play are the most useful. Sand and water play, a dolls' house and play telephones are the best means with preschool children.

Drawing, for instance asking the child to draw a person or their family, is useful in assessing the child's intelligence, fantasies and feelings. Children's drawings progress through recognisable stages:

- *scribbling* (2–3 years): the child enjoys the circular motor activity and the increasing hand control, and also tries to imitate the actions of others.
- *single lines* (4 years)
- *symbolic representations* (5–6 years): the child can now draw a person, consisting mostly of circles and ellipses to represent the head and the body with 'stick' lines as the arms and legs.
- *descriptive drawing* (7–10 years): the child now pays more attention to detail and details of clothing appear.
- *visual realism* (11 years onwards): the child now draws in profile and attempts a realistic representation. The child may also show some inhibition, preferring to draw designs rather than people.

Observation of the child while drawing allows the assessment of his motivation and self-esteem ('I am not very good at drawing') as well as his motor skills and co-ordination. The child's fantasies and feelings are often revealed by asking the child to make up a story about the drawing. Certain features of the drawing may be suggestive of underlying feelings. For instance:

- large drawing (aggressiveness) versus small drawing (insecurity, with-drawal, unhappiness)
- heavy pressure (tension, aggressiveness) versus light pressure (inade-quacy, timidity, low self-esteem)
- peripheral placing of drawing — insecurity, dependency
- omission of facial features — uneasiness
- prominence of one feature, e.g. ear or nose — possible handicap
- large eyes — anxiety or suspiciousness
- small eyes — guilt
- bared teeth — aggressiveness.

The validity of these interpretations has, however, not been subjected to objective analysis.

Finally, specialist toys such as anatomically correct dolls and Teach-a-body dolls are used in therapeutic work with sexually abused children and in preparation of children for painful investigatory procedures in hospital respectively.

These diagnostic assessment sessions with the child are likely to occur over several sessions. They can provide invaluable information about the child's view of the problem and be used to compliment the other aspects of the assessment. Clinicians do tend to distinguish between a diagnostic assessment and a therapeutic series of individual sessions, though the distinction is often blurred. Individual psychotherapy with children is discussed in Chapter 17.

*Family assessment*

The techniques are described in the family therapy section of Chapter 17.

## PSYCHOLOGICAL ASSESSMENT

Psychological assessment carried out by a child psychologist is an invaluable and integral part of the overall assessment of a child's problems in many situations. It can provide information about three aspects of development:

● intellectual ability
● educational attainments
● specific skills.

Assessment is usually based upon the administration of standardised assessment procedures. These tests are *norm-referenced* or *criterion-referenced*. The former compares the child's ability with other children of the same age, whereas the latter is on a pass/fail basis, for instance whether or not the child can tie his shoelaces. Ideally, the test items should have good discriminatory value (distinguish between children with different abilities), be predictable (give similar results when repeated) and valid (in agreement with other independent evidence). An important aspect of the assessment is that the tasks are carried out in a standardised fashion, thereby increasing their reliability and validity.

### Intellectual ability

Traditionally, the IQ (intelligence quotient) was defined as the mental age/chronological age X 100. More recently, the precise value of the IQ score has justifiably been given less importance, so that the overall assessment of the child's ability with a profile of his strengths and weaknesses is given much more emphasis.

*Developmental assessment in infancy and early childhood (Table 4.2)*

The commonly used tests are the Bayley Scales of Infant Development (Bayley 1969), the Griffiths Mental Development Scale (Griffiths 1954) and the Denver Developmental Screening Test (Frankenberg et al 1975).

*Intellectual assessment of school-age children (Table 4.3)*

The most popular test is the Wechsler Intelligence Scale for Children — Revised Form (WISC-R) (Wechsler 1974). This covers an age range of 6–16 years. Ten subtests are usually used, measuring different aspects of the child's abilities. The tests are usually divided into 'verbal' and 'performance' categories yielding a *verbal IQ* and a *performance IQ*. The

**Table 4.2**   Psychological tests of developmental and intellectual ability

| Test | Age range | Scales | Comments |
|---|---|---|---|
| Griffiths | 0–2 years | Locomotor<br>Personal/social<br>Hearing and speech<br>Hand/eye performance | Poor predictor of later intellectual ability |
| Bayley Scales | 0–2 years | Mental scale<br>Motor scale<br>Behaviour record | Scales yield mental and psychomotor development indices which correlate poorly with subsequent ability<br>Behaviour scale is not well standardised |
| Stanford–Binet | 2–24 years | Verbal reasoning<br>Abstract reasoning<br>Visual reasoning<br>Quantitative reasoning<br>Short term memory | Composite score (IQ equivalent)<br>Bias towards verbal items so inaccurate assessment of intellectual functioning in children with speech and language problems<br>Test administration is long (2 h) |
| McCarthy | 2.5–8.5 years | Verbal and perceptual performance<br>General cognitive<br>Memory<br>Motor | Increasingly popular as it is easy to administer and the child enjoys the test<br>Administration time is good (45–60 min) |
| Wechsler Intelligence Scale for Children (WISC) | 6–16 years | Verbal and performance subscales | See Table 4.3 |
| Wechsler Pre-School and Primary School Scale of Intelligence (WPPSI) | 4–6.5 years | Similar to WISC<br>Downward extension of WISC | Long administration time<br>Restricted age range |

'verbal' subtests commonly used are information, comprehension, arithmetic, similarities and vocabulary, while the 'performance' tests are picture completion, picture arrangement, block design, object assembly and coding. Each subtest has a mean score of 10, so that combining the 10 tests gives a 'full-scale' IQ of 100 with a standard deviation of 15. The normal distribution of the test scores means that it is possible to state that 66% of children will be within the IQ range 85–115, 95% within IQ range 70–130, 99% within IQ range 55–145.

Other tests used include the Stanford–Binet (Form L-M) (Thorndike 1973) and the British Ability Scales (BAS) (Elliott et al 1983).

**Table 4.3** WISC subscales

| SCALES | ABILITY |
| --- | --- |
| **Verbal** | |
| Information | Ability to retain and utilise general knowledge |
| Comprehension | Ability to reason about social situations |
| Arithmetic | Numerical ability |
| | Simple mental arithmetic problems |
| Similarities | A test of classification and abstract reasoning |
| Vocabulary | Definition of word meanings |
| **Performance** | |
| Picture completion | Visual scanning of pictures in order to discover the piece that is missing |
| Picture arrangement | Re-arrangement of a series of picture cards into a logical sequence to tell a story |
| Block design | Analysis of visually presented patterns and their reproduction by use of coloured blocks |
| Object assembly | Perceptual reasoning |
| | Requires construction of cardboard forms (e.g. manikin, horse etc) from its constituent parts |
| Coding | Speed of thought and perceptuo-motor functioning |

## Educational attainment

There are two commonly used reading tests, the Schonell Graded Word Reading Test (Schonell & Schonell 1950) and the Neale Analysis of Reading Ability (Neale 1958). The latter is more comprehensive but takes longer to administer. It provides information about speed, accuracy and comprehension of reading. The scores are transformed into reading ages in years and months, for instance 6 years 11 months.

Other attainment tests include the Schonell graded spelling test (Schonell & Schonell 1950). There is no satisfactory standardised test of mathematical skills, although appropriate subtests scores of the WISC-R and the BAS can be used as a guide to mathematical ability.

## Specific skills

The Reynell Developmental Language Scale (Reynell 1969), the Bender Visual Motor Gestalt Test (Bender 1938) and the Halstead–Reitan Neuropsychological Test Battery (Reitan & Woolfson 1985) are examples of tests to assess the child's acquisition of certain abilities and skills. They are often helpful with specific problems.

## Limitations of assessment

Caution should always be exercised in the interpretation of test results. It is wrong to attribute undue significance to a single result, most often done with the IQ score. Many factors influence test results, including fatigue, poor testing conditions and the use of inappropriate tests. The results should be evaluated in the context of the overall assessment and the report from the clinical psychologist. A great deal of harm, upset and distress can be done to a child when he is incorrectly classified or labelled as able or dull on the basis of an unreliable psychological assessment.

## ADDITIONAL INFORMATION

A distinctive feature of child psychiatry practice is the importance attached to obtaining independent evidence about the child's behaviour. This is for two reasons:

- A child's behaviour varies from one situation to another, so that it is helpful to have information about the child's behaviour in several situations
- Total reliance on parental accounts of the child's behaviour is unsafe, as it may be the parents who are disturbed rather than the child.

Consequently, an important part of assessment is to obtain reports from other professionals involved with the family such as schoolteachers, health visitors or family doctors. Another common practice is the use of questionnaires to supplement information provided by referrers and other more formal reports. Several questionnaires (Rutter et al 1970b, Richman et al 1982, Achenbach & Edelbrock 1983) have been devised to assess different age ranges and have satisfactory psychometric properties. The most commonly used questionnaires for school-age children in the UK are the Rutter Parents' and Teachers' Scales, also known as Rutter Scale A and Rutter Scale B respectively. These scales have established reliability and validity as well as classifying children into *neurotic or emotional, conduct or antisocial* and *mixed* categories.

## APPENDIX: SAMPLE FORMULATION

### Main problems

Joanne Harvey is a 12-year-old girl seen as an emergency in September 1992 on account of a 1-month history of weight loss, a 1-week history of refusal to eat food or take fluids together with increasing arguments with parents over food and school attendance. Further questioning reveals a gradual reduction in food intake over the summer holidays accompanied by increasing concern over the plight of starving people in Africa. Since her return to school Joanne has complained about her inability to complete her work satisfactorily. The family consists of Mr and Mrs Harvey and Joanne's 10-year-old brother, Gavin. Father is a civil servant and mother a part-time teacher with a history of postnatal depression. Joanne is described as a conscientious, intelligent girl with several close friends.

Examination shows a thin girl (10th centile for height, 5th for weight) with no other obvious abnormality. Joanne is downcast, avoiding eye contact and speaking in a quiet voice. She describes herself as tired and tearful, especially in the mornings, and despondent about her ability to cope with school work. She says that eating is difficult as it makes her feel sick and that other people can do without food, for instance the people in Africa, so that she should be able to do so as well.

## Differential diagnosis

The three main diagnostic possibilities are:

- primary organic disorder with psychological symptoms as a secondary response
- anorexia nervosa with secondary depressive symptoms
- depressive disorder with eating disorder as part of the affective disorder.

Despite the history of weight loss, physical examinations show no major abnormalities that would support a diagnosis of organic disorder, for instance malignancy, diabetes or thyrotoxicosis. Again, though the weight loss is a prominent symptom, the child's demeanour, her explanation for food refusal and her affect are not common in patients with anorexia nervosa. The most consistent explanation is that the primary diagnosis is depressive disorder with a secondary eating disorder.

## Aetiology

Aetiologically, three factors appear important in the onset of the depressive disorder:

- the maternal history of depression
- the premorbid personality traits of conscientiousness and perfectionism
- the demands of secondary schooling.

As a couple, the parents are gentle and unassertive, so that they may have been reluctant to put pressure on Joanne to eat regularly and to ensure that her dietary intake was satisfactory.

## Management

It is essential to exclude any underlying medical disorder by haematological screening, blood sugar test for diabetes and thyroid function tests. Assuming that these results are normal, the two main components of management are an adequate food and fluid intake and the commencement of antidepressant medication. This should be combined with individual sessions for Joanne and also some joint discussions with her parents. Amitriptyline, increasing from 25 mg to 50 mg and then 75 mg at night as soon as possible depending on side-effects, is the first choice antidepressant. Dosage should be increased until tolerance is reached and/or a beneficial response is evident. Joanne's parents should be given advice about the importance of adequate food and fluid intake and the strategies involved in managing this task. Review again in 1 week. Possibly consider in-patient assessment if improvement does not occur soon.

## Prognosis

Prognosis of this episode is reasonable on account of acute presentation and prominent physical symptomatology such as sleep disturbance. Long-term prognosis is guarded until Joanne's response to treatment is known. Early age of onset of depression is a bad prognostic sign.

# 5. Disorders in preschool children

## INTRODUCTION

The separation of a group of disorders by age rather than by type or syndrome is the most useful way to discuss psychiatric problems occurring in children aged 0–5 years. Developmental influences are so pervasive but also so variable that it is more sensible to think about disturbed behaviour in terms of developmental and chronological age rather than by the occurrence of specific behavioural syndromes. Except for rare but severe disorders such as pervasive developmental disorders, psychiatric disorders in the preschool age group are mostly deviations or delays from normality rather than identifiable psychiatric illnesses. The variation in developmental progress is such that it is often not possible to state with any certainty whether the behaviour is abnormal, for instance the precise limits of the normal separation response are not clearly established. Moreover, the child's behaviour and development are so influenced by his immediate surroundings, particularly that of the family, that his response in many circumstances may be easily understandable and therefore not pathological. Another reason to adopt a cautious approach to the interpretation of the child's behaviour is that the main source of information is usually the mother, who may be disturbed herself rather than the child. Finally, it should be noted that most problems in this age group are treated by general practitioners or paediatricians with only a small minority referred for specialist psychiatric advice.

This chapter discusses the following topics:

- behaviour problems
- feeding and eating difficulties
- sleep disorders
- disorders of attachment
- the psychiatric aspects of child abuse.

This last subject is discussed in this chapter as child abuse most commonly presents in this age group, though it certainly occurs in older children and adolescents, particularly in the form of sexual abuse. These latter aspects are covered in the chapter on adolescence.

Developmental disorders including encopresis, enuresis and specific learning and language disorders are considered in other chapters.

## AETIOLOGY

Four factors contribute to the occurrence of problems to a varying degree in the individual child:

- temperamental factors
- physical illness or handicap
- family psychopathology
- social disadvantage.

The New York Longitudinal Study (Thomas et al 1968) showed clearly that children with certain temperamental characteristics, particularly those with the 'difficult child' or the 'slow to warm up child' profile, were at a greater risk of developing behaviour problems. The presence of physical illness or handicap is also likely not only to delay developmental progress but also to cause parental anxiety, both of which increase the likelihood of behavioural disturbance. Parental psychiatric illness, marital disharmony and poor parenting skills are instances where disturbances in the parents adversely affect the child's behaviour. Moreover, several authors (Richman 1977, Brown & Harris 1978) have found high rates of depression among mothers with preschool children. Finally, social disadvantage such as poor housing or inadequate recreational facilities has been shown to increase the risk of disturbance among preschool children (Richman 1977).

## PREVALENCE OF PROBLEMS

Table 5.1 shows the prevalence of common behaviour problems among 3- and 4-year-olds in the general population (Richman & Lansdown 1988). The main problems are concerned with eating or sleeping difficulties and with bowel or bladder control. The latter two problems show a marked decline over the 1-year period. Affective symptoms such as unhappiness and relationship problems are infrequent, but when they arise, they are probably of some significance. Community studies (Richman et al 1975) indicate that 20% of children are regarded by their mothers as having problems, with 7% rated as severe. Richman and colleagues (1975) also found that there was a strong association between behaviour problems and language delay, 25% of children with language delay having significant behaviour problems. The most likely explanation for this association is that slow language acquisition leads to poor communication and social skills with increased frustration, so that behaviour problems arise.

Follow-up studies (Richman et al 1982) found that over 60% of the children originally identified as disturbed aged 3 continue to have problems aged 4, with nearly 60% still having problems aged 8. Persistent problems

**Table 5.1** Problem behaviours in 3- and 4-year-olds (Richman and Lansdown 1988)

| Behaviour | 3-year-olds (%) | 4-year-olds (%) |
|---|---|---|
| Poor appetite | 19 | 20 |
| Faddy eater | 15 | 24 |
| Difficulty settling at night | 16 | 15 |
| Waking at night | 14 | 12 |
| Overactive and restless | 17 | 13 |
| Poor concentration | 9 | 6 |
| Difficult to control | 11 | 10 |
| Temper | 5 | 6 |
| Unhappy mood | 4 | 7 |
| Worries | 4 | 1 |
| Fears | 10 | 12 |
| Poor relationships with siblings | 10 | 15 |
| Poor relationships with peers | 4 | 6 |
| Regular day wetting | 26 | 8 |
| Regular night wetting | 33 | 19 |
| Regular soiling | 16 | 3 |

were more common among boys who were below average intelligence, were rated as a severe problem aged 3 and were also described as overactive at that age. This study also found that problems were more likely to persist when there was marital discord, psychiatric disturbance in the mother or social disadvantage.

## COMMON PROBLEMS

This section discusses those problems that are particularly characteristic of the pre-school period while others, such as soiling, that occur in older children as well, are discussed in the relevant chapter.

### Temper tantrums

These usually arise when the child is thwarted, angry or has been hurt. They can occur in isolation or as part of a wider problem. They comprise a variety of behaviours, including screaming, crying, often resulting in collapse to the floor with the banging of the feet. The child can be aggressive towards other people around him, but rarely injures himself. Most tantrums 'burn themselves out', so that specific intervention is not necessary. If it is, then the following points are useful:

- If necessary, restrain from behind by folding arms around the child's body
- Minimise any additional attention to the child
- Only respond and praise when behaviour has returned to normal.

## Breath-holding attacks

These are common in preschool children, starting around the age of 12 months with peak frequency between the ages of 2 and 3. The episodes are normally precipitated by frustration or a minor upset or injury. This is followed by crying which increases in intensity until the child is extremely upset. Breathing then stops, usually in expiration, and the child may gradually become blue, especially around the lips. Usually the child spontaneously begins to breath again after about 30 seconds. Occasionally, however, the episode continues and in a very small number of children they may produce an epileptic seizure. The parents may inadvertently reinforce this behaviour by excessive attention and concern, so that some children even begin to use this behaviour as a means to alarm, or to express anger towards the parents. The best management is to deal with the situation as calmly as possible and minimise reinforcement for the behaviour. The prognosis in most cases is good.

## Thumb-sucking and nail-biting

These common habits are often the source of concern for parents. Thumb sucking is used by small children as a means of comfort and support at a time of stress. Most children spontaneously outgrow these habits. By themselves, they are not indicative of any underlying psychiatric disorder. Persistent thumb sucking may lead to malocclusion of the teeth.

## Eating disorders

These range in severity from a minor problem such as the finicky child to the severe disabling problem of *non-organic failure to thrive* (NOFTT). It is most unlikely that children will become nutritionally deficient from their poor eating habits, a point of reassurance for mothers. Minor problems will usually respond to patient and attentive listening to the parents' concerns, counselling and specific advice.

### Rumination disorder of infancy

This is defined by DSM-III-R as the repeated regurgitation of food in the absence of any gastrointestinal abnormality with failure to gain weight or

**Table 5.2**    Features of failure to thrive

**Common symptoms**
- Food refusal
- Vomiting
- Diarrhoea

**Growth**
- Less than third centile for height and weight

**Physical appearance**
- Thin, wasted baby, distended stomach, wispy, thin hair

**Developmental retardation**
- Generally delayed

**Behaviour**
- Apathetic
- Withdrawn
- Sad
- Expressionless face
- Irritable
- Indifferent

even a loss of weight. Onset is usually between 3 months and 12 months of age. In many cases, it is a reflection of the disturbed mother–child relationship.

*Non-organic failure to thrive (NOFTT) (Table 5.2)*

This usually manifests itself in the first year of life as persistent failure to gain weight. The child is below the third percentile for weight, with additional evidence of developmental and cognitive delay. Examination and investigation reveal no cause for the failure to gain weight. The infant is irritable, lethargic and apathetic. The most striking feature is the poor mother–child relationship, manifest by the critical and rejecting attitude of the mother towards the infant's feeding. This often occurs in the context of more widespread emotional and social deprivation with the individual characteristics of the child such as adverse temperamental factors and aversion to feeding also making a contribution. The clinical picture varies widely, more severe cases proving extremely intractable (Skuse 1985).

Admission to hospital is frequently necessary in order to ensure the child's safety and also to assess the mother–child relationship. Extensive support and counselling is the mainstay of treatment, though in many situations this is not successful. Alternative care arrangements for the child, including foster care and ultimately adoption, may be required in the most severe cases.

*Deprivation dwarfism*

This condition, first described by Powell et al (1967), occurs in the toddler and older child. It usually presents as idiopathic short stature. It shares many features of NOFTT, including developmental and cognitive delay, behaviour problems and abnormal eating habits. The latter include food searching, scavenging, hoarding and gorging. These are clearly evident when the child is observed at home or when admitted to hospital for investigation. The family circumstances are also similar to those in NOFTT with poor mother–child relationship and social/emotional deprivation. Long-standing modification of the family interaction patterns is often difficult to achieve and sustain, so that placement of the child in a new family may be the most sensible and realistic option.

### Pica

This is defined as the ingestion of inedible material such as dirt or rubbish. It is a normal transitory phenomenon during the toddler period. Persistent ingestion is found amongst mentally retarded, psychotic and socially deprived children. Lead poisoning, though always mentioned, is a possible but uncommon danger from pica.

## Sleep problems

The common problem is wakefulness at night, while other problems such as nightmares, night terrors, somnambulism and narcolepsy occur in older children (see Ch. 13).

### Wakefulness at night

Community studies have shown prevalence rates of 20% in 2-year-olds, 10% in 3-year-olds and 4% in 8-year-olds (Richman 1981, Eaton-Evans & Dugdale 1988).

*Clinical features.* The two most frequent problems are: reluctance to settle at night and persistent waking up during the night. Several factors contribute to the problems, including adverse temperamental characteristics in the child, perinatal problems, maternal anxiety and family stress. Clinically, it is important to distinguish those situations in which the sleep problem is the sole problem from those where it is part of a more widespread problem, which may be more difficult to change.

*Management.* It is useful to separate those factors responsible for the onset of the problem, for instance adverse temperamental characteristics, from those for the maintenance of the problem, for instance excessive parental concern or attention. Medication such as trimeprazine (30–60 mg at night), promethazine (15–30 mg at night) or chloral (500–1000 mg at night) is frequently prescribed, but is usually ineffective, with the additional dangers resulting from long-term usage. The only genuine indication for medication is to provide a brief respite for the parents and to ensure that the child has an uninterrupted night's sleep.

|  | Monday | Tuesday | Wednesday | Thursday | Friday | Saturday | Sunday |
|---|---|---|---|---|---|---|---|
| Woke up in the morning |  |  |  |  |  |  |  |
| Daytime nap |  |  |  |  |  |  |  |
| Went to bed in the evening |  |  |  |  |  |  |  |
| Went to sleep in the evening |  |  |  |  |  |  |  |
| Time(s) woke up |  |  |  |  |  |  |  |
| What you did |  |  |  |  |  |  |  |
| Time(s) went to sleep again |  |  |  |  |  |  |  |
| Parents' bedtime |  |  |  |  |  |  |  |
| Time(s) woke up |  |  |  |  |  |  |  |
| What you did |  |  |  |  |  |  |  |
| Time(s) went to sleep again |  |  |  |  |  |  |  |

**Fig. 5.1**  Sleep diary

The most successful management is a behavioural strategy. This involves the basic behavioural approach of a functional analysis of the problem together with an accurate diary record of the sleep pattern. Figure 5.1 shows the format of the sleep diary, while Table 5.3 summarises the main headings of the functional analysis. Further details of the behavioural treatment approach are provided in Chapter 17, and the book by Douglas & Richman (1984) provides a useful summary of suitable techniques. The key elements in a successful programme are as follows:

- joint parental participation (this is absolutely essential)
- agreement with parents about the goals of treatment, for instance acceptable bedtime or the duration of night-time crying before parental intervention
- explanation and implementation of operant techniques such as positive reinforcement, extinction, shaping and fading
- accurate recording of the programme
- regular review and modification of the programme.

Clinical experience shows this approach to be successful, especially where the sleep problem is the main source of concern.

---

**Table 5.3** Assessment schedule for sleep problems

---

**Details of the child**
- Age/sex/developmental history/previous medical history

**Family circumstances**
- Ages and occupations of the parents
- Age(s) of the sibling(s)
- Housing
  - type (house/flat/maisonette)
  - number of bedrooms
  - sleeping arrangements
- Current stress(es) for the family

**Child's current sleeping pattern**
- Child sleeps in own room/own bed or cot/shares with sibling
- Bedtime routine
  - What time does child begin to get ready for bed?
  - Is there a bedtime routine, for instance bath followed by story?
  - Any special ways to settle the child?
  - Does the child have a special toy or comforter?
- Record of sleep disturbance(settling/waking up at night)
- See sleep diary chart

---

## Separation anxiety and attachment disorders

DSM-III-R and ICD-10 have defined a new category of disturbance which they call *separation anxiety disorder* and *reactive attachment disorder* respectively. The main features are excessive separation anxiety and poor mother–child attachment. These categories constitute a recognition that the development of satisfactory social relationships is of prime importance during infancy and early childhood. By definition, the mother–infant relationship is poor and is characterised by 'anxious attachment' (child chronically anxious about mother's ability to reassure and calm) or 'avoidant attachment' (child avoids contact after separation due to previous rejecting, angry responses from the mother).

ICD-10 has also introduced another new category, *disinhibited attachment disorder*, to describe a general failure of some children to form selective attachments to individuals but instead to respond indiscriminately towards everyone. This pattern of behaviour is frequently seen in children whose early childhood was severely disrupted because of multiple care placements and/or residence in institutions. These children are disinhibited, overactive, emotionally labile and often aggressive. Placement in stable, secure environments on a long-term basis is the best way to resolve the problem. Placements with families often fail, however, as the child is unable to fulfil the adults' expectation of warmth and responsiveness, so that a small children's home may be a better solution for some children.

## PSYCHIATRIC ASPECTS OF CHILD ABUSE

Originally, the term 'child abuse' was restricted to the 'battered baby' syndrome (Kempe & Kempe 1978), but it has now been extended to include physical abuse, emotional abuse, sexual abuse and neglect. Recent enquiries and controversies, particularly the Cleveland affair (DHSS 1988), have highlighted the importance of this topic for all doctors involved in the care of children. It is also important to remember that different aspects of child abuse are frequently present in the same child and family, so that many of the comments about detection, management and treatment apply equally well to all aspects of child abuse. The main professional responsibility for child protection lies with the Social Services Department, though other professions are frequently involved at various stages in the individual case.

This section concentrates on the psychiatric aspects relating to infants and younger children, while Chapter 14 discusses the adolescent aspects. Several recently published books (Kempe & Kempe 1979, Jones 1982, Porter 1984, Bentovim et al 1988) provide very useful accounts of current practice on various aspects of child abuse.

### Prevalence

Accurate estimates are hard to obtain, mainly because of the variation in the diagnostic criteria, the population studied and the reluctance to disclose episodes of abuse. Mrazek & Mrazek (1985) quote prevalence rates of 3.4, 2.2 and 0.7 cases per 1000 per child per year for physical, emotional and sexual abuse respectively.

### Physical abuse (non-accidental injury; Mrazek & Mrazek 1985)

Diagnostic awareness and suspicion are the key elements in the detection and recognition of physical abuse. Three sets of factors, often present simultaneously, are found in many cases: predisposing factors in the child, risk factors in the parents and adverse social circumstances (Table 5.4). The most important point for clinical practice is, however, to recognise that child abuse can occur in all sections of society.

#### Management

Three separate stages can be identified in the investigation of suspected child abuse:

- the detection and disclosure phase
- child protection and legal considerations
- therapeutic and practical support for the child and family in the immediate and long term.

**Table 5.4**   Common features of abused children and their families

**Vulnerability factors in the abused child**
- Product of unwanted pregnancy
- Unwanted child in family
- Low birthweight
- Separation from mother in neonatal period
- Mental or physical handicap
- Habitually restless, sleepless or incessantly crying
- Physical unattractiveness

**High-risk factors in the parent(s)**
- Single parent
- Young
- Abused as children
- Low self-esteem
- Unrealistic expectations of child and his development
- Inconsistent or punishment-orientated discipline

**Adverse social circumstances**
- Low income or unemployment
- Social isolation
- Large family

These separate stages usually proceed one another in a sequential manner.

Stage 1 involves the Social Services Department and frequently general practitioners and/or paediatricians. Stage 2 involves the convening of a case conference to obtain a comprehensive assessment of the child's needs and the initiation of statutory measures of care, if necessary, to ensure the protection of the child. This stage is also concerned with decisions about pursuing criminal proceedings against the perpetrator of the abuse, who is often one of the child's carers. Stage 3 is the institution of a therapeutic plan to remedy the psychological sequelae of the abuse for the child and also to improve the quality of parenting. The latter includes practical help to lessen the burden of child care as well as specific advice and counselling on parenting skills.

The child psychiatrist can make a useful contribution in two ways:

- by acting as an outside consultant to other professionals and agencies working with the family on the various aspects of detection, management and treatment
- by providing individual and family therapy for the child, the parents or the family in particular instances depending upon the assessment.

In addition to its immediate effects, child abuse may have medium-term and long-term sequelae. Many abused children continue to be exposed to emotional abuse and neglect throughout their childhood, so that they often show symptoms of disturbance such as unhappiness, wariness, lack of trust, low self-esteem and poor peer friends. This childhood experience in turn predisposes abused children to become abusing parents as adults (Kempe

& Kempe 1978) and they are at greater risk of psychiatric disturbance as adults. Mullen et al (1988) found that women with a childhood experience of physical or sexual abuse were four times more likely to be disturbed as adults than non-abused women.

## Emotional abuse

This term has been introduced to describe the severe impairment of social and emotional development resulting from repeated and persistent criticism, lack of affection, rejection, verbal abuse and other similar behaviour shown by the parent(s) to the child over a long period of time. Affected children display a variety of symptoms including low self-esteem, limited capacity for enjoyment, severe aggression and impulsive behaviour. Many children also show the more specific features of the syndromes of NOFTT and deprivation dwarfism. Diagnosis is made through observation and interview of the parent(s) and child, separately and together. The parents rarely have a formal psychiatric disorder, though personality disturbance and a history of parental childhood deprivation are common. Management involves similar principles to those outlined for stage 3 of physical abuse.

## Sexual abuse (Ousten 1990)

This has become a topic of major public and paediatric concern in the late 1980s (DHSS 1988). A commonly used definition is: 'the involvement of dependent children and adolescents in sexual activities they do not truly comprehend, to which they are unable to give informed consent, or which violate the social taboos of family roles.'

Fundamental to child sexual abuse is the misuse of adult power. The range of activities includes fondling, masturbation, rape and buggery. The term also covers some activities not involving physical contact such as posing for pornographic photographs or films. The abuser is frequently known to the child and is often a member of the family.

The presentation of the sexual abuse varies widely depending on the nature of the abuse and on the relationship between the abused child and the perpetrator. Open disclosure or accusation is more likely when the offender is outside the family, whereas physical symptoms involving the anogenital region and/or emotional or behavioural disturbance are commoner when a family member is responsible. As with physical abuse, diagnostic awareness and suspicion are the key elements in the detection and recognition of the abuse.

### Investigation (Bentovim et al 1988)

Sensitivity and tact are clearly essential when conducting the examination and interview of the child during the initial investigation. Separate detailed questioning and interviewing of the parents are also necessary.

*Management (Bentovim et al 1988)*

The same principles apply in sexual abuse as in physical abuse. The role of the child psychiatry team is more directly relevant in sexual abuse, as interviewing skills, psychotherapeutic expertise and the use of special equipment, in particular anatomically accurate dolls (White et al 1986), are often necessary at the detection and also the treatment stages of management. Detailed accounts of this work, including the use of the anatomical dolls, are found in the book by the Great Ormond Street Child Sex Abuse Team (Bentovim et al 1988). The establishment of specialised assessment teams in every locality is another important recommendation of the Cleveland Enquiry (DHSS 1988).

## Neglect

This varies markedly, ranging from relative inadequacy and incompetence in providing safety, shelter, love and security for the child to the severe failure in the provision of basic essentials, often combined with emotional and social deprivation. Though more difficult to quantify than physical or sexual abuse, the condition is certainly more common, at least in its milder forms, than these other two forms of abuse. Additionally, it may be more long-lasting, with potentially more serious consequences for the child's development. It is often noticed and reported by relatives, neighbours, health visitors and teachers. Adverse social circumstances and poor parenting are usually found, and alternative family placement for the child is most suitable solution in the long term in many cases.

## Munchausen's syndrome by proxy (Meadow 1982)

This remarkable variant of physical abuse often occurs against the same background of parental psychopathology and social disadvantage as other forms of abuse. The essential feature of this syndrome is the fabrication of physical illness in the child by the parent(s), usually the mother. Common examples include factitious recurrent bleeding and the unstable control of diabetes or epilepsy. Extensive investigation and admission to hospital are carried out with fruitless results. It is only when the possibility of parental abuse is recognised that the explanation becomes apparent.

*Management*

As soon as the diagnosis is established, the parents should be confronted openly with this situation. The main priority is the protection of the child, including where necessary the removal of the child from the family home. The immediate and longer-term aims of treatment are similar to that for child abuse as the underlying psychopathology and social circumstances are similar. The role of the child psychiatrist is usually confined in most cases to offering counselling for the parents and/or family therapy when indicated.

## Outcome

Meadows's (1982) original series of 19 cases had a very variable outcome: two died; two continued to attend the doctor frequently; eight were removed from home and were thereafter symptom-free; and seven remained at home symptom-free. A recent review of 117 cases (Rosenberg 1987) found that 9% of cases had died, most commonly from suffocation or poisoning, with further episodes even after the diagnosis was made. There was also the involvement of siblings in some cases.

# 6. Pervasive developmental disorders

## INTRODUCTION

Earlier versions of DSM and ICD classified autism under the category of childhood psychosis, as it is a severe and disabling condition with clear-cut abnormalities. However, children with autism do not experience hallucinations or delusions, the characteristic features of psychosis. Moreover, unlike other psychotic disorders, the abnormalities in autism are present from early infancy, usually without a period of normal development. For these reasons, ICD-10 has renamed infantile autism as *childhood autism* and placed the disorder as an example of a new category called *pervasive developmental disorders*. Other pervasive developmental disorders include Rett's syndrome, disintegrative disorder and Asperger's syndrome. This chapter discusses the clinical features of these four pervasive developmental disorders.

## CHILDHOOD AUTISM

Kanner's (1943) original description of 11 children with 'an extreme autistic aloneness' has not been improved upon with its astute observation of 'an inability to relate in an ordinary way to people and to situations' and 'an anxiously obsessive desire for the maintenance of sameness'. Subsequently, opinions have fluctuated about the diagnosis, aetiology and treatment. Most authorities now agree that three features are essential to the diagnosis:

- general and profound failure to develop social relationships
- language retardation
- restricted repertoire of activities.

Usually, these abnormalities should be manifest before 30 months, with later-onset cases classified as *childhood-onset*.

### Prevalence

Community surveys (Lotter 1966, Wing & Gould 1979) have found prevalence rates of 2/10 000 increasing to 20/10 000 when individuals with

**Table 6.1**   Clinical features of childhood autism

**Impaired social relationships**
- Impaired attachment and bonding
- Lack of co-operative and reciprocal play
- Failure to use eye-to-eye gaze, facial expression, body posture and gesture to regulate social interaction
- Lack of empathy

**Language abnormalities**
- Delayed and deviant
- Impaired imitation and comprehension
- Echolalia, pronominal reversal and poor social use

**Restricted repertoire of activities**
- Preoccupation with stereotyped and restricted patterns of interest
- Specific attachments to unusual objects
- Adherence to specific non-functional routines or rituals
- Stereotypic and repetitive motor mannerisms involving hand/finger flapping or twisting, or complex whole body movements
- Preoccupations with part-objects or non-functional elements of play materials, for example the odour, the feel of the surface or the noise/vibration
- Distress over changes in small non-functional details of environment

**Other features**
- Symptoms usually present before 30 months
- 75% of children with childhood autism have IQ in retarded range
- Approximately 15% develop epilepsy during adolescence

severe mental retardation and some autistic features are included. Boys are three times more commonly affected than girls.

## Clinical features

Children usually present in the third year of life with developmental delay, particularly in language (Table 6.1).

### Impaired social relationships

Parental recollections of infancy often reveal that as an infant, the child was slow to smile, unresponsive and passive with a dislike of physical contact and affection. Contemporary social deficits include:

- failing to use eye-to-eye gaze and facial expression for social interaction
- rarely seeking others for comfort or affection
- rarely initiating interaction with others
- lack of empathy
- little interest in co-operative play.

The children are aloof and indifferent to people.

*Language abnormalities*

Language acquisition is delayed and deviant, with many autistic children (approximately 50%) never developing language. When language is present, abnormalities are many and varied, including:

- immediate and delayed echolalia (repetition of spoken word(s) or phrase(s))
- poor comprehension and use of gesture
- pronominal reversal (use of 'you' when 'I' is meant)
- abnormalities in intonation, rhythm and pitch.

*Restricted repertoire of activities*

Common abnormalities are:

- rigid and restricted patterns of play
- intense attachments to unusual objects such as stones
- unusual preoccupations and interests, for instance total rote recall of timetables or bus routes to the exclusion of other pursuits
- a marked resistance to any change in the environment or daily routine. Tantrums and explosive outbursts often occur when any change is attempted.

*Other features*

Autistic children often exhibit a variety of stereotypies including rocking, finger twirling, spinning and tiptoe walking. They are often overactive, with a short attention span. 70% of autistic children are in the retarded range of intelligence, with only 5% having an IQ of above 100. Occasionally, some have remarkable abilities in isolated areas, for instance computation, music or rote memory. 15% will develop epilepsy during adolescence, though it is not usually severe.

## Association with other conditions

Autistic behaviour occurs in some patients with a diverse group of conditions including rubella, phenylketonuria, tuberose sclerosis, neurolipidoses, infantile spasms and the fragile X syndrome (Rutter 1985b). More recently, Rett's syndrome, with its marked autistic features, has been described (see below).

## Aetiology

Most people favour a primary cognitive basis with an underlying organic basis for the following reasons:

- neurological abnormalities are common
- because of the association with epilepsy and various neurological syndromes
- because of the increased rate of perinatal complications
- because of the higher concordance rate in monozygotic compared with dizygotic twins (Rutter & Schopler 1978).

Application of new investigative techniques such as CAT scan, MRI and positron emission tomography have not revealed any consistent abnormality, though increased serotonin levels have been reported. The relationship between autism and the fragile X syndrome is also unclear, as the different rates in the various studies may be a reflection of the degree of mental handicap rather than of aetiological significance. A most interesting psychological perspective on the autistic deficit has been provided by the series of experiments described by Hobson (1986). Hobson concluded that the primary deficit in autism is a lack of empathy, that is, the inability to perceive and interpret emotional cues.

## Treatment

The explanation of the diagnosis is a vital first step in helping parents to accept the presence of handicap with the consequent lessening of the parental guilt about aetiology. Counselling and advice are likely to be necessary throughout childhood. Rutter (1985b) has suggested that treatment aims should have four components:

- promotion of normal development
- reduction of rigidity and stereotypies
- removal of maladaptive behaviour
- alleviation of family stress.

Behavioural methods, including operant conditioning and shaping (see Ch.17) are the most likely way to achieve some success with the first three aims, while counselling is important for the fourth. Special schooling, where the child's special social and educational needs are recognised, is very beneficial, sometimes on a residential basis. Drugs do not have an important part in management.

## Outcome

Many individuals with childhood autism are unable to live independently, only 15% looking after and supporting themselves as adults (Lockyer & Rutter 1969). Many are placed in institutions for the mentally handicapped though, in the UK, government policy is now directed towards community care. Autistic children with an IQ of at least 70 who receive appropriate special education and who come from middle-class families do better than

**Table 6.2**    Symptoms in Rett's syndrome by age

**First three years**
- Uneventful prenatal and perinatal history
- Normal development during first 7–12 months, e.g. sitting, fine motor skills
- Deterioration of behaviour and mental state
- Delayed onset of walking (25 months) or non-walking (50%)
- Truncal ataxia
- Deceleration of head growth

**Later childhood**
- Mental retardation, relatively stable, autistic-like behaviour
- Stereotypic hand movements (hand-wringing)
- Ataxic myoclonus-like movements; apraxic, shuffling gait; episodic hyperpnoea

**In adolescence**
- Spasticity, especially lower limbs; walking may be lost
- Scoliosis
- Vasomotor disturbances of lower limbs

**Variable age onset**
- Seizures

their less able counterparts. In most individuals, there is some improvement in social relationships as they grow older, but many are still very handicapped. Parents often find it helpful to join the National Society for Autistic Children, who are able to offer long-term advice and support.

## RETT'S SYNDROME (TABLE 6.2)

Rett (1966) described 22 mentally handicapped children, all girls, who had a history of regression in development and displayed strikingly repetitive movements of the hands. He thought that the children were autistic with progressive spasticity, and proposed that diffuse cerebral atrophy was the underlying cause. More recent reports (Hagberg et al 1983, Kerr & Stevenson 1985) have indicated that this syndrome is more common than previously believed, with a prevalence rate of 1/30 000 (1/15 000 girls).

### Clinical features

The condition, which has only been described in girls, shows a characteristic clinical picture: a period of normal development up to around 18 months followed by a rapid decline in developmental progress and the rapid deterioration of higher brain functions. Within the following 18 months, there is evidence of severe dementia, loss of purposeful use of the hands, jerky ataxia and acquired microcephaly. After this rapid decline, the condition may stabilise, with no further progression for some time. Subsequently, more neurological abnormalities appear, including spastic paraplegia and epilepsy.

## Aetiology

Rett originally believed that high levels of ammonia were responsible for the condition, though subsequent studies have not confirmed this observation. The most commonly proposed explanation is that it is due to a dominant mutation on one X chromosome, and that the condition is non-viable in males.

## Prognosis

The majority of children are left profoundly retarded with severe neurological impairments. Many succumb to intermittent infections or to the underlying neuropathological disorder.

## DISINTEGRATIVE DISORDER

### Clinical features (Corbett et al 1977, Rutter 1985b)

This term refers to a group of conditions characterised by normal development until around 4 years of age followed by profound regression and behavioural disintegration, loss of language and other skills, impairment of social relationships and the development of stereotypies. It can follow on from a minor illness or from more definite neurological disease such as measles encephalitis. The prognosis is poor due to the underlying degenerative pathology in many cases. Most individuals are left with severe mental retardation.

## ASPERGER'S SYNDROME/SCHIZOID PERSONALITY

This condition, originally described by Asperger (1944), shows some similarities to childhood autism in that there is an impairment of social relationships with a lack of reciprocal social interaction and a restricted, stereotyped repetitive repertoire of interests and activities. However, the children differ diagnostically from those with childhood autism in two important respects: there is no general intellectual retardation and the language development is normal. Other characteristics include male preponderance and poor motor co-ordination with marked clumsiness. The condition is in many ways a minor variant of childhood autism (Wing 1981) with the impairment in social relationships persisting into adult life.

The term *schizoid personality of childhood* was coined by Wolff & Chick (1980) to describe a small number of children with unusual but distinctive personality characteristics, similar in some ways to children with Asperger's syndrome. These 'schizoid' children are described as aloof, distant and lacking in empathy. Other features include:

- obstinate and aggressive outbursts when under pressure to conform, often at school

- undue rigidity
- sensitivity to criticism
- unusual interests to the exclusion of everything else.

More recently, Wolff (1991) has argued from follow-up studies of these children that they form a separate diagnostic category, the schizoid personality of childhood, similar to but distinct from childhood autism and Asperger's syndrome. As adults, Wolff (1991) found that they showed features of the schizotypal disorder.

## OTHER CONDITIONS

Many children with mental retardation show some autistic features. In clinical practice, it is often difficult to know whether they fulfil the criteria for pervasive developmental disorder in addition to that for intellectual retardation. It is clear that there is a wide diversity in the severity of these 'autistic features', so that it is often arbitrary whether the label 'childhood autism' is applied to these children. Many of them also show features of hyperactivity and aggression. For these reasons, ICD-10 has made two additional categories: *overactive disorder associated with mental retardation and stereotyped movements* and *pervasive developmental disorder unspecified.*

# 7. Schizophrenia and related conditions

## INTRODUCTION

*Psychosis* is a term frequently applied, often loosely, to describe serious disorders such as schizophrenia. Despite the slackness of its definition, psychosis is so embedded in psychiatric terminology that it is likely to remain in use for the foreseeable future. Consequently it is important to define its characteristics:

- severe and disabling
- marked social impairment
- qualitatively abnormal experience(s)
- lack of insight.

Psychotic conditions have a profound effect on the daily functioning of affected individuals during an acute episode as well as having long-term implications for social adjustment and well-being. The impairment affects social relationships, so that the individual is unable to maintain normal friendships, with consequent increasing isolation and withdrawal. This probably arises from the individual's own poor social skills as well as from other people's response to the his odd and unpredictable behaviour. Education and later employment are also adversely affected, as the individual lacks motivation and persistence to make a success of these tasks.

The term *qualitative abnormal experience(s)* indicates that an individual with a psychotic illness has some experiences that are outside the limits of normality and are by definition pathological. The two most common types of qualitatively abnormal experience are hallucinations and delusions (Table 7.1). A *hallucination* is a false sensory perception, that is, a sensory experience without any external stimulus. It has the same qualities as a normal perception in that it is experienced as being in the external world and has the usual perceptual features of depth, location and detail. Hallucinations may occur in any sensory modality including auditory, visual, olfactory or tactile. *Delusions* are false beliefs that are held with absolute conviction and are out of keeping with the cultural and educational background of the individual. There are two types of delusion, *primary* and

**Table 7.1**    Hallucinations and delusions

**Hallucination**
- Definition – A false sensory perception, that is a sensory experience without an external stimulus
- Features – Same qualities as an ordinary perception, that is perceived as coming from the external world with the normal features of location, depth and detail
- Modalities – Auditory, visual, olfactory or tactile

**Illusion**
- Definition – A misinterpretation of a sensory stimulus
- Modalities – Auditory, visual, olfactory or tactile

**Delusion**
- Definition – A false belief which is held with absolute conviction and is out of keeping with the cultural and educational background of the individual
- Two types, primary and secondary, are distinguished by the context in which they arise rather than their content

*secondary*, which are differentiated by the context in which they arise rather than by their content (see next section).

*Insight* refers to the individual's ability to recognise or appreciate whether he is ill or not. This self-appraisal of psychological functioning is lacking to a major extent during an acute psychotic episode, so that the delusional ideas and hallucinatory experiences are accepted as normal.

This chapter discusses the major group of illnesses associated with psychotic features, the schizophrenia(s) and related conditions.

## CHILDHOOD SCHIZOPHRENIA

Both ICD and DSM adopt the position that schizophrenia in childhood should fulfill the same criteria as that occurring in adult life. They do, however, recognise that the pattern and distribution of symptomatology may be different in childhood than in later life.

### Background

The 19th-century German psychiatrist Kraepelin (1919), was responsible for the division of psychoses into *functional* and *organic*. He made this distinction on the basis of his own studies into the long-term outcome of these conditions. He further divided functional psychoses into *dementia praecox* and *manic-depressive psychosis*, again because of their different prognosis. Dementia praecox, or schizophrenia as it was later to be known, was regarded as a serious, disabling condition affecting young adults (hence the term 'praecox') resulting in a gradual deterioration or degeneration of mental faculties. By contrast, manic-depressive psychosis did not show the same deterioration or loss of functions over time.

Bleuler (1911) coined the term *schizophrenia* or *group of schizophrenias* to describe those conditions previously known as dementia praecox. He chose this new term to emphasise the separation, or lack of cohesion and integration, between the various aspects of psychological functioning which is so characteristic of the disease. Mood, motivation, thinking and behaviour all function independently, often incongruously, producing the diagnostic abnormalities of thought, perception and movement.

Though Kraepelin and Bleuler acknowledged that schizophrenia could occur in childhood, the first accounts of psychosis in childhood were by De Sanctis (1906) and Heller (1930), who used the terms *dementia praecos-sisima* and *dementia infantilis* respectively. Potter (1933) also described the clinical features of schizophrenia presenting in childhood. Despite these accounts, there was little agreement about the nature of psychosis in childhood, a confusion probably exacerbated to some extent by Kanner's delineation of infantile autism (Kanner 1943).

These uncertainties have now been resolved by clinical studies involving the long-term follow-up and the comparison of the family characteristics of affected children (Volkmar et al 1988). The consensus of opinion is that childhood autism and childhood schizophrenia are distinct and separate conditions with little overlap in symptomatology, prognosis or family characteristics.

## Prevalence

Accurate figures are difficult to estimate, though the disease is very rare before middle childhood. Even in adolescence, the rate is probably less than 3/10 000. Summarising the results from four large studies, Volkmar et al (1988) found that there was a slight male predominance, low average intelligence (IQ around 85) and the children came from a lower socioeconomic background.

## Clinical features

The onset is often insidious or gradual in younger children, with a more florid or acute onset in older children and adolescents. The classical features of schizophrenia, a well-developed delusional system with auditory hallucinations and marked agitation, are easily recognised when present, though commonly the clinical picture is less clear, with a mixture of symptoms, often involving mood disturbance.

The following features are characteristic:

- thought disorder
- disorders of perception
- emotional disturbance
- motor or movement disturbance
- social impairments (Table 7.2).

**Table 7.2**   Clinical features of schizophrenia

**Disorders in the form of thinking**

- Thought block (the experience of the train of thought being suddenly stopped and followed by a new unrelated train of thought)
- Thought insertion (the experience that thoughts are being put into one's mind)
- Thought withdrawal (the experience that thoughts are being removed from one's mind)

**Disorders in the content of thinking (delusions)**

- Primary delusions
  - Delusional (autochthenous) idea – a false belief arising out of the blue with the quality of a 'brain wave'. Not explicable in terms of previous or current experiences
  - Delusional perception – an ordinary sensory stimulus is given a delusional interpretation, e.g. traffic lights changing to green
  - Delusional mood – a state of perplexity in which the individual feels that 'something is going on'
- Secondary delusions
  A false belief understandable in terms of preceding or current situation, for instance if a person is convinced that there is a plot to harm him, then it is reasonable to believe the man loitering outside the house is a member of the secret service

**Disorders of perception**

- Hallucinations – auditory hallucinations are commonest
- Illusions – sometimes occur in very agitated individuals

**Emotional disturbances**

- Emotional expression is inadequate with frequent fluctuations in expression
  - 'Incongruous' – inappropriate emotional expression, e.g. hilarity at death of close friend
  - 'Flattening' – limitation in the range of emotional expression

**Disorders of movement/mobility**

- Extreme agitation and impulsive outbursts, stereotypies and abnormal postures (catatonia)

**Social disabilities**

- May be gradual
- Withdrawal and isolation, with long-term adverse consequences on relationships and ability to function independently

*Thought disorder*

The thought disorder is of two types, form or content. Disorders of *thought form* are *thought block* (the experience that a train of thought stops abruptly and is followed by a new, unrelated train of thought), *thought insertion* (the experience that thoughts are being put into one's mind) and *thought withdrawal* (the experience that thoughts are being removed from one's mind).

Disorders of *thought content* are *delusions* which may be primary or secondary. A *primary delusion* has three features, all of which need not be present in each instance:

- delusional ideas
- delusional perception
- delusional mood.

The *delusional idea* arises 'out of the blue' or 'like a brain wave' and is not understandable in terms of the preceding mood or behaviour. It often starts with a *delusional perception*, a delusional interpretation of a normal perception, for instance when the traffic light turns green, this is a signal that the world has changed into a new order. *Delusional mood* is the state of perplexity in which the individual has a sense that some inexplicable change is happening, or that 'something is going on'.

By contrast, *secondary delusions* do not have an 'out of the blue' quality, but rather arise from or are understandable in the light of existing mood change or events in the individual's current environment. For instance, the patient's conviction that the man loitering outside his house is a member of the secret services may be understandable because the patient already has another delusional idea that the authorities are watching him because he has devised a new method of breaking into the national security computer network.

## Disorders of perception

Disorders of perception are *hallucinations* and *illusions*, the latter being a misinterpretation of a real perceptual stimulus. The most common type of perceptual abnormality is auditory hallucinations, while hallucinations in other sensory modalities are much less common. Occasionally, a very agitated patient can experience auditory or visual illusions.

## Disturbances of emotion

Disturbances of emotion include feelings of depression or excitement, but more characteristically there is a general inability to express emotions adequately. Classically, this is described as *emotional incongruity*, that is the expression of an emotion inappropriate to the circumstances, or 'flattening' of affect, that is the restriction in range of emotional expression.

## Motor or movement disturbance

Abnormal motor symptoms and signs include stereotypies, unpredictable and violent behaviour, facial grimacing and contortions and, rarely, catatonic behaviour in which the individual assumes an abnormal posture.

## Social impairments

Abnormalities in social functioning, for instance withdrawal and social isolation, may be the first symptoms of the disease, and their persistence a major source of long-term disability.

**Table 7.3**    Abnormalities in children with schizophrenia

| Study | Number of children | Thought disorder (%) | Delusions (%) | Auditory hallucinations (%) | Visual hallucinations (%) |
|---|---|---|---|---|---|
| Kolvin et al 1971 | 33 | 60 | 58 | 82 | 30 |
| Green et al 1984 | 24 | 100 | 54 | 79 | 46 |
| Volkmar et al 1988 | 14 | 93 | 86 | 79 | 28 |
| Russel et al 1989 | 35 | 40 | 63 | 80 | 13 |

Finally, Table 7.3 summarises the main clinical findings from some recent review series of children with schizophrenia. The results show that auditory hallucinations and thought disorder are very common features in children with schizophrenia, results which support the view that schizophrenia in children and adults should have the same diagnostic criteria.

## Differential diagnosis

Two features, the impairment of consciousness and the occurrence of prominent affective symptoms, may give rise to some diagnostic confusion. The presence of clouding or alteration in consciousness is strongly suggestive of an underlying organic condition such as a postictal epileptic confusional state or a drug-induced state. Consequently, a neurological assessment including investigations and/or a toxicological screening is sometimes important. Furthermore, temporal lobe epilepsy is associated with an increased risk of schizophrenia (Ounsted et al 1986), so that this may need to be considered in the differential diagnosis. A mixture of affective and schizophrenic symptoms is a common presentation in older children and adolescents, making it extremely difficult initially to distinguish between a schizophrenic, a hypomanic and a mixed affective episode. The subsequent course and/or the recurrence of symptoms are probably the best diagnostic guide in the long term.

## Aetiology (Kendell & Zealley 1993)

Clearly, genetic and environmental factors are both involved in the development of the disease. The evidence for a major genetic contribution, mainly from adult studies, is threefold:

- The first degree relatives of patients with schizophrenia have a 12% risk of developing the illness compared with the general population risk of 1%

- There are higher concordance rates for monozygotic than for dizygotic twins
- The fostered or adopted children of parents with schizophrenia have a similar risk of developing the disorder as those who remain with their schizophrenic parents.

The contribution of environmental factors is less clear-cut. Studies in the 1960s and 1970s proposing that deviant communication patterns, particularly the 'double bind' hypothesis of Bateson and his colleagues (1956), were a major contributory factor to the onset of schizophrenia have now largely been abandoned. The most likely explanation for any odd communication patterns present is that they represent a secondary response by the parents to the presence of a disturbed child within the family or possibly a reflection in a minor form of the child's condition (Leff et al 1982). The role of life events in childhood schizophrenia has not been studied systematically, but is probably less relevant.

## Treatment (Table 7.4)

The same treatment principles that are applied to adults are relevant to children and adolescents, with the important additional consideration of education and later on employment. The three major components of treatment are:

- medication
- individual and family counselling
- the provision of specialised educational resources.

### Medication

In the acute phase, treatment with major tranquillisers, for example chlorpromazine or haloperidol, is the mainstay of treatment. It is essential

**Table 7.4**  Treatment of childhood schizophrenia

**Drug treatment**
- Major tranquillisers (phenothiazines or butyrophenones) are the main treatment agents
- Extrapyramidal side effects (acute dystonic reactions and parkinsonian symptoms) are common
- In the longer term, maintenance treatment with a depot preparation, e.g. fluphenazine decanoate, is very useful

**Individual and family support**
- Crucial to work collaboratively with child and family from outset
- Parents need long-term support to enable them to cope with unpredictable and erratic behaviour

**Educational resources**
- Child often needs specialised individual help following discharge from hospital
- Employment prospects are an important determinant of long-term outcome

to monitor for possible extrapyramidal side effects, particularly acute dystonic reactions or parkinsonian symptoms (see Ch. 17 for more details). It is often also necessary to admit the child or adolescent to a psychiatric in-patient unit in order to institute medication and to observe the child's behaviour more closely. The major tranquillisers are usually effective in reducing the 'positive' symptoms such as hallucinations or delusions, but less so with the 'negative' symptoms such as apathy, inertia or poor motivation. It is sometimes necessary to continue medication on a long-term basis because of persistent symptomatology, so that a switch to maintenance treatment with an intramuscular depot preparation of the major tranquilliser is the best solution.

## Child and family

The child and family need individual and group support from the outset in order to enable them understand the illness and minimise the social handicaps. Clearly, it may be difficult to work with the child initially, but it is essential to work collaboratively with the parents from the outset. The long-term support of the family by a member of the nursing staff from the in-patient unit is extremely useful, not only in ensuring that medication is taken on a regular basis but also helping the parents cope with the unpredictable and erratic behaviour of their child.

## Education

The child may require specialised educational advice and help following the acute episode in order to give him the best opportunity to benefit from educational provision. In the long term, the likelihood of obtaining employment is a key factor in the subsequent successful outcome.

## Outcome

Evidence about the long-term outcome is limited by the quality of follow-up studies. A 20-year follow-up of 57 children diagnosed as schizophrenic in childhood (Eggers 1978) showed that 20% had complete remission, 30% improved and 50% had a moderate or poor outcome. Unfavourable outcome was associated with early onset (younger than 10 years) and poor premorbid personality adjustment. Table 7.5 summarises the important prognostic factors from available follow-up studies.

## ORGANIC PSYCHOTIC STATES

Acute and chronic neurological disorders can produce wide ranging psychiatric symptoms, so that an underlying organic basis must be excluded

**Table 7.5**    Prognostic features in childhood schizophrenia

**Good prognostic features**
- Good premorbid adjustment
- Above average intelligence
- Acute onset related to stress
- Good home circumstances and relationships
- Family history of affective disorder

**Bad prognostic features**
- Poor premorbid personality adjustment, e.g. schizoid
- Insidious onset
- Younger age
- Incomplete response to medication
- Unsatisfactory home circumstances and relationships
- Positive family history
- Long duration of symptoms

**Note**
- 'Positive' symptoms such as delusions and hallucinations have little prognostic value
- 'Negative' symptoms such as flattening of affect indicate poor outcome

for many psychiatric syndromes. Three clinical types of presentation with an organic basis are recognised:

- acute confusional states or delirium-like states
- psychotic reactions
- the irreversible deteriorating intellectual conditions or dementias.

Each produces a distinctive pattern of mental state abnormalities.

## Acute confusional state or delirium states (Table 7.6)

*Clinical picture*

The presentation is often dramatic, with marked and frequent fluctuations in the individual's condition. The level of consciousness varies widely from slight alteration of consciousness to complete disorientation and delirium. Orientation for time, place and person is impaired. Attention is ill-sustained, with prominent visual illusions and hallucinations. The individual is usually agitated, frightened and suspicious.

*Aetiology*

These conditions are particularly common in young children with infectious diseases associated with high fevers such as measles or with some pneumonias. The same presentation in the older child or adolescent is most likely to be due to accidental or intentional ingestion of various drugs, including prescribed drugs such as tricyclic antidepressants or illicit drugs such as heroin or cocaine. Glue and solvent sniffing produce a similar acute

**Table 7.6**   Acute confusional/delirium states

**Clinical features**
- Consciousness – drowsiness, disorientation, poor attention and concentration, fluctuating level of consciousness
- Behaviour – restless and agitated
- Illusions and hallucinations (usually visual)
- Mood – suspicious, anxious and frightened

**Causes**
- Infections – measles or pneumonias
- Intoxications – antidepressants, alcohol and hallucinogens
- Metabolic – hepatic or renal failure
- Epilepsy – during or after a seizure
- Head injury
- Intracranial – infection and tumours
- Cardiac/respiratory diseases – cardiac or respiratory failure

confusional state. Very rarely, a non-infective agent, for instance acute intermittent porphyria, is responsible.

*Treatment*

The main aim is to identify, if not already known, the underlying cause for the acute confusional state and to treat it accordingly. Psychological aspects of management include nursing in a well-lit side room, if possible, and a consistent approach from the nursing staff in their contact with the patient and in their organisation of the ward routine. Sedation, especially at night, may occasionally be necessary.

**Psychotic reactions**

Some neurological conditions can occasionally produce a clinical picture similar to an acute schizophrenic episode with hallucinations and delusions. These include:

- some cerebral infections, especially encephalitic conditions
- repeated epileptic seizures
- withdrawal states from alcohol or amphetamine dependence.

Features suggestive of an organic basis for the episode are a history of epilepsy or drug abuse, clinical symptoms of disorientation in time and place, and visual rather than auditory hallucinations.

*Management*

This involves neurological assessment and investigation to determine whether there is an underlying neurological lesion.

## Dementias (see also Ch. 6)

Dementia, the irreversible loss of cognitive skills, is a rare condition in childhood, only usually arising from neurodegenerative diseases. The clinical presentation varies but usually involves neurological, cognitive or behavioural symptoms, alone or in combination, in a progressive manner. Neurological symptoms include weakness, spasticity, epilepsy, involuntary movements and the loss of bowel or bladder control. Cognitive deterioration is shown by loss of reading and language skills. Behavioural abnormalities may be prominent, with the child showing marked autistic features. When the latter occurs, it is probably more appropriate to classify the illness as a disintegrative disorder.

### Aetiology

Causes are many, including metabolic, infective and degenerative. The most crucial diagnostic point is often the initial recognition that the child is gradually declining and progressively losing skills. Extensive neurological investigation is the key to accurate diagnosis.

### Prognosis

The underlying pathology determines the outcome, but this is usually gloomy with some children dying and the remainder 'burnt out', leaving a very intellectually impaired and neurologically compromised child. The child is likely to require long-term specialist nursing care and support.

# 8. Mood disorders

## INTRODUCTION

This chapter discusses those syndromes in which mood disturbance is the major abnormality with other symptoms such as withdrawal or overactivity seen as secondary to the primary disturbance of mood. Historically, the classification of these disorders has been controversial, terms such as endogenous versus reactive, neurotic versus psychotic, unipolar versus bipolar being used in a bewildering and confusing fashion. The new ICD classification avoids the problems of earlier schemes based on aetiology or symptoms by simply classifying the disorders in terms of the major mood disturbance (Table 8.1).

This chapter has the following sections:

- depression as a symptom during childhood and adolescence
- depressive disorders
- bipolar affective disorder
- suicide and attempted suicide.

## DEPRESSION AS A SYMPTOM/SYNDROME (TABLE 8.2)

Depression has been recognised as a syndrome in adults for a long time because of its characteristic constellation of symptoms, response to treatment and outcome. The depressed mood or *dysphoria* has qualities other than just simple sadness or unhappiness. Rather, it includes the inability to derive pleasure or satisfaction from daily life (*anhedonia*) or to be able to respond emotionally to ordinary events. Other features of the syndrome are cognitive disturbances, behavioural changes and alterations in physiological functions. The cognitive disturbances are primarily cognitive distortions around oneself (self-blame, self-reproach, guilt and worthlessness), the world (helplessness and despair about one's life situation) and the future (hopelessness and despondency about the future). The behavioural changes range from marked agitation to withdrawal and stupor, while the physiological changes are poor appetite, weight loss and disturbed sleep pattern. Finally, the consistent pattern of treatment response and prognosis is further evidence for the validity of the syndrome.

**Table 8.1**   Classification of mood disorders

| Syndrome | Main features | Other features |
| --- | --- | --- |
| Manic episode | Elevated mood | Increased activity or physical restlessness<br>Increased talkativeness<br>Difficulty in concentration or distractibility<br>Decreased need for sleep<br>Increased sexual energy |
| Bipolar affective disorder | Mood elevation and/or depression during course of illness | Episodes of hypomania and depression occur at different stages of illness, often close together, followed by periods of normality |
| Depressive disorder | Depressed mood, loss of energy and enjoyment, and decreased energy or increased fatigue | Impaired concentration and attention<br>Reduced self-esteem and self-confidence<br>Ideas of guilt and unworthiness<br>Pessimism about future<br>Ideas of injury or self-harm<br>Disturbed sleep and diminished appetite |
| Recurrent depressive disorder | Repeated episodes of depression, with periods of normality between episodes | See depressive disorder |
| Persistent mood disorders | Long-term minor fluctuations in mood (hypomania or depression) not sufficiently severe to be a discrete episode | Less severe symptoms of hypomania, depression or mixture of both |
| Other mood disorders | Mood disorders which do not fit neatly into the above categories | Usually not severe |

**Table 8.2**   Depression as a symptom

- Transient mood state, especially among adolescents
- Symptom in other psychiatric disorders – for instance chronic anxiety, conduct disorder or anorexia nervosa
- Symptom found as frequent accompaniment of many chronic illnesses, e.g. diabetes, asthma or postviral infections, e.g. infectious mononucleosis
- Major symptom of a depressive disorder with the following features as well:
  - Low self-esteem
  - Suicidal ideas
  - Persecutory ideas
  - Disturbances of eating and sleeping
  - Obsessional ideas and behaviour
  - Symptoms of bipolar affective disorder

The position with children is less clear. While Graham (1974) expressed doubts about whether a depressive syndrome existed in children, much research of the past 15 years has been carried out to prove firstly that the syndrome does exist and secondly that it can be assessed accurately by interview and questionnaire.

## Age trends in depressive symptomatology

Most authorities agree there is a definite increase in the frequency of depressive symptoms from early childhood into adolescence. They are, however, reluctant to accept that depressive disorder occurs in young children, for several reasons. First, children do not have the cognitive ability to form an evaluative appraisal of themselves and their circumstances, a necessary prerequisite for depressive ideas. Secondly, a central feature of depressive symptomatology is the sense of loss or failure, a concept that depends on the ability of the child to think about times past and times future, a cognitive skill beyond young children.

### Preschool period

Psychoanalytic and attachment theories attribute considerable significance to the infant's response to separation and loss. For instance, Klein (1932) described 'the depressive position' as a reparatory attempt by the infant to undo the harm caused by its early aggression, while Bowlby (1969) discusses the 'protest, despair and dejection sequence' in response to separation. Spitz (1946) used the term *anaclitic depression* to describe the infant's response to the emotional deprivation found in extremely unstimulating and unsatisfactory institutional upbringing. These authors do no necessarily regard these responses as pathological, but rather as a part of the normal developmental process or as an understandable response to adverse circumstances. General population studies of preschool children (Richman et al 1982) have shown that depression and unhappiness are not often reported by mothers, with prevalence rates of 5% approximately. Even when such symptoms do occur, most clinicians usually regard them as a reflection of the poor mother–child relationship rather than an indication of mood disorder in the child.

### Middle childhood

Clinical practice and research evidence show that depressive symptoms become more common in this age group, though very often other symptoms, particularly anxiety, are also present. The Isle of Wight study of 10-year-olds (Rutter et al 1970b) found that 10–12% were rated as miserable by their parents or teachers, 13% appeared depressed during the clinical interview and 9% were preoccupied with depressive topics. Despite these ratings however, only three children out of 2000 were given a primary diagnosis of depression, indicating that depressive symptoms are usually seen as a feature of another syndrome or as a secondary response to another disorder. Pearce (1978) found that depressive symptoms occurred in about 10% of prepubertal children referred to a psychiatric out-patient department. McConville et al (1973) studied changes in symptomatology in a group of clinically depressed children between the ages of 6 and 13 years. Sadness and unhappiness were the most common symptoms between the ages of 6 and 8 years, while reports of feeling restless, of being unloved and of being used unfairly by others predominated between the ages of 8 and 11 years. After the age of 11 years, guilt was a noticeable feature, with children saying that they had been wicked, that they deserved to die because of their badness or that they wished to be reunited with a deceased love one.

*Adolescence*

When Rutter et al (1976) reassessed the children in the original Isle of Wight study at the age of 14–15 years, two major differences were apparent — the large increase in frequency of depressive symptomatology and the altered sex ratio of depressive symptomatology. Clinical interview revealed that 40%, 20% and 7% respectively reported feelings of misery and depression, self-deprecation and suicidal feelings at one time or another. There were 9 cases of depressive disorder and a further 26 cases of mixed affective disorder. Pearce (1978) also demonstrated a large increase in depressive symptomatology, 25% approximately, during adolescence. Rutter (1988), in a further analysis of Pearce's 1978 data, found that there was a striking increase in depressive symptomatology among postpubertal boys compared with prepubertal boys. The explanation for these changes in the frequency of depressive symptoms during adolescence is not known, though endocrine changes and/or psychological maturation during puberty may well be responsible.

## DEPRESSIVE DISORDERS

Both ICD and DSM now state that depression in children should have the same features as that in adults. Two major categories are recognised, *depressive episode* and *recurrent depressive disorder*, referring to a single and repeated episodes respectively. The symptoms should last for a minimum of 2 weeks in the absence of alcohol or drug abuse with no evidence of hypomanic symptoms. Table 8.3 shows the clinical features of depressive disorder; usually a minimum of two core and two additional features should be present.

**Table 8.3**    Clinical features of depressive disorders

**Core features**
- Abnormal depressed mood for minimum of two weeks
- Marked loss of interest or pleasure in almost all activities
- Decreased energy or increased fatigue

**Additional features**
- Loss of confidence and self-esteem
- Unreasonable feelings of self-reproach and guilt
- Suicidal ideas or thoughts of death
- Poor concentration and indecisiveness
- Psychomotor agitation or retardation
- Sleep disturbance
- Loss of appetite

**Note:** A minimum of four features should be present including two core features

## Aetiology

There is no adequate theory for childhood depression. There was some support for the two main theories, genetic and environmental. Evidence for a *genetic* component comes from twin studies, adoption and family studies, though the size of the effect is not known. *Environmental* theories range from the traditional psychoanalytic, such as the loss of a loved object, to the stressful effects of adverse life events (Goodyer et al 1985) and finally to cognitive theories.

Two variations of the latter are Seligman's model of learned helplessness (Seligman 1975) and Beck's cognitive distortion model (Beck et al 1979). Seligman proposes that when the individual perceives that his environment is unpredictable and that he has little opportunity to influence events, he becomes despondent, 'gives up' and behaves with learned helplessness or depression. Beck's model of depression regards the individual's negative view of himself, the world and the future as the cause of the depression, though clearly these cognitions could be seen as a consequence of the depressed mood rather than the cause. Finally, biochemical studies for abnormalities in noradrenaline metabolism or with the use of the dexamethasone suppression test (Carroll 1982) as a biological marker for depression, have so far proved disappointing.

## Assessment

This involves detailed and sensitive interviewing of the child, usually alone, as well as assessment of the child and family. Family assessment is useful for two reasons:

- The child's behaviour can be seen in the context of current family functioning
- The other sources of stress for the child or family may be identified.

Physical symptoms are frequently found among depressed children, though the findings are not specific as anxious children often have physical symptoms as well. The differential diagnosis must involve the distinction between normal sadness or unhappiness, other psychiatric conditions with depressive symptomatology, for instance anorexia nervosa, or physical illnesses such as infectious mononucleosis or influenza.

Recently, several semi-structured interviews and questionnaires have been developed to provide a more standardised rating of depression. Popular instruments are the Kiddie Schedule for Affective Disorder and Schizophrenia (K-SADS) (Chambers et al 1985) and the Childhood Depression Rating Scale Revised (CDRS-R) (Poznanski et al 1984). The K-SADS is a modification of the adult version of the Schedule for Affective Disorders, which in turn is based upon the research diagnostic criteria (RDC) of Spitzer & Endicott (1978). The CDRS-R is a modified version of the Hamilton Depression Rating Scale (Hamilton 1960) that rates the severity of depression based upon information obtained from the child, parent, teacher and clinician.

## Treatment

A comprehensive package is most likely to be most effective. Components include drug treatment, individual and family therapy and the reduction or lessening of stressful circumstances. The relative emphasis and sequence of treatments is dependent upon assessment.

Drug treatment is most likely to be effective with children who are most severely affected and have disturbance of physiological functions such as appetite, sleep or weight. Unfortunately, few well-designed drug trials into treatment of depression have been carried out. Tricyclic antidepressants, traditionally imipramine for retarded depression and amitriptyline for agitated depression, are the most commonly prescribed antidepressants, with dosage modified according to the age of the child. Autonomic side effects such as dry mouth are often troublesome. Benefits should be evident within 3 weeks on adequate dosage and treatment should be discontinued after that time if there is no improvement.

The purpose of individual therapy varies widely depending on the assessment and therapeutic style of the clinician. The common aims of all individual approaches are:

- to establish a trusting relationship with the child
- to enable the child or adolescent to feel understood and accepted
- to allow the child or adolescent to disclose his concerns and anxieties, including suicidal thoughts.

Beyond these core aims, the therapeutic approach is varied, ranging from the psychodynamically insight-orientated psychotherapy to the cognitive–

behavioural. Generally, the more intensive individual treatment is carried out with older children and adolescents.

Treatment involving the family is often undertaken mainly in order to improve communication within and between members of the family rather than to treat family dysfunction specifically. Family sessions are extremely useful at the start of treatment as a way to discuss events of emotional significance that may have happened recently but have not been talked through, for instance a family illness or bereavement. These sessions also provide the opportunity to discuss ways to reduce any overt sources of stress or anxiety for the child. Common sources of stress include lack of friends, bullying or teasing at school and the child's sense, usually distorted, of academic failure at school.

## Depressive symptoms in other disorders

Depressive symptoms are frequently found in other psychiatric disorders and also in physical disorders. This poses two sorts of question: is the depression primary or secondary in these other psychiatric disorders; and are the physical symptoms a covert expression of an underlying depressive disorder, the so called *depressive equivalent* or *masked depression*. The answer to these questions are not clear cut, but some consensus exists. First, 'depressive equivalent' and 'masked depression' are unsatisfactory terms, as it is impossible to define their characteristics with any certainty. Secondly, many individuals with 'masked depression' often describe other depressive symptoms as well, so that the diagnostic problem is reduced. Thirdly, though clinicians prefer a single diagnosis to account for all symptoms, there is no doubt that the two disorders can occur simultaneously, that is, co-morbidity is a real phenomenon. Finally, in many cases, individuals with two distinct symptom clusters often have an outcome and/or a response to treatment characteristic of one disorder rather than the other, so that the primary diagnosis becomes clearer.

### Other psychiatric syndromes

Many childhood disorders can have depressive features. The two most common conditions with frequent dysphoric features are anxiety states and conduct disorders. Comparison of the three main diagnostic groups in the Isle of Wight study (Rutter et al 1970b), emotional, conduct and mixed disorders, showed that children with mixed symptoms resemble children with conduct disorder rather than children with emotional disorder with respect to sex ratio, family characteristics, intelligence and learning difficulties. This has been interpreted as suggesting that the affective symptoms are secondary to the primary disturbance of behaviour. In other words, the child becomes depressed and unhappy in response to his aggressive and antisocial behaviour.

The Isle of Wight study also showed that anxiety and dysphoric symptoms are frequently present together. The most sensible way to distinguish between the two conditions is the intensity and frequency of the two symptoms and their relative onset in the course of the illness. Follow-up studies indicate that the majority of individuals with mixed anxiety and dysphoric symptoms are more likely to have anxiety rather than depression if they are psychiatrically ill as adults (Zeitlin 1986).

*Physical disorders (see also Ch.9)*

Many physical disorders have associated psychological symptoms. 'Psycho-somatic' medicine is based upon the premise that psychological disturbance can manifest itself by physical symptomatology (Lask & Fosson 1989). Infectious mononucleosis and influenza are illnesses with a recognised increased risk for subsequent depression. It is however far less clear whether *myalgic encephalitis* (ME) is a definite syndrome with an underlying and unrecognised depressive basis.

## BIPOLAR DISORDER (MANIC-DEPRESSIVE PSYCHOSIS)

ICD and DSM use similar criteria for the diagnosis of bipolar affective disorder whether in children or adults. The following list summarises the main diagnostic points of ICD and DSM:

- The disorder is characterised by repeated, i.e. at least two, episodes in which the subject's mood and activity are significantly disturbed. This disturbance consists on some occasions of an elevation of mood with increased energy and activity (*mania* or *hypomania*), and on others of a lowering of mood with decreased energy and activity (*depression*)
- Recovery is usually characteristically complete between episodes
- Manic episodes usually begin abruptly, lasting from 2 weeks to 4–5 months, while depressive episodes last longer.

The term *manic-depressive disorder* or *psychosis* is now used mainly as a synonym for *bipolar disorder*.

## Prevalence

Anthony & Scott (1960), applying a strict set of ten criteria, were sceptical that mania or hypomania occurred in childhood. More recently, Weller et al (1986) conducted an extensive review of 157 case reports of psychotically ill children and concluded that hypomania was more common that previously recognised. Despite these comments, there is no doubt that it is extremely rare during childhood.

**Table 8.4** Clinical features of hypomanic/manic episode

**Core features**
- Mood is elevated, expansive or irritable over a sustained period of time
- Irritability often a prominent feature

**Other features**
- Increased activity or restlessness
- Increased talkativeness (manic episode has pressure of speech and flight of ideas)
- Difficulty in concentration or distractibility
- Decreased need for sleep
- Increased sexual energy
- Spending sprees or other types of recklessness
- Increased sociability or over-familiarity
- Inflated self-esteem or grandiosity

## Clinical features

Hypomanic and depressive episodes are equally common as a first manifestation of bipolar illness, but subsequent episodes are more likely to be hypomanic than depressive. The depressive episodes show similar features to other depressive illnesses except that they tend to be more severe, with pronounced disturbance in physiological functioning and frequent suicidal thoughts.

The main feature of the hypomanic episode is an elevated, expansive or irritable mood; the other aspects are understandable in terms of the elevated mood (Table 8.4). The common features are:

- increased physical activity or physical restlessness
- increased talkativeness
- difficulty in concentration or distractibility
- less need for sleep
- increased sexual energy
- mild spending sprees or other types of recklessness or irresponsible behaviour
- increased sociability or over-familiarity.

A manic episode causes severe disruption to the individual's life. The increased talkativeness becomes a 'pressure of speech' with flight of ideas (rapid switching of ideas based on a literal rather than logical association, for instance rhyming or punning). The social disinhibition and recklessness can have a devastating effect on the individual's life. Cases with early onset have a worse prognosis, being associated with more frequent episodes, rapid cycling of moods and a greater risk of suicide.

## Differential diagnosis

Though uncommon, several organic conditions can mimic a hypomanic episode. These are summarised in Table 8.5.

**Table 8.5**    Differential diagnosis of hypomanic/manic episode

- Infections
  e.g. Encephalitis
- Endocrine
  e.g. Hyperthyroidism
- Neurological
  e.g. Repeated seizures
      Head injury
      Stroke
- Brain tumours
  e.g. Glioma
      Meningioma
- Medication
  e.g. Steroids
      Antituberculous drugs
- Substance abuse
  e.g. Alcohol
      Drug abuse (amphetamines/hallucinogens)

## Aetiology

A genetic predisposition is the most favoured explanation, mainly from studies of adult patients. Family studies have shown that first degree relatives are 10 times more likely than people in the general population to develop an affective disorder.

## Treatment

An organic basis for the episode must be considered and excluded as necessary. A depressive episode should be managed in a similar manner to other depressive episodes, that is by means of tricyclic antidepressants, individual and family support. ECT may need to be considered for the severely depressed and/or suicidal patient.

The hypomanic episode is often harder to manage as it usually requires in-patient admission, measures to ensure the safety and protection of the patient and also drug treatment. The most useful drug for the acute episode is haloperidol (dosage 0.05 mg/kg/d in three divided doses). It is usually necessary to supplement this medication with anti-parkinsonian drugs such as benzhexol or orphenadrine. Acute dystonic reactions such as oculogyric crises or acute torticollis are more likely with children when treatment is first begun. Consequently, it is essential to closely observe the introduction of the medication.

Lithium carbonate is also effective in the acute episode, though its effect has a slower onset. Lithium is more useful as a prophylactic medication for individuals who have had several episodes. Its introduction should be carefully supervised and monitored. There have, however, been few controlled trials of the effectiveness of lithium in the prevention of further episodes in children or adolescents, although it has been shown to be less effective among individuals with rapid cycling disorder, a feature common among children and adolescents with bipolar affective illness. Other drugs such as carbamazepine, sodium valproate and clonazepam have been reported in the treatment of previously drug-resistant manic episodes in adults. There is however not sufficient evidence available to evaluate their efficacy with children and adolescents who have bipolar affective illness.

## Prognosis

Most individuals usually recover from the acute episode. For individuals with repeated episodes, the poor prognostic features include:

- the absence of a precipitating factor
- a family history of recurrent illness
- the continuation of some symptoms between acute episodes.

Finally, Carlson et al (1977), in a 20-year follow-up of adolescents with mania, reported that 60% of patients had a good social outcome, 20% had significant impairment and 20% were chronically ill.

## SUICIDE AND ATTEMPTED SUICIDE

Suicide is the act of killing oneself intentionally, whereas *attempted suicide* or *parasuicide* is the deliberate attempt to harm oneself, with a non-fatal outcome. Some individuals who kill themselves probably do not intend to die, whereas other individuals who make an unsuccessful attempt may still be determined to die. Motivation or intent is the key element in the understanding of this behaviour as the individual's intent varies along a continuum from absolute determination at one end to transient impulsivity at the other.

### Characteristics of suicide (Table 8.6)

Suicide is extremely rare below the age of 12 with an increase during adolescence to approximately 30/1 000 000/year (Shaffer 1974, McClure 1984). It is more common in males, with no social class trend. Males tend to use violent methods such as shooting, hanging or jumping from high buildings or bridges, while females have a preference for self-poisoning. Shaffer (1974) identified four types of personality characteristics in children and adolescents who commit suicide:

- irritable and over-sensitive to criticism
- impulsive and volatile

**Table 8.6** Profile of suicidal behaviour

**Prevalence**
- Childhood – extremely rare
- Adolescence – 30/1 000 000/year

**Sex**
- More common in males (whereas attempted suicide is more common in females)

**Method**
- Usually violent in males (shooting, hanging or jumping from high buildings or bridges)

**Personality characteristics**
- Irritable and over-sensitive
- Impulsive and volatile
- Withdrawn and uncommunicative
- Perfectionist and self-critical

**Family history**
- Some evidence of increased psychiatric morbidity in the family

**Precipitating factors**
- Most common factor was 'disciplinary crisis'

- withdrawn and uncommunicative
- perfectionist and self-critical.

He also found that there was some evidence for increased psychiatric disturbance within the family and that a 'disciplinary crisis' was the most common reason precipitating the suicide.

## Attempted suicide

### Clinical features

Attempted suicide is uncommon in children before adolescence, but the rate rises to 4/1000/year in the 15–19 years age group. Females are three times more likely than males to make an attempt, with an excess in the lower socioeconomic groups. Not surprisingly, the families show evidence of marital disharmony and parental psychiatric ill health, particularly maternal depression and paternal personality disorder. In addition, poor communication patterns within the family and inconsistent parental discipline are common features. About 50% of the children and adolescents show some evidence of definite psychiatric disorder, particularly depression. Chronic physical ill health is sometimes a feature. In older adolescents, there is often a history of alcohol or drug abuse and running away from home. Social isolation and poor peer relationships are also common.

### Circumstances of suicide attempt

The most common method is an overdose of non-opiate analgesics such as aspirin or paracetamol, probably because of their easy availability. The severity of the overdose varies markedly from a few tablets taken impetuously to swallowing the contents of a whole bottle of analgesics. The attempt often follows a row with a boyfriend or a serious dispute with the parents over discipline. The individual may have threatened to take an overdose on previous occasions and about 50% have consulted their general practitioner in the month prior to the overdose.

*Assessment of future suicidal risk (Table 8.7)*

After the patient has recovered from the physical consequences of the attempt, it is important that a careful assessment of the situation is carried out and that plans are made for providing further help when indicated. A useful approach is to interview the child or adolescent alone, followed by a separate interview with the parents and, finally, a joint interview with the parents and the child. It may be necessary to have several meetings before a final decision is made about future care. The sequence of the interviews may vary, but it is essential that a careful assessment is made of the child's or adolescent's mental state in order to assess his suicidal risk.

The following aspects are important in the assessment interview(s):

- establishing rapport with the patient and family
- understanding the suicidal attempt
- uncovering current problems
- investigating the background
- establishing the mental state and current attitude of the patient to suicide
- discussing resources and coping strategies
- arranging future plans and contact.

It is essential at the outset that the interviewing doctor explains to the patient and the parents the purpose of the interview, that is, to understand the circumstances surrounding the overdose and to identify whether further help or contact with psychiatric services are necessary. A clear account of the suicidal attempt, including an understanding of the circumstances and the motivation, is the main purpose of the assessment. Detailed questioning about the events prior to the attempt are necessary as well as a 'blow by blow' account of the event itself. This includes the degree of planning, the presence or otherwise of other people at the time of the event, motives, suicide note, action taken after the event and the precipitating circumstances. Clarification of the current difficulties for the patient and family is important, particularly the patient's relationship with his parents. The patient may also have problems with peer relationships or at school.

The assessment of the patient's intentions about further suicidal attempts and of his current mental state, particularly for the presence of depressive symptoms, is one of the main purposes of the interview. It is important to enquire whether the overdose has altered the child's or family's attitude to

**Table 8.7**    Assessment of attempted suicide

---

**Interview** child separately, parents separately and child and family together. A series of interviews may be necessary

**Establish rapport**
- Explain purpose of interview (circumstances of the attempt and need for help)

**Understanding attempt**
- Detailed account of 48 hours prior to attempt
- Event itself
  - planning
  - motives
  - nature of attempt
  - social isolation
  - suicide note
  - action after event
  - contemporaneous alcohol consumption

**Current problems**
- Child
  - friendships/relationships
  - school
- Family
  - marital problems
  - parental psychiatric disorder
  - erratic parental discipline

**Background**
- Relevant personal & family history

**Physical health**
- Previous attempts

**Current suicidal intent and mental state**
- Depressive symptoms
- Attitude to future
- Attitude to further attempts

**Coping strategies and resources**
- Willingness of parents and child to resolve difficulties and improve communication
- Capacity for change
- Alteration of circumstances at home and school

**Future plans and contact**
- Agree whether further help necessary
- Agree on future contact

---

their current difficulties and their resolve to improve the situation. The interviewer should also make some assessment of the coping strategies and the capacity for change within the family in order to make a more realistic judgement about the future. Finally, the interviewer should obtain some agreement about future plans and further contact between the patient and family and the relevant professional agencies.

*Treatment*

This depends on the assessment and clinical judgement. The majority of children and adolescents do not require specialist psychiatric follow-up, though clearly they must know how to contact psychiatric services in order to arrange further help when necessary. The indications for more specialised help include:

- the seriousness of the attempt
- the presence of definite depressive disorder and persistent suicidal ideas
- poor family circumstances and social support
- limited capacity of the family for change.

A small number may require in-patient psychiatric care, particularly the older adolescent. Follow-up psychiatric contact often involves individual counselling for the child or adolescent as well as family sessions where the aim is to improve communication and the ability to resolve disagreements. Contact with the school is helpful in some circumstances.

*Outcome*

Few systematic follow-up studies are available, though clinical impression suggests that those with definite psychiatric disorder and adverse social or family circumstances are more likely to be 'repeaters'.

# 9. Emotional disorders

## INTRODUCTION

This chapter discusses those disorders in which the primary abnormality is one of 'emotions'. Emotion is the preferred term as it encompasses a wide range of feelings characterised by the subjective sense of distress. Anxiety is the central feature in this group of disorders. It may be expressed overtly as in anxiety states or covertly as in somatisation or hysterical conversion states. Other emotional or affective components of the disorder present in many cases are distress, crying, sadness, self-consciousness, social withdrawal and shyness. This group of disorders is clearly similar to the traditional adult category of *neurotic disorder* with a further subdivision into anxiety and phobic states, obsessional disorder and hysterical conversion disorder or somatisation categories.

The usefulness of this categorisation was demonstrated by Hewitt & Jenkins (1946) who found a broad distinction could be made between those disorders characterised by subjective distress, unhappiness and anxiety with those where antisocial or deviant behaviour resulting in conflict with other people or society was the main feature. These authors saw emotional disorders as arising from excessive parental pressures on the child resulting in the development of anxiety symptoms. By contrast, conduct disorder stems from the inadequate socialisation of the child by incompetent or neglectful parents and/or exposure to deviant role models from within the family or from the peer group in the community. These two groups of disorders, known as *emotional disorder* and *conduct disorder* respectively, differ with respect to aetiological factors, family characteristics, personal history and outcome (Table 9.1).

The Isle of Wight study (Rutter et al 1970b) confirmed the value of this categorisation into emotional and conduct disorders with their distinctive background, clinical and outcome features. This study also established two further points of general importance: the existence of a third major category, the *mixed disorder*; and the mixed pattern of symptomatology among children with emotional disorders.

Children with mixed emotional and conduct problems were more similar to children with conduct disorder than to those with emotional

111

**Table 9.1**   Characteristics of emotional and conduct disorders

| Characteristic | Emotional disorder | Unsocialised (aggressive) conduct disorder | Socialised (delinquent) conduct disorder |
|---|---|---|---|
| Child's behaviour | Anxious<br>Socially inhibited | Oppositional<br>Aggressive | Stealing<br>Vandalism |
| Family | Small size<br>Over-involved | Large size<br>Ineffective discipline | Large size<br>Ineffective discipline |
| Parental style | Intrusive | Parental rejection | Neglect<br>Deviant role model |
| Schooling | Conformist | Poor scholastic progress | Poor scholastic progress plus truancy |
| Outcome | Good | Variable | Variable |

disorder. The mixed symptomatology of the emotional disorders meant that there was much less differentiation into clear-cut adult neurotic categories such as depression or obsessional/compulsive disorder. More recently, Achenbach & Edelbrock (1983), using sophisticated statistical techniques, proposed two main categories of disorder, an 'internalising' and an 'externalising' group. The former comprises over-controlled behaviour with anxiety and social withdrawal symptoms, corresponding to emotional disorder, whereas the latter has under-controlled behaviour with inattention, overactivity and aggression, comparable to conduct disorder.

ICD and DSM adopt the principle that emotional disorders in childhood are similar to those occurring in adults unless there are specific features that require separate categorisation. ICD has a broad category called *neurotic, stress-related and somatisation disorders* with a separate specific subcategory in the childhood section called *emotional disorders with onset specific to childhood*. By contrast, DSM has separate categories for *anxiety states, somatisation* and *obsessional disorder* with further categories for *anxiety disorders* and *adjustment disorders of childhood*.

This chapter discusses emotional disorders under the following sections:

- anxiety and phobic states
- obsessional disorders
- conversion disorders, dissociative states and somatisation disorders
- reaction to severe stress and adjustment disorders.

Anxiety disorders specific to childhood and adolescence are discussed in the section on anxiety and phobic states, while the stress related disorders are included in this chapter as the major feature of these disorders is the symptom of anxiety.

**Table 9.2**    Manifestations of anxiety

**Cardiovascular**
* Palpitations
* Tachycardia
* Flushing or pallor

**Respiratory**
* Shortness of breath
* Increased respiratory rate

**Skin**
* Blotching
* Increased perspiration

**Muscular and skeletal**
* Tremor
* Muscular tension

**Gastrointestinal**
* Nausea
* Abdominal pain
* Diarrhoea

**Other physical**
* Headache
* Dizziness
* Fainting
* Chest pain

**Psychological**
* Appears tense, frightened and panicky
* Described by others as nervous or highly-strung

**Behavioural**
* Appears edgy in social situations
* Over- and under-reacts
* Reluctant to engage in risky activities or
  alternatively indulges in reckless behaviour

## ANXIETY AND PHOBIC STATES

As discussed in Ch.2, anxiety is central to the understanding of emotional disorder in general and of anxiety and phobic states in particular. It can manifest itself directly through physical symptoms such as palpitations or dry mouth as well as psychological symptoms such as fear or apprehension (Table 9.2). Anxiety is also proposed as the underlying reason for the development of obsessional and somatisation or hysterical conversion disorders. A *phobia* is a specialised form of anxiety which is directed towards a specific object or situation. The phobia is pathological because

* it is excessive with respect to the situation or object
* it cannot be explained or reasoned away
* it leads to avoidance of the feared situation (Table 9.3).

**Table 9.3**   Childhood phobias

**Definition**
A phobia has the following features:

- Out of proportion and excessive to the demands of the situation
- Cannot be reasoned or explained away
- Leads to avoidance of feared situation or object
- Beyond voluntary control

**Common fears during childhood**

*Preschool period*
- Unfamiliar people and situations
- Fear of dark, imaginary monsters or animals

*Middle childhood*
- Fearful of ridicule from peers and embarrassing social situations

*Adolescence*
- Appearance
- Fear of failure
- Social situations, e.g. parties

Despite its psychopathological potential, anxiety is not necessarily pathological, indeed it is often protective and adaptive. Anxiety is an appropriate response in many situations including dangerous or frightening situations, novel or new situations or from the operation of conscience. If the child overcomes his anxiety and is able to manage the situation successfully, the child's confidence, competence and sense of mastery increase considerably, with beneficial effects on maturity. Several factors affect the outcome including the child's temperament, age and previous experience of similar situations.

The concept of emotional maturity is useful in understanding the process whereby the child is able through the maturation of cognitive skills and from experience to learn to cope with progressively more complex and stressful situations. Inevitably, the child suffers some setbacks but, providing the gains outweigh the failures, he should progress towards increasing independence and self-confidence. Major factors which hinder the child's progress are:

- adverse temperamental traits such as poor adaptation to new situations
- over-protective and over-anxious parents
- previous traumatic experience such as failure to cope with a stressful situation. The consequence of this failure is that the child is less confident and becomes reluctant to face new challenges and novel situations.

Psychodynamic and social learning theories propose radically different explanations for the development of the maladaptive responses to anxiety. Psychodynamic theory states that pathological anxiety arises from a conflict between unconscious, hostile feelings on the one hand and affectionate feelings on the other. For instance, if the child has aggressive feelings towards his father whom he also loves, he becomes fearful of his father and this subsequently generalises to all men in positions of authority. By contrast, social learning theory maintains that three elements are necessary for the appearance of maladaptive anxiety

- exposure to a fearful situation
- avoidance behaviour to escape from the feared situation
- anxiety reduction consequent on the completion of the avoidance behaviour.

The anxiety reduction is the crucial element in the development and maintenance of the avoidant behaviour. The major consequence of this avoidance behaviour is the increasing restriction and limitation that it imposes on the individual's daily life. Hence the behaviour is maladaptive. In common with the psychodynamic explanation, the key element is the generalisation of an appropriate response to anxiety to other situations where it is disabling and excessive.

## Anxiety states

### Clinical features

Anxiety is the most common emotional disorder, with a prevalence rate of 2.5% in the Isle of Wight study (Rutter et al 1970b). The disorder manifests itself with physical and psychological symptoms. The child is shy, timid, over-dependent on parents and mixes poorly with other children. The fears are often exaggerations or extreme examples of normal fears, often involving harm or loss to the family, death or some other disaster. The child has difficulty getting off to sleep at night, with the sleep pattern interrupted by frequent wakening and nightmares. Common physical or somatic symptoms are abdominal pain, diarrhoea, palpitations, dry mouth and headaches with restlessness, agitation and tension. Panic attacks may also occur. These consist of an acute onset of extreme fear and dread with a sense of doom and gloom. This is accompanied by marked sweating, palpitations and dry mouth, feeling faint and shaking. These episodes are extremely disabling, the child becoming apprehensive and wary in situations which resemble the previously frightening experience. The severity of the anxiety state may fluctuate quite markedly, with exacerbations at times of stress, for instance starting or changing school.

### Predisposing factors

Several factors usually combine and interact with each other in most instances.

*Temperamental traits.* Children with 'difficult' and 'slow to warm up' temperaments are more likely to develop anxiety states.

*Parental attitude and behaviour.* Over-solicitousness and over-involvement by the parents generates excessive dependency and anxiety in the child, thereby reinforcing the anxiety level in many situations. Parental over-anxiety can have many causes, including parents' own childhood experience, co-existing parental anxiety state and the 'special child syndrome'.

*Special child syndrome.* This describes children who are treated in an over-protective manner by their parents. The 'specialness' may arise in several circumstances:

- the child is much valued or wanted, for instance following a period of infertility or may be of the preferred sex
- threat to child's life during pregnancy or early life, for instance miscarriage or neonatal problem
- 'anxious' attachment between the mother and child.

*Stress.* Many childhood experiences are inevitably distressing and stressful, for instance admission to hospital, parental illness or disability and the start of school. The parental ability to regulate and to minimise undue stress is crucial to the healthy adjustment of the child.

## Treatment

Several approaches may be used, often in parallel or in sequence.

*Reduction of stress.* Clearly, attempts should be made to lessen or moderate the stress whenever possible.

*Individual counselling.* This is often useful to give the child the opportunity to understand the basis for anxiety and also to teach the child some strategies for anxiety management.

*Parental counselling.* Again, parents may need considerable help and support to reduce their intrusive and over-dependent behaviour. Persuading the parents to allow the child more independence and autonomy is an important component of the treatment programme.

*Family therapy.* It is sometimes useful to see the whole family, particularly when the child's anxiety is symptomatic of more general dysfunction within the family group.

*Drug treatment.* Anxiolytic drugs, for instance diazepam, are not commonly used except for specific circumstances and then only in the short term.

## Phobic states

As discussed earlier, phobias are quite common. Pathological fears often rise from ordinary fears that are exacerbated by parental and/or social reinforcement. It is the avoidance behaviour associated with the phobia that makes the behaviour maladaptive. It leads inevitably over time to increased restriction and limitation of the child's activities. Animal and insect phobias tend to be most common in younger children whereas social phobias and anxieties begin around adolescence. Agoraphobia is uncommon during childhood and only begins to occur with any frequency during late adolescence and early adult life.

*Treatment (see Ch. 17)*

Behavioural methods are the most successful approach. The most popular method is *desensitisation*, which has two components, a) graded exposure to the feared object or situation and b) relaxation training. The rationale behind this approach is that continued exposure to the feared stimulus reduces the anxiety associated with the stimulus, thereby decreasing avoidant behaviour.

The success of the method often depends upon the ability of the therapist to devise a treatment programme that achieves gradual exposure without inducing too much anxiety. Relaxation training is used in parallel with the graded exposure. This involves training the individual to recognise the symptoms of anxiety and secondly, to develop techniques for anxiety reduction. The techniques comprise tension and relaxation of muscles in sequence in conjunction with controlled breathing exercises. Occasionally, anxiolytic drugs are used in conjunction with this behavioural approach.

Another exposure treatment method is *implosion* or *flooding* which involves persuading the patient to remain in the feared situation at maximum intensity from the start, the reverse of desensitisation. The rationale is, however, similar to that for desensitisation in that continued exposure is assumed to weaken the association between the feared situation and intolerable anxiety. Implosion has been compared with jumping into a swimming pool at the deep end, whereas desensitisation is getting your feet wet gradually from the shallow end. Implosion clearly demands trust and confidence between the therapist and patient if it is to be successful.

Finally, *modelling*, or exposure to someone coping without stress in the feared situation is another behavioural treatment approach.

## Outcome of anxiety and phobic states

Follow-up of the Isle of Wight study (Graham & Rutter 1973) showed that the prognosis is generally good, with over two-thirds remitting in a 4-year period. Often the stress that produced the anxiety or phobic reaction disappears or resolves. The child's increasing maturity is another beneficial factor in the favourable prognosis. As adults, this group of children have a slightly greater risk of developing neurotic disorder (Berg 1970).

**Table 9.4**   School refusal

**Clinical features**
- Final common pathway for expression of social or separation anxiety
- Most frequent at start of school, change of school and beginning of secondary school
- Good academic attainments
- Conforming at school, oppositional at home
- Fear of illness or injury to other family members
- Often precipitated by loss or threat of loss to self or other family members

**Mechanisms**
- Separation anxiety whereby child and/or parent is fearful of separation
- Specific phobia about some aspect of school attendance, for instance mixing with other children
- Indication of more general psychiatric disturbance such as depression or low self-esteem

**Treatment**
- Early return to school
- Short-term treatment with anxiolytics (sometimes)
- Desensitisation for specific phobic aspects of school attendance
- Family therapy and case work
- Occasionally, in-patient assessment for intractable non-attendance

## School refusal/school phobia (Hersov & Berg 1980) (Table 9.4)

This term refers to the child's irrational fear of school attendance. It is also known as the *masquerade syndrome* (Waller & Eisenberg 1980) as it can present in a variety of disguises, including abdominal pain, headaches and postviral fatigue.

### Clinical features

The child is reluctant to leave home in the morning to attend school (in contrast to the truant, who leaves home but does not arrive at school). The condition usually develops gradually, often following a genuine reason for absence from school such as a minor physical illness. The problem is most noticeable after weekend or holiday breaks. Ultimately, the problem becomes acute and the child adamantly refuses to go to school despite persuasion and support. This often produces a dramatic conflict between the supportive parent(s) and their defiant child, with the parents' powerlessness to exert effective authority strikingly apparent.

School refusal occurs most commonly at the commencement of schooling, change of school or beginning of secondary school. Boys and girls are equally affected. Typically, most school refusers have good academic attainments and are conformist at school, though oppositional at home. In older children and adolescents, the problem may well become chronic and intractable, particularly when parents have abandoned attempts to enforce school attendance.

Most cases can be understood in terms of the following three mechanisms, often in combination:

- separation anxiety, where the child and/or the parent are fearful of the unavoidable separation caused by attendance at school
- specific phobia about some aspect of school attendance, such as travelling to school or mixing with other children, or some part of the school routine, e.g. certain subjects, often games or physical education, or assembly
- an indication of more general psychiatric disturbance such as depression or low self esteem, more common among adolescents.

More recent studies (Kolvin et al 1984, Last et al 1987) have shown that many children with school refusal often have signs of more widespread disturbance, for example separation anxiety syndrome in younger children and depression in adolescents.

*Treatment*

The initial essential step is to recognise the condition itself, that is, to avoid unnecessary and extensive investigations for minor somatic symptoms or to advise prolonged convalescence following minor illness. For the acute case, early return to school, with firm support for the parents and liaison with the school, is the most successful approach. For the more intractable cases, extensive work with the child and parents along with a graded return to school is advisable. A specific behavioural programme for the phobic elements may be necessary as well as the use of anxiolytic drugs in some instances. The chronic problem often requires a concerted approach, sometimes involving a period of assessment and treatment at a child psychiatric in-patient unit. Many clinicians also use family therapy to tackle the major relationship problems that exist in many cases.

*Outcome*

Two-thirds usually return to school regularly, while the remainder, usually adolescents from disturbed families, only achieve erratic attendance at school at best. Follow-up studies into adult life have found that approximately one-third continue with neurotic symptoms and social impairment (Hersov & Berg 1980).

## Anxiety states specific to childhood and adolescence

ICD and DSM now recognise that some anxiety states are no more than an extreme example of developmental variation rather than a qualitatively abnormal behaviour. Consequently, it is more sensible to classify these conditions separately from other anxiety states. Separation anxiety and over-anxious disorder fall into this category.

### Separation anxiety disorder

As separation anxiety is a normal phenomenon in small children, this disorder should only be diagnosed when it is sufficiently severe and persistent to impair markedly the child's social functioning. Moreover, the symptoms should not be part of a more generalised disturbance of emotional or personality development. The major symptoms concern the excessive preoccupation with and worry about separation and/or the possible harm when the child is separated from his major attachment figures. The condition is diagnosed most frequently in younger children. So far, the validity of this separate category is not known.

### Over-anxious disorder

The main features are:

- excessive and unrealistic worries about one's own social competence, with marked self-consciousness and need for reassurance
- inability to relax
- somatic complaints such as headaches or abdominal pain.

Additionally, DSM specifies that the symptoms must be present for at least 6 months with no evidence of a more generalised anxiety state or other psychiatric disorder. Again, the diagnostic validity of this syndrome is not yet known.

## OBSESSIONAL DISORDERS (TABLE 9.5)

### Definition

An *obsession* is a recurrent, intrusive thought that the individual recognises to be irrational but cannot ignore. The important phenomenological distinction between an obsession and a *delusion* is that the individual has insight into the irrational nature of the former, whereas this does not occur with the latter. This distinction is, however, often less clear with children. A *compulsion* or *ritual* is the behaviour(s) accompanying these ideas, the aim of which is to reduce the associated anxiety. Figure 9.1 shows the pathway through which obsessional symptoms can develop. Anxiety, arising from parental over-protection and/or individual predisposition, elicits indecisive or perfectionist behaviour leading to the development of compulsions or rituals. The compulsions produce a temporary relief in anxiety so that they are reinforced and thereby self-perpetuated.

**Table 9.5** Obsessional disorders in childhood

**Definition**

*Obsession*: a recurrent, intrusive thought that the individual recognises is irrational but cannot ignore

*Compulsion*: a behaviour(s) carried out to reduce the anxiety associated with the obsessional idea, usually repeatedly

**Clinical course**

- Usually begins in middle childhood, often with fluctuating course
- Common themes of obsessional ideas
    - cleanliness
    - washing/dressing
    - contact/contamination with disease/illness
    - foreboding sense of doom
- Mood disturbance, usually depressive, common
- Family members involved in rituals

**Treatment**

- Treatment of any mood disturbance (e.g. depression)
- Identify any precipitating stress
- Enlist help of family and school
- Behavioural techniques, e.g. response prevention

Bender & Schilder (1940) coined the term *impulsion* to describe a variety of behaviours such as constantly looking at an object, preoccupation with a single idea or object, hoarding of objects or counting of numbers repeatedly. The behaviour occurs in mainly younger children aged between 4 and 10. The important phenomenological distinction between an obsession and an impulsion is the absence of resistance with an impulsion. There is some evidence that a proportion of children with impulsions subsequently develop definite obsessional disorder.

*Clinical features*

Most children display obsessional symptoms to a minor degree, for instance avoiding cracks between paving stones or not walking under ladders. These have no significance unless the behaviour begins to interfere with everyday activities. This interference manifests itself as increasing amounts of time taken over daily routines such as washing, dressing or the checking of homework. Common obsessional rituals are hand washing and dressing. Obsessional thoughts often have a foreboding quality, for instance that 'something could happen' to a parent or sibling or that the child might die or get run over. Recently, fear of HIV infection or the AIDS syndrome has become a theme of obsessional thoughts. The rituals, though maladaptive, are maintained because they produce temporary reduction in anxiety.

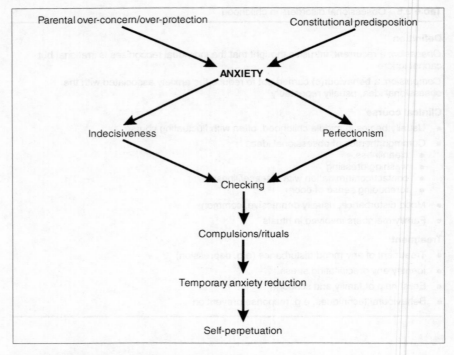

**Fig. 9.1**   Development of obsessional symptoms

Commonly, the child involves other members of the family in the performance of the rituals so that the child assumes a controlling role within the family.

The disorder is rare, with a community prevalence rate of 0.3%. It is commoner in older children and adolescents and can have an acute or gradual onset. The child is likely to be quiet, reserved and somewhat perfectionist. Affected children frequently show anxiety and depressive symptoms, with anorexia nervosa, Tourette's syndrome and schizophrenia as possible alternatives in the differential diagnosis with the older child.

*Aetiology*

The relative contribution of genetic, constitutional and environmental factors is not yet known. The contribution of the family to the development of the disorder is not in doubt, though whether this operates through genetic mechanisms or through the exposure of the child to deviant role models is unclear. While anxiety reduction provides psychoanalytic and social learning theories with an explanation for the persistence of the obsessions and compulsions, the two theories do not satisfactorily account for the initial occurrence of the symptoms. At the present time, an individual formulation highlighting the role of different causative factors is the most useful way to understand the aetiology of the disorder.

## Treatment

A combined approach involving behavioural, drug and family counselling is likely to be the best approach. Behavioural methods, particularly response prevention strategies, are successful in reducing the obsessional thoughts and ritualistic behaviour. Response prevention consists of training the child to become aware of the cues that trigger the obsessional idea or compulsive ritual and then using distraction techniques to interrupt the obsessional idea or to make the performance of the ritual impossible. Medication, commonly clomipramine, is helpful for anxiety or depressive symptoms. The involvement of other family members, whether specifically for family therapy or in assisting the child to eliminate the rituals, is essential. In some cases, the condition is so severe that in-patient admission is necessary.

## Outcome

The prognosis for a single episode is good, though a recent follow-up study on children with severe disorder (Flament et al 1990) showed that less than one-third of the 27 patients were symptom free at follow-up. Overall, most studies have shown that two-thirds of children make a good recovery, with the remainder continuing to have problems, usually in a fluctuating fashion.

## CONVERSION DISORDERS, DISSOCIATIVE STATES AND SOMATIC DISORDERS

The latest versions of ICD and DSM show major changes in an attempt to simplify these categories, though whether this is entirely successful is debatable. ICD has grouped the previously separate conversion and dissociative states into one category, *dissociative disorder*, and added a new category, *somatoform disorder*, which includes somatisation disorder and hypochondriacal disorder. The new ICD-10 dissociative categories thus include dissociative amnesia, dissociative motor disorders and dissociative anaesthesia and sensory loss. DSM's approach is similar, with new categories of *dissociative disorders* and *somatoform disorders*, though conversion disorder is included in the somatoform category rather than the dissociative category.

A major problem with the terms 'conversion' and 'dissociation' is that they refer to psychological processes or mechanisms of questionable value, especially when applied to children. Despite this criticism, psychiatrists continue to use the terms, so that this section discusses conversion disorders, dissociative states and somatisation disorders together. *Hypochondriacal disorder*, where the individual believes that he has a serious underlying physical disease despite repeated negative findings on investigation and repeated reassurance, has only been rarely described in childhood, so that it will not be discussed further.

## Conversion disorders

### *Clinical features*

This condition is uncommon in childhood, and very rare before the age of 7 or 8 years. The main feature of conversion disorder is the development of physical symptoms, usually of the special senses or limbs, without any pathological basis, in the presence of identifiable stress and/or affective disturbance. Common symptoms include blindness, paralysis, aphonia, anaesthesia for part(s) of the body, seizures and motor inco-ordination.

The traditional psychoanalytic explanation for the disorder is in terms of primary and secondary gain. The primary gain of the symptom is that the emotional conflict is kept out of consciousness and the secondary gain is the avoidance of stressful situations. The emotional conflict is said to be converted into physical symptoms which are less threatening to the individual than the underlying psychological conflict. For example, a person who has an inner conflict about the expression of rage or anger may develop aphonia or paralysis of an arm following an argument with someone. The aphonia or paralysis symbolises the conflict and also enables the individual to avoid expressing anger.

Alternative explanations for the disorder are the concepts of *abnormal illness behaviour* (Pilowsky 1969) and *the sick role* (Parsons 1951). The latter emphasises the social context in which illness occurs: ill people are freed from obligations; dependency is encouraged; more attention is paid by parents, other family members and by doctors. Abnormal illness behaviour is the situation where the individual persists with and exaggerates the symptoms of the illness despite apparent recovery. Here, the underlying uncertainty and anxiety about the illness result in the patient being reluctant to abandon the symptoms. The concepts of the sick role and abnormal illness behaviour have proved extremely useful in the design of treatment programmes (see below) where the emphasis is upon minimising the advantages of the sick role and ignoring the signs of illness behaviour.

It is extremely dangerous to diagnose conversion disorder solely by the exclusion of organic disease, as follow-up studies of children originally diagnosed as conversion reactions have found that a substantial minority subsequently develop definitive organic disease, most notably amblyopia (Caplan 1970). Misdiagnosis is most likely when physical signs are absent and coincidental emotional upset is present (Rivinus et al 1975). There should always be positive psychological reasons to explain the development of symptoms. Common reasons include:

● major life events or stresses for the child

- a major stress affecting other family member(s)
- an underlying depressive disorder.

Minor degrees of these disorders are extremely common and frequently occur as a transitory phenomenon during the course of many illnesses. As discussed earlier, the term 'abnormal illness behaviour' has been used to describe this situation. This term has many similarities to the phrase 'functional overlay', an expression used by adult physicians to describe the situation where the patient exaggerates or prolongs symptoms during the course of an illness.

### Treatment (Dubovitz & Hersov 1976)

Successful treatment depends upon the recognition that the symptoms are 'real' for the child — psychic pain is as distressing as physical pain. The following principles are important:

- Remember that anger and confrontation are unhelpful
- Find out the parental explanation of the problem, physical or psychological
- Enlist parental co-operation with the treatment programme
- Adopt a firm, sympathetic approach with little attention to the symptom per se
- Avoid rewarding the symptom
- Devise a graded rehabilitation programme where necessary
- Allow the child to give up symptoms with a good grace — this often involves providing the child with some face-saving reason for improvement
- Identify and treat any affective disturbance
- Adopt an optimistic approach to the resolution of the problem.

### Outcome

This is usually good for the individual episode unless there is a very slow or insidious onset. Long-term adjustment is, however, less clear as adequate follow-up studies are not available.

## Dissociative disorders

These conditions are extremely uncommon in childhood, so they will only be briefly described here. Their defining feature is the restriction or loss of consciousness and self-awareness due to psychological causes. This is usually accompanied by disturbance of memory, sensation or movement. Like conversion disorders, the definition implies a psychological basis for the disorder, namely underlying anxiety. The two commonest syndromes are dissociative amnesia and dissociative fugue. The main feature of the former is a loss of memory which is not explained on an organic basis or by normal forgetfulness. The amnesia is usually centred on a traumatic or distressing event such as an accident or bereavement. The loss is partial, selective and varies on a daily basis. Dissociative fugue shows the same features of memory loss, but in addition the patient makes a purposeful journey of which he has no subsequent recollection.

## Somatisation disorder (Lask & Fosson 1989)

### Clinical features and management

Many children complain of somatic symptoms which do not have a pathological basis. Common symptoms are abdominal pain, headaches and limb pains and the community prevalence rate is approximately 10% (Apley & MacKeith 1968, Faull & Nicol 1986). This condition is usually managed by general practitioners, though it sometimes results in a referral for a specialist opinion. Management involves the minimum necessary investigation to exclude any pathology, the identification of any stressful circumstances and a sensitive explanation of the basis for the symptoms. The prevention of restrictions and the active encouragement of normal activities are essential.

When somatic symptoms are persistent, chronic and involve several systems of the body, ICD and DSM use the term *somatisation disorder*. While it is doubtful whether this disorder occurs in childhood, there is no doubt that persistent unexplained physical complaints are a common reason for children being taken to see the doctor. In many cases, there is clear evidence of underlying anxiety or recent stressful events.

Minuchin and colleagues (1975) proposed that there is a distinctive pattern of interaction among families where the child has persistent somatic symptoms, the so-called psychosomatic family (Table 9.6). The purpose or 'meaning' of the somatic symptoms is to prevent the family from discussing their emotional and/or conflictual problems which would engender too much anxiety and be too stressful. The psychosomatic family has four distinctive patterns of interaction:

- enmeshment
- over-protection
- rigidity
- avoidance of conflict.

Enmeshment is shown by the excessive closeness, lack of privacy and blurring of interpersonal boundaries between family members. The over-protectiveness of the parents towards the child is shown by their excessive concern about the child's health and safety. The parents therefore inhibit the development of independence and autonomy in

**Table 9.6** Characteristics of Minuchin's psychosomatic families

**Common symptoms**
- Abdominal pain
- Headaches
- Limb pains

**Patterns of interactions**
- Enmeshment or excessive closeness
  Lack of privacy and blurring of interpersonal boundaries
- Over-protection
  Excessive concern for each other's health and safety
- Rigidity
  Aversion to change and inability to adapt to the child's changing developmental needs
- Lack of conflict resolution
  Fearful of overt expression of hostile feelings so that disagreements are avoided and conflicts unresolved

their child so that the child is not allowed to participate in activities outside the home such as team sports or Scouts/Guides. The family's rigidity is shown by the parents' strong aversion to change coupled with their inability to respond to the changing developmental needs of the child. This is particularly noticeable at times of transition during the child's life, for instance starting school or entering adolescence. The excessive aversion to conflict means that the family devotes much effort to avoiding disagreement or friction. This occurs because the family is fearful of the possible damaging consequences arising from open expression of conflict or disagreement. Consequently, conflict is rarely addressed or resolved within the family.

Although the underlying psychopathology is often more severe in many cases of somatisation disorder, the principles of management outlined by Dubovitz & Hersov (1976) for conversion disorders would apply, that is, minimise restrictions, promote rehabilitation and avoid rewarding the symptom. Minuchin (Minuchin et al 1978, Minuchin & Fishman 1981) has also written extensively about the application of family therapy techniques for psychosomatic families (see Ch. 17).

## REACTION TO SEVERE STRESS AND ADJUSTMENT DISORDERS

This group of disorders arises in response to an exceptionally stressful event or a significantly adverse life change. The clinical features of the different syndromes vary considerably, with a preponderance of affective symptoms in most cases. Table 9.7 summarises the factors determining the individual's response to stressful life events.

**Table 9.7**  Determinants of response to acute stress

| Variable | Effect |
|---|---|
| Age | Depends on type of stressor, for instance separation with preschool children and social occasions such as parties or dances with adolescents |
| Sex | Boys more vulnerable |
| Temperamental characteristics | 'Slow to warm up' and 'difficult' style more vulnerable |
| Previous experience | Prior successful coping enhances resilience and ability to manage new stresses |
| Family | Resourcefulness and coping skills of parents are crucial. For instance, the parents of 'psychosomatic' families may exaggerate and worsen stresses for the child |

## Adjustment disorder

### Definition

This is a maladaptive response occurring within 3 months of an identifiable psychosocial stressor. The maladaptive response must be of sufficient severity to impair daily activities such as schooling, hamper social relationships and be greater than expected given the nature of the stressor. Finally, the reaction must not last longer than 6 months.

### Clinical features

By definition, the symptoms vary with ICD and DSM recognising more than six categories. Clinical practice shows that anxiety and depressive symptoms, often combined, are the most frequent categories. Common stressors include parental divorce, unemployment, family illness or family move.

### Predisposing factors

Age has different effects depending on the type of stressor. For instance, separation is more upsetting for the younger child than for the adolescent, whereas a loss or change of heterosexual relationship is far more important for an adolescent than for the younger child. Boys are also more vulnerable to the adverse effects of stress than girls (Rutter 1981). Temperamental characteristics such as 'difficult' or 'slow to warm up' style probably influence susceptibility as well. Again, the child's previous experience and repertoire of coping skills affect the response to the current stressor. For instance, if the child has successfully coped with adversity in the past, his resilience and ability to withstand the present situation are enhanced.

Finally, the family, particularly the parents, can magnify or minimise the impact of a stressor, depending on their resourcefulness and coping style.

*Outcome*

By definition, the disorder can only last for 6 months, after which time the diagnostic category must change. The more important clinical consideration is not the change in diagnostic category, but the adverse effect that chronic or repeated stresses can have on the child's long-term adjustment.

## Post-traumatic stress disorder (Yule 1991)

The recent 'epidemic' of disasters which have involved British children (the capsize of the *Herald of Free Enterprise*, the sinking of the cruise ship *Jupiter*, the Pan-Am Lockerbie air crash and the crushing disaster at the Hillsborough football stadium) have made clinicians acutely aware of this syndrome. Clinicians are now familiar with the wide symptomatology often found and have also become involved in treatment programmes to reduce the distress in the immediate aftermath and also in the longer term.

*Definition*

This disorder arises following exposure to a stressful event of an exceptionally threatening or catastrophic nature that would cause pervasive distress in almost anyone. The events include accidents or disasters as well as more personal traumas such as witnessing murder, rape or torture.

*Clinical features*

Table 9.8 summaries the main symptoms of the syndrome. These include:

- 'flashbacks' (the repeated re-enactment of the event with intrusive memories, dreams or nightmares)

**Table 9.8** Common symptoms of post-traumatic stress disorder (PTSD)

**General symptoms**
- 'Flashbacks' (re-enactment of event with intrusive memories)
- Detachment and 'numbness' about ordinary daily life
- Hyperalertness and increased vigilance
- Avoidance of activities or places reminiscent of traumatic event
- Mixed anxiety and depressive symptoms

**Specific symptoms**
- Foreshortened view of future ('only plan for today')
- Survivor guilt (self-reproach about own survival while companions died)
- Acute panic reactions

- a sense of detachment, 'numbness' and emotional blunting
- irritability, poor concentration and memory problems.

Following disasters, many survivors often experience an increased awareness of danger, a foreshortened view of the future ('only plan for today'), a feeling of 'survivor' guilt (self reproach about own survival while companions died) and acute panic reactions.

Yule (1991) indicates that between 30% and 50% of children show significant psychological morbidity following disasters, with symptoms persisting for several months (Yule et al 1990).

### Individual vulnerability factors

Important modifying factors are probably age, previous experiences, current life situation and availability of help. Though cognitive immaturity may protect the child from appreciating the implications of the disaster, it may also be disadvantageous as the child may not be given the opportunity to talk about the event. The child's previous experience of stressful events and their outcome, successful or otherwise, is likely to influence the response to the disaster. Similarly, co-existing adverse circumstances such as family disharmony or school problems reduce the child's capacity to cope with the new situation.

### Management

Though most research is anecdotal rather than systematic, the available evidence (Yule 1991) suggests that post-disaster 'debriefing' sessions on an individual or group basis are helpful. Specific counselling sessions to help the child deal with phobic, anxiety or depressive symptoms are frequently necessary as well as helpful. Cognitive/behavioural approaches are particularly suitable for these types of problem.

## Epidemic/mass/group hysteria

This term refers to the simultaneous 'outbreak' of somatic symptoms without a pathological basis in a group of people living in close proximity. It is of interest to child and adolescent psychiatrists because it has been described most frequently amongst school-age children and adolescent girls (McEvedy et al 1966).

Common symptoms include headaches, dizziness, fainting, nausea, vomiting and abdominal pain. The episode usually occurs in a boarding school or hospital. Characteristically, the episode begins when one girl has a fainting or collapsing episode. Soon other girls are affected, with rapid spread throughout the group. The initially affected girl is often a dominant or prominent member of the group, whereas those affected later on are more likely to be dependent and suggestible. The episode often arises at a time of considerable physical and/or psychological stress for the group. Physical stresses include heat, exertion and fatigue, while psychological stresses are low morale, anxieties about sexual matters such as pregnancies, imminent examinations or the death of a classmate.

## Management

The following principles are important:

- Recognise phenomenon promptly
- Avoid extensive investigations for pathological agents
- Explain the basis of the behaviour to the group (for instance the recent stress)
- Isolate affected individuals from one another and from the rest of the group
- Adopt a calm approach to the situation and maintain the normal routine of the group.

### Outcome

With suitable management the situation usually resolves quickly with few long-term sequelae.

# 10. Conduct disorder

## INTRODUCTION (ROBINS 1991)

Conduct disorder is usually defined as persistent, antisocial or socially disapproved of behaviour that often involves damage to property and/or aggression towards other people and is unresponsive to normal control or authority.

Most children at some time or other commit some antisocial behaviour. Three features characterise the behaviour of the conduct-disordered child:

- the range, frequency and severity of the disturbed behaviour
- disregard for and contravention of normally accepted standards of behaviour
- failure to modify or desist from the antisocial behaviour despite persuasion or punishment.

The distinction between the normal and the abnormal or between the acceptable and non-acceptable is often blurred, with an element of social and cultural value judgement inevitably attached to the evaluation of the behaviour. Clearly, what is acceptable as normal for a child living in a developed Western urban area in the late 20th century is different from what is normal for their contemporaries living in the Third World or for their predecessors earlier in the century. Despite the arbitrary nature of the assessment, there is usually other evidence to suggest that the child's adjustment is not satisfactory. Many children with conduct disorder are unpopular, socially isolated and with few close friends. The disturbance in social relationships may be a cause or a consequence of the antisocial behaviour, and results in considerable impairment of the child's daily life.

## CLASSIFICATION (TABLE 10.1)

Traditionally, a broad distinction has been made between socialised and unsocialised antisocial behaviour (Jenkins 1969). Children with *socialised conduct disorder* show persistent antisocial behaviour but are well integrated and accepted within their peer group. Their behaviour is often acceptable to their parents and also similar to that of their friends. They often express

133

**Table 10.1**   Classification of conduct disorder

| ICD-10 | DSM-III-R |
|---|---|
| **Conduct disorders** | **Disruptive behaviour disorders** |
| Confined to the family context | Attention-deficit hyperactivity disorder |
| Oppositional defiant disorder | Oppositional disruptive disorder |
| Unsocialised conduct disorder | Conduct disorder |
| Socialised conduct disorder | Solitary |
| | Group |
| | Undifferentiated |
| **Mixed disorders of conduct and emotions** | |

remorse or regret for their misdemeanours and also wish to change their behaviour. By contrast, children with *unsocialised antisocial* behaviour are not integrated with their peers, express little regret for their actions and are unpopular with peers and adults. Unsocialised antisocial behaviour is of more serious significance as it is often a solitary activity against a background of parental rejection or neglect and poor peer relationships. In many ways, children with socialised conduct disorder have acquired moral or ethical values but the wrong ones, whereas those with unsocialised conduct disorder have not acquired any values at all.

Despite the popularity of the socialised and unsocialised categories, research evidence (Rutter et al 1970b, Wolff 1985) indicates that children with conduct disorder do not fall neatly into these categories. Indeed, considerable overlap is the norm. The Isle of Wight study (Rutter et al 1970b) showed that not only was there a wide range of behavioural symptoms but also that many children had emotional or neurotic symptoms in addition to the behavioural problems, the so-called *mixed category*. Children in the mixed category were also more similar to children with conduct disorder than to children with emotional disorder, so that the emotional symptoms in the mixed category are therefore regarded as secondary to the primary disorder of conduct.

ICD's solution (Table 10.1) to the classification difficulties is to retain the clinically useful categories of socialised and unsocialised conduct disorder, but also add a separate category of *mixed disorders of conduct and emotions*. DSM-III-R (Table 10.1) adopts a more agnostic approach by categorising conduct disorder within the larger category of *disruptive behaviour disorders* with further subdivisions into *solitary, group* and *undifferentiated*. DSM-III-R stipulates that at least three behaviours should be present for a minimum period of 6 months to meet the diagnostic criteria (Table 10.2). Unfortunately, there is no clear evidence at the moment to decide whether the ICD or DSM approach is preferable.

Both ICD-10 and DSM-III-R have introduced a new diagnostic category, *oppositional defiant or disruptive disorder*. This disorder occurs most

**Table 10.2**    DSM-III-R diagnostic criteria for conduct disorder

- Disturbance of conduct lasting at least 6 months during which at least three of the following have been present:
- Has stolen without confrontation from a victim on more than one occasion
- Has run away from home at least twice
- Often lies
- Deliberately engages in fire-setting
- Often truants from school
- Has broken into someone's house, a building or a car
- Deliberately destroys property
- Is physically cruel to animals
- Has forced someone into sexual activity
- Has used a weapon in more than one fight
- Initiates physical fights frequently
- Has stolen during confrontation with victim
- Is physically cruel to people

commonly in younger children, especially in the preschool period. The defining features are defiant, oppositional and provocative behaviour in the absence of other antisocial symptoms. Children with the disorder tend to be angry and resentful, with a low frustration tolerance, resulting in frequent tantrums and outbursts. The key discriminating factor is the lack of other antisocial behaviour. While clinical practice suggests that this category may be useful, it is unclear at the moment whether it is sufficiently distinctive to warrant separate categorisation.

*Delinquency* is the legal term referring to a young person who has committed a criminal offence. Clearly, the term can only be applied to children who are sufficiently mature to appreciate the nature of their deviant behaviour and also have reached the age of criminal responsibility. Delinquency is a common feature of antisocial disorder in older children and adolescents. Stealing, vandalism, arson, breaking and entering into property and fire-setting are common examples of delinquent behaviour (see later section). Delinquency is about 10 times more common in boys than girls and much delinquent behaviour either goes undetected or is not reported officially.

## CLINICAL FEATURES

### Prevalence

The Isle of Wight study (Rutter et al 1970b) found that conduct disorders, including the mixed category, accounted for over two-thirds of disorders and that boys were more than three times more likely to be affected than

**Table 10.3**   Common symptoms of conduct disorder

| | |
|---|---|
| Temper tantrums | Overactivity |
| Motor restlessness | Oppositional behaviour |
| Irritability | Lying |
| Wandering away from home/school | Aggressiveness |
| Learning difficulties, especially reading retardation | Stealing |
| Mood changes | Poor self-esteem |
| Poor peer relationships | Truancy |
| Delinquency (M:F 10:1) | Vandalism |
| Bullying | Arson |

girls. Other studies (Rutter et al 1975a, Offord et al 1987) have found similar prevalence rates, with the same sex ratio.

## Symptomatology

Conduct disorder manifests itself in many ways depending upon the age and sex of the child. Common symptoms (Table 10.3) are:

- aggression
- stealing
- lying
- vandalism
- arson and fire-setting
- truancy
- breaking into and entering property
- drug and solvent abuse.

The problem(s) are frequently confined within the family during the preschool period but often extend into the school in middle childhood. During adolescence, they involve the community, particularly when delinquent behaviour predominates.

### Aggression

As a symptom, this is a common cause for referral throughout childhood and adolescence. It is also a major reason why children with conduct disorder are unpopular, have few friends and are socially isolated. In the preschool period, the aggression is frequently directed towards other children, often when the child is frustrated, thwarted or in a rivalrous situation with another child. Temper tantrums and overactivity are frequent accompaniments. Aggression towards adults is less common, though children often become angry with their parents when the latter are insistent over certain routines such as eating or sleeping. Destructive behaviour such as tearing wallpaper, breaking furniture or damaging toys is indicative of more serious disturbance. Usually this is a reflection of parental neglect or rejection.

School-age children frequently become involved in fighting with other children. Verbal aggression through the use of nicknames and name-calling is another means by which children attack and annoy each other. Bullying is a common behaviour pattern of some conduct-disordered children. Despite their apparent enjoyment of such behaviour, most children who bully tend to be unhappy and are shunned by their peers. Cruelty to animals is much less common, though, when it occurs, it is indicative of more serious disturbance.

Overt aggression is less frequent among older children and adolescents, but their physical size and strength make the outcome for an individual outburst more serious. Adolescents are, however, more likely to engage in fights on a group basis. A small number of adolescents have episodic 'explosive outbursts' or 'blind rages' accompanied by a total loss of control with damage to themselves, other people or property. Often epilepsy is suggested as a possible basis for these episodes, but clinical experience shows that this is extremely uncommon.

*Stealing*

Most children have on occasion taken things that do not belong to them. Stealing becomes pathological when it is persistent and wide-ranging despite reprimand, disapproval and punishment. It is not sensible to think about children 'stealing' until around the age of 6 or 7 years, as children do not have an adequate concept of personal property or of the necessity to obtain permission prior to borrowing things until that age.

Usually, the child steals from other children, often at school, and also from shops when in the company of other children. The 'stealing' of food from the refrigerator is a not uncommon complaint of rejecting and neglectful parents about their preschool child. Rich (1956) categorised the psychological basis of stealing into three groups:

- 'comforting' stealing
- 'marauding' offences
- 'proving' offences.

'Comforting' stealing occurs when the child attempts to obtain through the theft a material reward to compensate for the lack of emotional affection shown by the parents. 'Marauding' offences are committed by older children when they steal from shops on a group or a gang basis. These children have few other symptoms of conduct disorder and fall within the socialised delinquency category. 'Proving' offences usually involve the older adolescent who carries out a daring exploit such as the theft of a car in order to improve his status or prowess within the group or with himself.

A frequent consequence of stealing is the necessity to lie in order to prevent detection. In many cases, the child's explanation is so patently incorrect that the confronting adult should be aware of the danger of humiliating the child by prolonged questioning. The psychoanalytic explanation for the child's flat denial is that an admission of responsibility would involve such a sense of guilt and shame that it is not acceptable, hence the denial.

## Lying

All children tell lies at some time or other. Most commonly, this is to avoid a reprimand or punishment for some misdeed or to prevent embarrassment. Many children with conduct disorder use lies to cover up their misdemeanours, often unsuccessfully, thereby compounding the problem. Persistent lying is a source of annoyance and anger to parents, teachers and to other children, so that the child who tells lies is labelled as untrustworthy, leading to further social isolation and rejection. A small minority of children fabricate elaborate stories and fantasies in a 'Walter Mitty' fashion. For some children, this is a reflection of emotional deprivation, while in others it is an maladaptive attempt to gain friendship.

## Truancy

This is the deliberate avoidance of school attendance. Two patterns are common; the child leaves home but does not arrive at school, spending the day wandering round the town alone or in the company of other truanting pupils; or the child spends part of the day at school and then 'skips' away from school at a convenient time, again either alone or with other children. This behaviour pattern usually begins in middle childhood, often becoming a major problem during adolescence. Motivation for the behaviour is not that the child is anxious or phobic about some aspect of schooling, but rather that the child dislikes or is resentful about the school curriculum or discipline. Truants often have definite learning difficulties and poor educational attainment.

The problem often goes undetected for a considerable time, leading to mutual recrimination between the parents and the school about the latter's failure to recognise the problem earlier. In many cases, the parents often overtly or covertly 'turn a blind eye' to the problem, believing that the school has little value for their child and is responsible for the child's poor interest or enthusiasm. Truants often show other symptoms of conduct disorder and frequently engage in other antisocial or delinquent behaviour when they play truant. Fogelman et al (1980) found that up to 20% of adolescents are absent from school for no apparent reason at any one time during their final school year.

The solution to the problem is fraught with difficulty as it requires the co-operation of the child, the parents, the school and the education department. Berg (1985) advocates the use of the juvenile justice system to enforce school attendance through the use of 'adjournment proceedings'. This procedure involves regular attendance at court by the child and parents to monitor school attendance.

## Specific delinquent behaviours

*Vandalism.* This is the deliberate, wanton damage or destruction of property. It occurs commonly in older children and adolescents and it is often carried out as a group activity. It often represents the expression of hostile, aggressive feelings about the adult world or a response to pent-up frustration over the lack of opportunity to release normal aggressive feelings in a socially acceptable manner. The latter is more likely among boys in socially deprived areas such as the council estates of large inner cities. Graffiti writing is particularly likely in anonymous, poorly supervised places such as the stairways of high-rise flats, subways or bus shelters.

*Breaking into and stealing property or taking and driving away cars.* These are common activities of juvenile delinquents, usually operating in pairs or in a group.

*Fire-setting.* This is an uncommon but serious symptom. It occurs throughout childhood and adolescence, with a distinctive psychopathology dependent upon the child's age. Many young children go through a stage of exploratory behaviour with matches or lighting small fires. In turn, most children respond and cease to engage in the activity following parental caution and reprimand. Persistent deliberate fire-setting is usually a sign of serious disturbance, reflecting the aggressive and hostile feelings of the child towards his parents. *Arson*, the intentional damage of buildings by fire, is a rare phenomenon, but with potentially catastrophic consequences for life and property.

Jacobson (1985a, b) and Gaynor & Hatcher (1987) have summarised the clinico-demographic characteristics and the psychopathology of fire-setters respectively. Their main findings were as follows:

- It is five times more common in boys than girls, more so in younger children
- There are two peaks at the ages of 8 and 13 years
- Most fire-setters had severe conduct disorder with marked aggressive and antisocial behaviours
- There was a high rate of specific reading retardation
- 50% of cases were associated with family discord.

*Drug abuse (see Ch. 14).* This is sometimes a symptom in older children and adolescents with severe conduct disorder.

**Table 10.4**   Causative factors in conduct disorder

**Family factors**
- Marital/parental disharmony
- Parental violence
- Lack of affection and rejection
- Ineffective and inconsistent discipline
- Large family size

**Individual characteristics**
- Genetic
- Temperamental
- Intelligence
- Physical illness

**Community influences**
- Peers
- Schooling
- Neighbourhood

## Associated features

*Reading difficulties (see Ch. 13)*

Research findings (Rutter et al 1970b, Offord et al 1987) have found a consistent relationship between reading failure and conduct disorder. *Reading backwardness* refers to a reading attainment at least 2 years below the chronological age, while *specific reading retardation* is a reading attainment at least 2 years below the chronological age even after adjustment for overall intelligence. For example, a 10-year-old of average intelligence with a reading age of 7.5 years would fulfil the criteria for specific reading retardation. Similarly, a 10-year-old child of superior intelligence with a reading age of 10 years also shows signs of specific reading retardation.

The direction of the association between specific reading retardation and conduct disorder is unclear, though most people favour the sequence of reading failure leading to disillusionment with school and subsequent delinquent behaviour. The delinquent behaviour is regarded as providing some satisfaction for an otherwise unhappy child. Alternatively, it has been proposed that temperamental characteristics such as impulsivity are responsible for both the conduct disorder and poor educational progress (Table 10.4).

## ASSOCIATED DISORDERS

As mentioned earlier, DSM-III-R classifies conduct disorder as part of the general category of disruptive behaviour disorders. The latter also includes *attention-deficit hyperactivity disorder*, which frequently has antisocial or conduct disorder symptoms as well. For example, Shapiro & Garfinkel (1986) found that a mixed pattern of conduct and attention-deficit

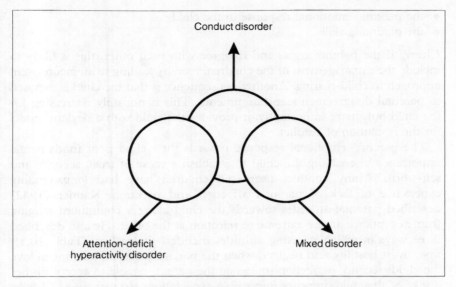

**Fig. 10.1**   Symptom overlap between conduct disorder, attention deficit disorder and mixed disorder

symptoms was more common than conduct or attention-deficit symptoms alone. Again, many children with conduct disorder have affective or emotional symptoms. Consequently in clinical practice, there is considerable overlap between attention-deficit hyperactivity syndrome, mixed disorders and conduct disorders. Fig 10.1 shows a convenient way to represent this overlap. Despite the similarity of the symptom profile in many cases, diagnostic practice should strive to retain discrete diagnostic categories whenever possible.

## CAUSATIVE FACTORS

Table 10.4 summarises the factors that contribute to the development of conduct disorder with the relative contribution of each factor varying between individuals. The three main categories are:

● family factors
● individual characteristics
● community influences.

### Family factors

The family is the most important factor in the development and maintenance of conduct disorder. Crucial aspects of family life are:

● the parents' relationship

- the parents' emotional response to the child
- the parenting skills.

Clearly if the parents argue and disagree with each other, this is likely to include their management of the children, thereby leading to an inconsistent approach to child-rearing. Another consequence is that the child is exposed to parental disagreements and arguments. This is not only distressing for the child but, more importantly, it provides the child with a deviant model for the resolution of conflict.

The parents' emotional response towards their child is of fundamental importance in enabling the child to establish a sense of trust, security and self-worth. Many conduct-disordered children have had long-standing experience of lack of parental affection and rejection. Kanner (1942) described parental attitudes towards the child along a continuum ranging from acceptance at one extreme to rejection at the other. He also described three ways in which rejecting attitudes manifest themselves (Table 10.5): first, overt hostility and neglect, when the parent makes no attempt to love the child; second, perfectionism, when the parent, unable to accept his/her dislike of the child, imposes impossible expectations, so that the child fails, thereby allowing the parent to be critical of the child; third, compensatory over-protection, where the parent is over-solicitous and concerned about the child in order to prove to him/herself and to other people that he/she is a good parent. Not surprisingly, as the child grows older, he often rebels against this attitude.

Deficient parent skills are important causes of conduct disorder. Ineffective and inconsistent parental control are frequently found in families with conduct-disordered children. The inconsistency results in an attitude to discipline which is alternately punitive and lax. In consequence, the child is exposed to conflicting standards which prevent the child from acquiring

**Table 10.5**  Kanner's scheme of maladaptive parental attitudes towards their children

| Type of rejecting behaviour | Description |
| --- | --- |
| Overt hostility | Parent dislikes the child and expresses resentment openly |
| Perfectionism | Parent is unable to accept his/her dislike of the child so imposes impossible restrictions. Consequently the child fails, allowing the parent to be critical of the child |
| Compensatory over-protection | Parent is over-solicitous and concerned about the child in order to prove to him/herself and to others that he/she is a good parent |
| **Other attitudes**<br>Non-rejecting over-protection | The child is an example of the 'special child syndrome', where the child has been especially wanted and/or has survived serious illness |

a coherent sense of moral values and also learning the ground rules of acceptable behaviour.

Finally, large family size is frequently associated with conduct disorder. The most likely explanation is that parents are unable to provide adequate supervision and care for the large number of children.

## Individual characteristics

The individual characteristics of the child influence the risk of conduct disorder in several ways. Important aspects are:

- genetic factors
- temperament
- intelligence
- physical illness or disability.

Although there is some evidence for the inheritance of adult criminality (Vandenberg et al 1986), this is much less so for antisocial disorder in childhood. Despite this, it is likely that *genetic factors* influence the risk of conduct disorder through their effects on temperament and cognitive development.

Adverse *temperamental characteristics* such as impulsivity, overactivity, restlessness and a prevailing negative or disgruntled mood are more common among children with conduct disorder.

*Low intelligence*, specific language and learning difficulties also increase the risk of conduct disorder. The child with below average intelligence is more likely to have a restricted repertoire of socially appropriate learning strategies, so that the risk of antisocial behaviour is increased. Poor language development and skills limit the child's ability to resolve conflicts verbally, so that an oppositional or aggressive response is more likely. Specific learning difficulties, especially reading, increase the child's frustration and disillusionment with schooling, thereby predisposing to school-based behavioural problems.

*Physical illness or disability* can have direct and indirect influences on the likelihood of conduct disorder. If the physical illness involves the central nervous system, as for instance in epilepsy or cerebral palsy, this can have direct adverse effects on cognitive function and temperamental characteristics such as attention, concentration and impulsivity. Caution is, however, necessary in the interpretation of the association between abnormal behaviour and neurological damage, as there is little evidence that most children with conduct disorder have demonstrable signs of brain damage. Changes, if present, are too subtle to be recognised with currently available imaging techniques such as computerised axial tomography (CAT) or magnetic resonance imaging (MRI). The indirect effects on behaviour arise from the secondary changes in self-esteem and mood associated with physical illness or disability.

## Community influences

Community influences are increasingly important for the older child and adolescent. Peer group values, especially when socially deviant, often pressurise the child into antisocial and delinquent behaviour in order to gain and retain acceptance within the group. Similarly, the poor provision of adequate community resources, common in large urban council estates, promotes a peer group ethos of anti-authoritarianism and disregard for property.

Rutter et al (1979) also found a definite association between delinquency, behaviour and school ethos. For example, schools where the emphasis was on a structured timetable, high teacher commitment and active rewards for desirable behaviour had the best outcomes. The presence of learning difficulties is also likely to exacerbate the child's problems in school.

## ASSESSMENT

The general principles of assessment are applicable to children with conduct disorder, though the mode and purpose of the referral often determine the subsequent therapeutic options. In many cases, the parents and child are clearly reluctant participants in the assessment process. Parental oppositionality, anti-authoritarian attitudes and failure to accept responsibility can severely restrict the chances of establishing a treatment contract. Sometimes however, the major problem is the unwillingness or lack of co-operation from the child or adolescent in the assessment process. For these reasons, in many cases contact with the child psychiatry service is restricted to the provision of an assessment and of recommendations about future needs. The latter role is likely when the referral has been made officially through the child justice system.

Table 10.6 lists the special features that may need to be considered in the assessment of conduct disorder. Three sections are listed, general physical state, psychiatric status and social assessment. The presence of any neurological abnormality should be noted and investigated when necessary. Special sense deficits in vision or hearing can exacerbate schooling difficulties. Children with short or tall stature often displace their frustration about their size by the development of aggression or other antisocial behaviour. Aggression from the physically strong and mature adolescent is a frequent source of conflict.

Psychiatric assessment should focus on the following:

- any additional affective features
- current self-esteem
- the capacity to form relationships
- the identification of any specific learning difficulties.

**Table 10.6** Specific features of conduct disorder assessment

**General physical state**
- Neurological status
- Stature

**Psychiatric state**
- Mood disturbance
- Additional affective symptoms (anxiety, depression)
- Self-esteem
- Intelligence level and educational attainments
- Reading retardation
- Presence of specific disorder amenable to treatment (e.g. enuresis)

**Social assessment**
- Family attitudes
- Family communication patterns
- Family models
- School functioning
- Peer relationships and models
- Community influences

The presence of significant additional affective symptoms may require treatment in its own right. Similarly, chronic low self-esteem may be helped with a cognitive-behavioural treatment approach. The assessment of the individual's ability to form relationships is important as this has an influence on the likely outcome and on the child's ability to benefit from some treatment options. The recognition of remedial conditions such as reading retardation or enuresis can be beneficial in gaining the co-operation of the child and family. Finally, the family's attitude, the presence of school difficulties and the availability of community resources determine the priorities for treatment intervention.

## TREATMENT

Treatment options vary markedly depending on assessment. Most treatment programmes are devised on an individual basis with the child and family. Key factors influencing the treatment choice are the family's motivation, the presence of educational or physical problems and the range of symptomatology. For instance, the occurrence of neurotic symptoms such as anxiety or depression may be an indication for individual work with the child. Table 10.7 summarises the principles underlying treatment approaches (see Ch. 17 for more detailed discussion of treatment methods).

Working with the family can involve parental counselling and/or the whole family. Patterson (1982), who has worked extensively with the families of conduct-disordered children, has emphasised the following general points:

- Establish and enforce a clear set of ground rules for household activities such as mealtimes, chores and bedtimes

**Table 10.7**   Treatment options for conduct disorder

- Work with the family
  - Counselling for the parents
  - Family therapy for the whole group
- Behaviour modification
  - Symptom management, for instance aggression
- Remedial education
- Treatment of physical problems
- Help with socio-economic disadvantage
  - Support for rehousing
- Removal from home including reception into care and/or residental schooling when necessary

- Monitor the child's behaviour closely to increase the parents' awareness of the child's feelings
- Ensure consistent, contingent response to behaviour, i.e. rewards for good behaviour, sanctions for bad
- Devise strategies to defuse crises, so preventing further escalation of problems.

Direct work with the child and family is commonly carried out in one of three ways:

- parental counselling
- family therapy
- behaviour modification.

The main aim of parental counselling is to enable the parents to implement the general principles of management outlined above. By contrast, family therapy is particularly useful as a method to define more clearly the roles and responsibilities within the family, to improve communication patterns and to devise tasks to modify the maladaptive patterns of family interaction. Behavioural techniques involving the co-operation between the parents and the child are most useful in the management of specific symptoms such as temper tantrums or aggressive outbursts. Careful behavioural analysis, close supervision of the treatment programme and the devising of suitable reinforcers and rewards are essential for a successful outcome.

Educational and school problems such as learning difficulties, non-attendance and disruptive classroom behaviour are extremely common among children with conduct disorder. The role of the child psychiatry team is dependent on the availability of other resources such as educational psychology, school counsellors and education-based social workers. The provision of remedial programmes for learning difficulties is often necessary and beneficial. Classroom-based behavioural programmes can be useful provided that realistic goals are established and the programme has a clearly defined life-span. Consultation and discussion with teaching staff are often a valuable means to improve staff morale and to reduce despondency. In many cases, conduct-disordered children benefit by transfer to special units within the school or to a special school. Residential schooling has also been extensively used in the past, though the gloomy long-term outcome, particularly when the children return home at the end of schooling, has brought about a reappraisal of the value of this form of intervention.

Some children with conduct disorder have remedial medical conditions such as impaired hearing or vision that can be greatly helped by referral to specialist medical services. Similarly, referral for occupational therapy or physiotherapy assessment and treatment is often useful for children who are clumsy and uncoordinated. Finally, support with rehousing applications is a practical way to help the many families whose problems are exacerbated by inadequate and unsatisfactory housing.

## OUTCOME

The long-term outcome is extremely varied depending on the range and diversity of the antisocial behaviour. Circumscribed antisocial behaviour, for instance that is confined to home or school, has a good prognosis, whereas extensive and varied symptomatology has a more gloomy outcome. While most children with conduct disorder do not have major disorders in adult life, it is nevertheless true that individuals with severe personality disorders usually displayed antisocial disturbance during childhood (Farrington 1978). When disturbance continues into adult life, the most common diagnosis is personality disorder, though other conditions such as neurotic disorder also occur. The most influential long term follow-up study has been that described by Robins (1966) involving children with conduct disorder referred to a child guidance service. This study found that approximately one-third had serious psychopathic disorder as adults compared with 4% of other clinical referrals and with 2% of the general population. A major reason for the poor outcome in this study was probably that most children had severe social and psychological deprivation as well as behaviour problems. The most important conclusion from follow-up studies is that the outcome is extremely variable and general optimism or pessimism is rarely warranted.

# 11. Disorders of elimination

This chapter discusses both enuresis and encopresis as they sometimes occur together, have similar clinical features and share common treatment approaches.

## ENURESIS

### Definition and terminology

Enuresis is the involuntary passage of urine, in the absence of physical abnormality, after the age of 5 years in a child of normal ability. It can be nocturnal and/or diurnal (by day). Lifelong bed-wetting, though not usually every night, is called *primary enuresis*, whereas when there has been a 6-month period of dry beds at some stage the term *secondary* or *onset enuresis* is used. Diurnal enuresis is much less common than nocturnal, but more common in girls and in children who are psychiatrically disturbed.

### Prevalence

Depending upon definition (commonly defined as a frequency of at least once per week), approximately 10% of 5-year-olds, 5% of 10-year-olds and 1% of 15-year-olds have nocturnal enuresis. A small number of individuals continue to be enuretic into adult life. Boys are twice as likely as girls to be enuretic, and enuresis is slightly more common in working-class children than other social groups.

### Psychiatric disorder

The presence of nocturnal or diurnal enuresis per se does not mean that the child has psychiatric disorder. The majority of children with nocturnal enuresis are not psychiatrically ill, though a substantial minority, approximately 25%, has signs of psychiatric disturbance. Diurnal enuresis is more frequently associated with psychiatric disturbance. The psychiatrically disturbed group of children with enuresis fall into two categories: those children where enuresis is one feature of a more widespread disturbance,

**Table 11.1**   Acquisition of dryness

| Age | Skill |
| --- | --- |
| Newborn | Empties bladder intermittently (not continuous dribbling) |
| 1.5 years | Has a word for wetness, e.g. 'wee' or 'piddle' |
| 2 years | Tells parents when wet |
| 2.5 years | Tells parents of need to urinate, but unable to delay micturition |
| 3 years | Can delay micturition long enough to use toilet, though 'accidents' common |
| 4–5 years | Child is interested in lavatories and wishes privacy for urination |

**Note:**
- Girls are usually ahead of boys
- Dryness by day usually precedes dryness by night
- Some measure of parental approval and avoidance of annoyance are helpful
- The value of some techniques, for instance 'lifting' the child when the parents go to bed, are difficult to prove, but they may be useful as they increase the child's and the parents' motivation and interest

and those where parental and/or the child's concern about enuresis generalises into other aspects of the child's life.

## Acquisition of dryness

Table 11.1 summarises the sequence in the acquisition of dryness. The development of dryness follows an orderly pattern in most children. Fashions about the ideal time to commence toilet training change over time and vary between cultures. The most crucial elements are probably to show approval for success and to minimise disapproval and despondency for failures or 'accidents'.

The newborn empties his bladder regularly but intermittently according to the volume and pressure of urine in the bladder. Around 18 months, the child can tell the parents of the need to urinate but is unable to delay micturition. Prompt production of a 'potty' is essential. The 3-year-old child can usually delay micturition for sufficiently long to ensure the usage of the toilet, though 'accidents' are frequent, especially when playing. Between 4 and 5 years, the child becomes interested in lavatories and wishes some privacy for urination. The child is also now able to micturate on request, for instance prior to outings. Girls usually acquire continence before boys, and dryness by day usually precedes dryness by night.

## Clinical features of enuresis

The majority of children with enuresis are seen by general practitioners and health visitors. Common reasons for paediatric referral are:

**Table 11.2**   Causative factors in nocturnal enuresis

**Individual Factors**
- Genetic
- Low intelligence
- Psychiatric disorder
- Urinary tract infection
- Small functional bladder capacity

**Environmental factors**
- Stressful life events
- Large family size
- Social disadvantage

- the persistence of the problem
- special features such as day-time wetting
- the failure of simple measures
- family anxiety about the problem.

Investigation is usually confined to the exclusion of renal disease, diabetes or occasionally, when appropriate, nocturnal epilepsy. Most paediatricians would initiate treatment themselves unless there was some contraindication, for instance underlying psychiatric disorder. Enuretic children referred to child psychiatry departments usually have psychiatric disorder and/or are treatment-resistant.

## Aetiology

### Nocturnal enuresis

Two sets of factors have been identified, individual and environmental (Table 11.2). 70% of enuretics have a positive family history, supporting the idea that there is a genetic component in the attainment of night-time continence. Low intelligence with delayed developmental progress impairs the acquisition of maturational skills such as dryness at night. Psychiatric disorder also impedes the child's ability to acquire new skills. Urinary tract infection and small functional bladder capacity make it more difficult for the child to achieve success. Stressful life events inevitably increase the child's anxiety, thereby inhibiting new skill acquisition. Large family size, social disadvantage and institutional upbringing all reduce the amount of individual attention that the child receives, so that the child's progress towards night-time continence is hindered.

### Diurnal enuresis

Similar factors are operative for day time wetting with the additional burden of psychiatric disorder which is present in many cases.

**Table 11.3**   Assessment and management of nocturnal enuresis

---

**History**
- Family history of nucturnal enuresis
- Previous treatments
- Sleeping arrangements
- Concurrent encopresis

**Examination**
- Back and lower limb reflexes
- Urine specimen to exclude renal failure and diabetes
- Mental state of child

**Treatment**
- Minimise handicap
- Accurate diary record of nocturnal enuresis
- Enuresis alarm
- Other treatments (for instance tricyclic antidepressants)

---

## Assessment and management

### Assessment

Table 11.3 summarises the key points in the assessment and management of nocturnal enuresis.

The presence of a positive family history is often a useful indication of the long-term outcome. Previous treatment strategies and the reasons for their failure are useful indicators of motivation and of the likely success of future treatment approaches. The attitudes of the child and family are central to the establishment of a therapeutic alliance between the clinician and the family. Unhelpful features are:

- parental criticism of and hostility towards the child
- parental unwillingness to participate actively in the treatment programme
- major disturbance in the parent–child relationship.

The sleeping arrangements, for instance whether the child has his own bed and room, are important as treatment with the enuresis alarm is likely to disrupt not only the child's sleep but also that of other family members. It is also wise to make sure that the child does not have encopresis as well. Checking that physical causes for the enuresis have been excluded is important. The mental state assessment of the child is valuable in determining his attitude to the problem, his motivation and also whether there are other features of his psychiatric state that require treatment in their own right.

### Management

It is important to exclude any physical basis for the enuresis by history, examination and, if necessary, investigation of the renal tract. Most clinicians would consider that specific treatment, in addition to reassurance

| Day of the week | First week | Second week | Third week | Fourth week | Fifth week |
|---|---|---|---|---|---|
| Monday | | | | | |
| Tuesday | | | | | |
| Wednesday | | | | | |
| Thursday | | | | | |
| Friday | | | | | |
| Saturday | | | | | |
| Sunday | | | | | |

**Fig. 11.1**    Star chart system for nocturnal enuresis

and advice, is only indicated when the child is around 6 years old. The decision to treat is influenced by parental attitudes and motivation as well as by the restrictions and limitations imposed by the enuresis on the child's daily life. An important consideration, which should be discussed with the child and family, is the possibility of treatment failure, as the latter may lead to further recrimination and despondency.

The initial stage of the treatment plan is as follows: explain to the parents and child

a.   the maturational basis of the problem
b.   the likelihood of spontaneous improvement
c.   the necessity to avoid invoking laziness or blame as the basis for the problem.

The second stage is to get the child to keep a diary of the pattern of night-time dryness/wetness. This is usually done with a star chart (Fig. 11.1). This consists of a daily record of dry nights with a star placed on the sheet for each dry night. A common practice is to use a single blue star for each dry night with three consecutive dry nights meriting a gold star. The star chart system has three main functions:

● to provide an accurate record of the problem
● to test the motivation and co-operation of the child and family
● to act as a positive reinforcement for the desired behaviour, that is a dry bed.

There are many variations of the star chart technique, including smiley faces and farmyard charts. The stars are usually sufficiently rewarding for 6–7-year-olds, though in addition a small monetary reward may be attached to each star, say 5p or 10p.

*Enuresis alarm.* This is an effective means of eliminating nocturnal enuresis, but it requires patience, co-operation and persistence to succeed. The alarm works on the principle that it goes off when the electrical current is completed by the child passing urine. The rationale of the technique is that the child should inhibit the release of urine when the bladder is full, initially to the sound of the alarm and then independently. The newer mini-alarms are so compact that the sensor slips inside an absorbent pad placed in underpants or knickers with the alarm clipped on to the top of the pyjamas or nightdress (Fordham & Meadow 1988). The method can be extremely disruptive to other family members, especially if it wakes them but not the enuretic child. Ideally, the child should have his own bedroom. When the alarm sounds, the child should get out of bed and go to the toilet. This pattern may initially occur two or three times per night, causing disruption, loss of sleep and irritability. Another problem is the false alarm rate. This is usually caused by excessive sweating short-circuiting the alarm. The aim of the training is to enable the child to inhibit bladder relaxation and/or to awaken the child when bladder distension occurs. Training, if successful, should be producing definite improvements by 1 month. The enuresis alarm programme should be combined with the start chart record to improve motivation and monitor progress accurately.

*Drug treatment.* Tricyclic antidepressants such as imipramine or amitriptyline (25–50 mg at night) are often effective in producing short-term improvement in enuresis. They are frequently prescribed by family doctors and to a lesser extent by paediatricians. The mode of action is unknown, though it is most unlikely to be a reflection of the antidepressant action. A more likely explanation is that there is a local effect produced by the tricyclic drug on synaptic transmission in the bladder. If the tricyclic drug is effective, the beneficial effect is usually apparent within 2 weeks. This rapid improvement is another indication that the efficacy of the tricyclic drug is not due to its antidepressant effect, as the latter only becomes evident after a period of at least 2 weeks on medication. The major drawback with the use of tricyclic drugs is that there is a high rate of relapse when treatment is discontinued. Consequently, commencement of drug treatment implies a commitment to treatment for several months. This is a practice many paediatricians feel is unwarranted for such a benign condition. Another concern with tricyclic usage is the possible accidental or occasionally intentional overdose of the drug by other siblings, with a potentially fatal outcome. A more sensible use of medication is to confine its usage to those occasions when the child is away from home and might be embarrassed by the enuresis, for instance at school camp or on holiday.

*Bladder training.* This involves training the child to defer micturition for increasing periods of time during the day. This technique is mainly used for diurnal enuresis. The rationale is that training increases the bladder capacity, which is thought to be small in some children with diurnal enuresis, an opinion that is not necessarily generally accepted. The training usually occurs when the parents can supervise the programme, for instance during school holidays. It involves the child gradually extending the time between micturitions in a graded sequence from half an hour up to 4 hours during the course of the training. Anecdotal evidence suggests that this can have a beneficial effect on nocturnal enuresis as well, presumably through the enlarged bladder capacity.

## Outcome

Outcome is extremely favourable for uncomplicated enuresis, with only around 1% of children still enuretic aged 15 years. Unfortunately, it is not possible to predict which child will become dry or when this will occur. Unfavourable prognostic signs for nocturnal enuresis are the presence of additional psychiatric symptoms and also diurnal enuresis.

## ENCOPRESIS

### Definition and terminology

Encopresis is the inappropriate passage of formed faeces, usually in the underclothes, in the absence of physical pathology after 4 years of age. Most children are normally clean by their fourth birthday. Soiling, the passage of semi-solid faeces, is often used interchangeably with encopresis. Symptoms vary markedly in severity, ranging from slight staining of the underclothes through to encopresis and the smearing of faeces on the floor, walls or furniture.

### Prevalence

Encopresis is uncommon, having a community prevalence rate of 1.3% and 0.3% among 10-year-old boys and girls in the Isle of Wight study (Rutter et al 1970b). Psychiatric disturbance is common in children with encopresis. Enuresis may also occur as well. There is no marked social class differential.

### Clinical features (Fig. 11.2)

These vary widely, with a broad division into two categories, a retentive or non-retentive group and a primary or secondary group. Children with retentive encopresis defaecate infrequently, leading eventually to overflow incontinence, while the non-retentive group defaecate regularly but inappropriately, usually in the underclothes. The primary or continuous group of children with encopresis have never had a period of being 'clean', in contrast to the secondary or discontinuous group who have had periods of continence interspersed with periods of encopresis.

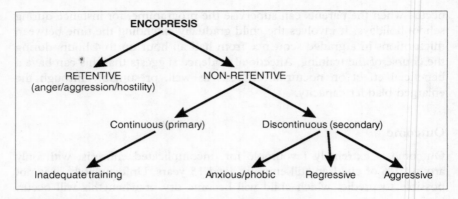

Fig. 11.2   Types of encopresis and their psychopathology

Clinically, three patterns of presentation are common:

- the child with primary encopresis
- the child with retentive encopresis
- the child with secondary encopresis.

Children with primary encopresis often come from chaotic, disorganised and socially disadvantaged families where reliable and regular toilet training is uncommon. The child does not experience the right conditions to acquire the habit of regular toileting, so that he often has diurnal enuresis as well as encopresis. The encopresis usually becomes a problem in the year prior to schooling when parents and/or nursery staff express concern about how the child will manage at school. Often, the child has additional problems such as developmental or language delay and behaviour problems, which make the resolution of the problem more difficult. The other presentation of primary encopresis is the child who is anxious or phobic about some aspect of toileting or toilet training — for instance, he is fearful when sitting on the toilet or is afraid of remaining in the bathroom. The child is less likely to have other symptoms such as developmental delay or behavioural disturbance, and usually comes from a more stable family background. The impasse between the mother and the child results in the mother requesting help from the family doctor in the period prior to the commencement of schooling.

Children with retentive encopresis usually present at an older age as they have been toilet-trained and have been clean for a variable length of time. There is sometimes a previous history of constipation or occasionally of an anal fissure. The latter is a small tear on the rim of the anus that can make defaecation painful, especially when it first develops. This painful experience is said to make the child apprehensive about defaecation, though clinical experience suggests that this is not in fact a common feature.

Regardless of the earlier history, the child with retentive encopresis subsequently resorts to hiding his soiled pants to avoid detection. This in turn leads to further acrimony between the mother and the child when the offending and offensive articles are eventually discovered, often hidden in drawers. The foul odour and stink from the child leads to further recrimination from the parent(s) as well as teasing and social rejection from peers.

The initial phase of the retention can go undetected for several months as there is no evidence of any problem at this stage. During this time, the faeces become impacted and hard, distending the large bowel. Eventually however, liquid faeces begin to pass around the mass of impacted faeces and leak out at the anus, giving the false impression of diarrhoea. The terms *constipation with overflow* and *spurious diarrhoea* are applied to this phenomenon. Once this has become established, the child has little control over bowel movements, so that constant soiling and encopresis are the rule.

Traditionally, the explanation for retentive encopresis has been that it represents a reaction by the child to the coercive, rigid toileting practices of the parents who are in turn rigid, tidy and obsessional individuals. The encopresis is regarded as an expression, often unconsciously, of anger and hostility towards the controlling parent. Changes in social attitudes towards toilet-training in the last 30 years have made this explanation less plausible. Despite this reservation, there is little doubt that encopresis generates considerable anger and resentment with mutual hostility between the parents and the child in many cases. Whether the resentment is a cause or a consequence of the encopresis is often unclear.

Discontinuous encopresis is commoner in the older child. Two types, regressive and aggressive, have been described. Regressive encopresis arises as a response to some external stress which may be acute or long-standing. As discussed in Chapter 3, regressive behaviour is a common response in children at times of stress or anxiety. Acute stresses include starting school, the birth of a sibling, family illness or a change of house or neighbourhood. Long-standing stresses include disturbance in family relationships and social disadvantage. Aggressive soiling often occurs in the context of disturbed parent–child relationship and poor family functioning, the encopresis being symptomatic of more generalised psychiatric disturbance. Children with discontinuous soiling sometimes hide or secrete their soiled pants, making matters considerably worse. The more disturbed child, often in the younger age group, may smear faeces on walls or furniture and sometimes soils his pyjamas and bedclothes. These behaviours provoke even more anger and further punitive responses from the parents.

## Aetiology

The preceding section indicates that several factors contribute to the development of encopresis, ranging from inadequate toilet training to seriously disturbed parent–child relationship. Often, children with encopresis have other symptomatology, so that it is important to decide whether the encopresis is the main clinical problem or merely part of a more widespread disturbance. There is often no single common pattern, and the factors discussed below have varying importance in the individual child.

### Individual characteristics

Children with developmental delay or below-average ability are likely to find toilet-training harder to master than other children. Specific phobia or anxiety about the toilet may be important in some cases, while more generalised aggression, oppositionality and defiance are present in other cases. Occasionally, the encopresis is symptomatic of an underlying depressive condition.

### Parental factors

Most parents are likely to be angry and annoyed with a child who soils regularly. Whenever possible, it is useful to decide whether the disturbance in the parent–child relationship is primary or secondary, that is, whether it is a cause of or a response to the encopresis. If the encopresis is thought primarily to reflect a disturbance in the parent–child relationship, this disturbance may be solely confined to the encopresis. More usually however, it may an indication of generalised parental neglect, rejection or hostility towards the child. Rarely, the parental attitude is of only marginal importance in the development of the problem.

### Family factors

Family dysfunction, expressed by poor communication and disorganisation, usually manifests itself in behavioural disturbance rather than encopresis, but occasionally the latter does occur. If this does happen, the affected child becomes the focus for the underlying resentment and hostility, thereby exacerbating the problem.

### Psychosocial factors

Chronic social adversity and acute stresses can be responsible for the failure to become toilet-trained adequately, i.e. for primary encopresis, or alternatively for the loss of toileting skills following an acute stress, i.e. for secondary regressive encopresis.

## Treatment (Table 11.4)

Given the wide range of severity and psychopathology associated with encopresis, it is only possible to outline general principles of assessment and

**Table 11.4**  Assessment and management of encopresis

**Aims**
- Promotion of bowel habit
- Improvement of parent–child relationship

**Assessment**
- Exclude physical disease by history, examination and investigation (if necessary)
- Previous treatments
- Parents' and child's attitude to problem

**Management**
- Dietary
  - Modify diet to ensure adequate intake of dietary fibre to increase faecal bulk
- Medical management
  - Bowel washout and/or enemas may be necessary initially
  - Drugs
    - motor stimulant (senna laxatives)
    - bulk agents (lactulose)
    - suppositories are often useful as well
- Psychological management
  - Behavioural (star chart)
  - Individual psychotherapy
    - enlist co-operation
    - show concern
    - develop trust
  - Parental counselling/family therapy
    - modify attitudes
    - hostile interactions
    - secondary problems

management. Individual clinical features determine the mixture and emphasis of the treatments used.

The first stage is to exclude a physical basis for the problem by history, examination and, if necessary, investigation. The family doctor and/or the paediatrician are likely to have carried out this assessment prior to referral to the child psychiatry service. Organic causes for diarrhoea or constipation are the main focus for investigation, though positive findings are unlikely. Traditionally, medical textbooks have emphasised the importance of excluding Hirschsprung's disease in the differential diagnosis of severe constipation. Hirschsprung's disease, the absence or relative scarcity of the nerve cells in the bowel wall controlling muscular contraction and muscle tone, does lead to severe constipation, but this usually presents with symptoms at a much earlier age than encopresis.

The next stage is to find out the measures that parents and other professionals have tried to resolve the problem and their degree of success. The parents' understanding and explanation of the encopresis are important as it may be necessary to devote some time to the modification of their hostile and critical attitudes. Similarly, the child's views of the problem and the parent–child relationship influence considerably the choice of treatment strategies.

Treatment has two aims: the promotion of a normal bowel habit, and an improvement in the parent–child relationship. These are achieved in three ways:

- dietary measures
- medical measures
- psychological treatment(s).

### Dietary measures

Many children have diets with a poor quantity of fibre, so that constipation is common. Children with retentive encopresis benefit by an increased dietary fibre content, thereby producing more bulky faeces. The problem is to persuade the parents and the child to modify their dietary habits in order to produce a long-lasting change.

### Medical measures

These are essential in the management of children with retentive encopresis, though less so in non-retentive encopresis. It is preferable for the medical treatment to be carried out separately from the psychiatric management, so that a joint paediatric–psychiatric team approach is best. Long-standing retentive encopresis has two important consequences that influence management: the volume of hard impacted faeces is large and difficult to remove easily; and the grossly dilated bowel has lost its muscle tone so that, even when the faeces are finally cleared out, the bowel is so flaccid that retention of any quantity of faeces is difficult.

The first stage in management is to ensure that the bowel is completely emptied of faeces, as otherwise the behavioural programmes are doomed to fail. This may necessitate bowel washouts, micro-enemas such as sodium alkylsulphoacetate and even manual removal of faeces. Examination and X-ray of the abdomen are necessary to check whether the procedures have been successful. Subsequent management is directed towards ensuring that the child can produce a sizable and discomfort-free bowel action on a regular basis. Drugs can usefully assist this process in some circumstances. For instance, senna laxatives stimulate bowel contraction and tone, dioctyl sodium sulphosuccinate softens the faeces and lactulose increases faecal bulk. These drugs are usefully combined with the behavioural programme described in the next section. Finally, suppositories can be used to relieve the constipation which often happens during the initial stages of the programme.

*Psychological interventions*

These include behaviour modification, individual psychotherapy, parental counselling and family therapy. Whatever approach is used, the establishment of a therapeutic alliance between the child, parents and therapist is essential. This involves the therapist showing concern and understanding towards the child as well as enlisting the co-operation of the parents in the treatment programme.

**Behaviour modification.** The object is to train the child to produce a normal bowel movement on a regular basis when using the toilet. The most useful approach is to 'shape' or gradually alter the child's behaviour until it approximates to the desired behaviour. Detailed discussions with the parent and the child are essential to find out the child's current behaviour and attitude towards toileting. This can be done during the joint sessions with the parents and the child or in the context of a family meeting. Careful baseline record-keeping of the frequency of the encopresis and an agreed strategy for the management of each encopretic episode by the parents and the child is necessary before starting the treatment programme. A star chart is an easy way to record this baseline information. The initial starting point for the programme is dependent on the individual assessment of the child. A common starting point would be for the child to go and to remain in the bathroom for 10 minutes after each meal. This would then be extended to include sitting on the toilet and then finally to producing a bowel action while on the toilet. The pace and staging of the programme vary considerably, but success is dependent on the ability to devise stages that represent graded progress while also continuing to motivate the child. Small successful steps are much better than unpredictable leaps. Finally, the behavioural programme is often combined with the drug treatment.

**Individual psychotherapy.** This can be used as an adjunct to the behavioural approach or as the main therapeutic strategy. The therapist must display clearly to the child a concern for and an understanding of the child's behaviour and a willingness to encourage the expression of feelings that may include some critical of the parents. Prolonged individual work is indicated when the primary cause of the encopresis is the aggressive, hostile and angry relationship between the child and his parent(s) and when joint sessions with the parents and the child would be destructive and counter-productive.

**Parental counselling.** This is commonly used in conjunction with the behavioural programme. The purpose is to modify unhelpful attitudes, for instance that the child is lazy or unconcerned about the problem. The parents may also be unaware that the chronic nature of the problem means that the child is unlikely to be aware of the sensations connected with either defaecation or the inhibition of defaecation, thereby compounding the difficulty. Similarly, a consistent but non-punitive response to the soiling combined with a positive reward in response to success is another example of a beneficial attitude change.

*Family therapy.* This may be a useful approach, particularly when the encopresis reflects poor communication, the inadequate expression of feelings and a lack of structure within the family system. As family therapy has become more popular, it has now replaced individual psychotherapy and parental counselling as the treatment of choice in many situations (see family therapy section in Ch. 17).

*Hospitalisation.* Admission to a child psychiatric unit may be necessary when out-patient contact has been unsuccessful. Wherever possible, it is preferable to admit to a child psychiatric unit rather than a paediatric ward as the more extensive psychiatric expertise of the child psychiatry unit is likely to produce better results both in the short term and in the long term. Close co-operation and collaboration between the parents, the child and the in-patient staff are necessary to ensure that a long-lasting resolution of the problem is achieved.

## Outcome

Most follow-up studies (Belman 1966) have shown that encopresis as a symptom does not usually persist into adult life. It is very likely, however, that when encopresis is indicative of more generalised disturbance the latter may manifest itself in other symptomatology, for instance aggression or other antisocial behaviour, unless the predisposing factors have been resolved. Finally, occasional case reports of persistence into adult life have been published (Fraser & Taylor 1986).

# 12. Overactivity syndromes and hyperkinetic disorder

## INTRODUCTION

Originally, the hyperkinetic or overactivity syndrome was seen as the prototype for syndromes attributable to 'minimal brain damage' (Strauss & Lehtinen 1947). This theory proposed that minor abnormalities or anomalies of brain structure and function produced a stereotyped clinical picture characterised by hyperactivity, distractibility, impulsivity, perseveration and cognitive defects. This was said to mimic to a lesser degree the well known effects of definite brain damage or insult. Subsequently, Clements & Peters (1962) coined the term 'minimal brain dysfunction' (MBD) to describe those children who were said to show the behavioural characteristics of children with brain damage but with no evidence of brain damage on investigation. These two terms became extremely popular as a means to describe a large group of disturbed children whose behaviour was characterised by overactivity, restlessness and oppositional or aggressive behaviour. Unfortunately, the theory was extended in such a way that the reasoning became tautological. For instance, certain behaviours were said to be pathognomonic of brain damage. Many writers (Bax & MacKeith 1963, Taylor 1986) have exposed the conceptual flaws underlying the usage of these terms, so that they have now been rightly abandoned.

The overactivity syndromes highlight the difference between DSM North-American-based diagnostic practice and the ICD system used in the UK (see Taylor 1985 for a British perspective and Schacher 1991 for a North American view). The syndrome(s) also demonstrate the dangers of the premature application of classification procedures when the rationale for such a procedure is not clearly established. Important sources of confusion between the North American and British approaches are:

- inadequate definition of terminology
- uncertainty as to whether pathological hyperactivity is a discrete or continuous variable
- the co-existence of additional symptoms suggestive of other disorders, most noticeably conduct disorder.

163

Clinicians and research workers have found it difficult to define clearly the meaning of such terms as 'attention deficit', 'impulsivity' or 'overactivity', so that it is difficult to compare the results from the various studies. Similarly, it is often unclear whether hyperactivity is a discrete or continuous variable, so that uncertainty exists about the definition of 'caseness'. The importance attached by British child psychiatrists to the term *pervasive hyperactivity*, that is, overactivity present in all situations, as opposed to *situational hyperactivity* (overactivity present in some but not all situations), illustrates this problem clearly. Moreover, if the overactivity variable has a continuous distribution in the population, the criterion for abnormality may not be obvious.

Finally, many children with overactivity show symptoms of other disorders, commonly conduct disorder. The ICD solution to this problem is to decide on the basis of symptomatology whether conduct disorder or hyperactivity is the primary diagnosis. By contrast, DSM allows the clinician to use more than one diagnostic category. Unfortunately, current knowledge does not provide the information to decide which of these two approaches is correct.

## TERMINOLOGY

The terms *overactivity or hyperactivity, attention-deficit disorder* and *hyperkinetic syndrome* are often used synonymously, so that it is important to define their use in each instance.

### Overactivity and/or hyperactivity

This refers to excessive motor activity and restlessness present in some but not all situations. About one-third of children are described by their parents as overactive while 5–20% of school children are so described by their teachers. The overactivity ranges in severity from normal childish exuberance to the severe and disabling hyperkinetic syndrome. Numerous studies, reviewed by Taylor (1986), have shown a big difference in the prevalence rates between the USA and the UK — USA: 10/100 children; UK 1/1000. The most likely explanation for this is probably a difference in terminology rather than a true difference in prevalence. British psychiatrists tend to limit the term *hyperkinesis* to the small number of children with hyperkinetic syndrome with the remainder classified as *conduct disorder* (since many conduct-disordered children have overactivity as an important feature of their disturbance).

Table 12.1 shows a convenient way to classify overactivity or hyperactivity. A broad distinction can be made between normal variation and pathological causes. Children vary markedly on the temperamental dimension of activity level, so that some children at the extreme end of the

**Table 12.1**   Clinical types of overactivity/hyperactivity

**Normal variation**
- Temperamental deviation
- Cognitive impairment

**Pathological causes**
- Hyperkinetic disorder
- Hypomania
- Anxiety state
- Conduct disorder
- Organic conditions
  - thyrotoxicosis
  - Sydenham's chorea
  - lead intoxication
  - mental retardation, for example phenylketonuria or rubella
- Response to some drugs, for instance barbiturates or benzodiazepines

continuum are quite overactive. Similarly, children with cognitive or intellectual impairment tend to be more active than other children.

Pathological causes can be divided into

- psychiatric
- organic
- abnormal drug response.

Among *psychiatric* causes, besides being a defining feature of hyperkinetic disorder, overactivity also occurs in hypomania, anxiety states and in children with conduct disorder. The latter is the most important alternative diagnosis to hyperkinetic disorder in clinical practice. Thyrotoxicosis, chorea and lead intoxication are possible *organic* causes for overactivity, while children with phenylketonuria and rubella are often overactive. Finally, some *drugs*, particularly barbiturates and benzodiazepines, can induce overactive behaviour when prescribed for children.

## Attention-deficit disorder

This term has been used extensively in North America to describe a large group of children (approximately 5–10% of the population) whose principal abnormalities are a short attention span and distractibility. Characteristically, the children are overactive in some situations, are aggressive and have learning difficulties. The prime abnormality of the disorder was thought to be a defect in attention and vigilance processing within the brain. A major weakness of this explanation, however, is the absence of any convincing experimental evidence to support it. Another disadvantage is that the category would include some children who are inattentive for other reasons, for instance children who are daydreaming or excessively anxious.

**Table 12.2**   DSM-III-R criteria for attention-deficit hyperactivity disorder (ADHD)

The individual should display at least eight of the behaviours listed below for a minimum period of 6 months
- Fidgetiness
- Cannot remain seated when expected to do so
- Easily distracted
- Unable to await turn in game or group situation
- Frequently blurts out answer before question is finished
- Has difficulty in persisting/completing tasks
- Ill-sustained attention
- Poorly sustained tasks
- Frequent shifts of behaviour between activities
- Unable to play quietly
- Talks excessively
- Interrupts and intrudes on other people
- Unable to listen to what is being said
- Frequently loses items necessary for activities or tasks at home and at school
- Reckless and dangerous behaviour with little foresight about serious consequences

**Note:**
- The above behaviours must be more frequent than in other children of the same age and cognitive ability
- Onset before 7 years
- No other features of pervasive developmental disorder

DSM-III-R has recognised the difficulties with this terminology, so that the disorder has now been renamed *attention-deficit hyperactivity disorder* (ADHD) and included as one of the three categories of disruptive behaviour disorder. Table 12.2 lists the diagnostic criteria adopted by DSM-III-R.

This approach assumes that there is a core abnormality which is responsible for the wide range of disturbed behaviour.

### Hyperkinetic syndrome

In the UK, this category is restricted to the small number of children (less than 0.1%) who have severe pervasive hyperactivity, are restless and distractible and have a short attention span. These criteria are very similar to those proposed by ICD-10 (Table 12.3). The latter states that hyperkinetic disorder should be present from an early age, occur in most situations and have the cardinal features of impaired attention and overactivity which manifest themselves in a wide variety of situations. In addition, children with hyperkinetic syndrome are reckless, impulsive and prone to accidents. They also often find themselves in trouble, mainly because they break rules without thinking of the consequences rather than from a deliberate intention to be defiant. They are socially disinhibited, showing a lack of caution or reserve with adults. Behaviour can be aggressive at times, with marked mood swings. Other associated features are a male predominance (at least 3:1), low intelligence, learning difficulties and often

**Table 12.3**   ICD-10 criteria for hyperkinetic disorder

Core abnormalities of attention and overactivity which manifest themselves at home and away from home in the following ways:
- Short duration of spontaneous activities
- Failure to complete tasks
- Frequent changes between activities
- Poor persistence at task
- High distractibility
- Motor restlessness
- Fidgetiness
- Excess activity in situations where composure expected
- Difficulty in remaining seated when required

Other common features include:
- Recklessness and impulsivity
- Accident proneness
- Social disinhibition with lack of caution or reserve
- Labile mood

**Note:**
- Onset before age of 6 years
- Duration of at least 6 months
- IQ above 50

some signs of neurological impairment. The hyperactivity is at its peak between the ages of 3 and 8 years.

ICD further divides hyperkinetic syndrome into that characterised solely by disturbance of activity and attention and that with additional conduct disorder. The latter is a recognition of the frequent co-existence of conduct disorder symptoms in children with hyperkinetic syndrome. In order to warrant inclusion in this category, the individual must fulfil the criteria for conduct disorder as well as those for hyperkinetic disorder.

The convergence of diagnostic criteria in the latest versions of ICD and DSM makes it possible to discuss the syndromes of hyperkinetic disorder and attention-deficit hyperactivity disorder together.

## HYPERKINETIC DISORDERS (ATTENTION-DEFICIT HYPERACTIVITY DISORDER)

### Prevalence

The variation in diagnostic criteria, methods of assessment and population studied makes it difficult to obtain the 'true' prevalence rate from previous studies. For instance, Taylor (1986) found a 20-fold difference in prevalence rates between the UK and the USA, 0.06% and 1.2% respectively. Similarly, the most recent comprehensive community survey of hyperkinetic disorder from North America, the Ontario Child Health Study (Szatmari et al 1989a, b) found a prevalence rate of 6%. The high prevalence rate found in the study is probably accounted for by the use of questionnaires to determine the presence of disorder. This study also showed the following features about the diagnostic habits of North American child psychiatrists with respect to attention-deficit hyperactivity disorder (ADHD):

- The peak prevalence was between 6 and 9 years
- It was three times more common among boys
- ADHD was the most common diagnosis between 4 and 11 years (whereas conduct disorder was more common among adolescents 12–16 years)
- 40% of children with ADHD had the additional diagnosis of conduct disorder
- Only 15% were pervasively hyperactive
- Only 20% were in contact with psychiatric services.

While it is possible that there are real differences in prevalence rates between the two populations, the most likely explanation is the different diagnostic practices between clinicians in the USA and those in the UK.

## Aetiology

Several factors, operating in combination, are probably responsible for the development of the disorder. Constitutional factors such as genetic or perinatal insult increase the predisposition, while environmental factors such as parenting behaviour determine the severity, persistence and outcome of the disorder.

### Genetic

Though early studies found strong links between parental personality disorder and childhood hyperactivity, these studies failed to distinguish between hyperactive children with or without conduct disorder. Clearly, the presence of the latter could be the common factor explaining the close association between childhood hyperactivity and parental personality disorder. Recently, more convincing evidence of a genetic contribution has come from the studies of August & Stewart (1983) and Goodman & Stevenson (1989). The former found that a significant minority of the fathers of the ADHD children had the syndrome when they were children, while the latter found that monozygotic twins were more alike than same-sex dizygotic twins on objective measures of attentiveness and parent and teacher ratings of hyperactivity. The parent and teacher ratings in this study were derived from the Rutter Scale subscores for hyperactivity, so that it is unlikely that most children would have fallen within the strict definition of hyperkinetic syndrome. It is more likely that the results are a reflection of the genetic contribution that temperamental factors can make to overactivity.

## Temperament

Thomas & Chess (1982) found that overactivity in later childhood was preceded by similar behaviour in early infancy, a finding consistent with the constitutional role of temperament in the development of the hyperkinetic disorder. Their studies do not, however, answer the question of whether this continuity is simply a reflection of the stability of the activity level dimension over time or a more specific indication for a constitutional component to the hyperkinetic syndrome.

## Brain injury

Children with definite neurological disorders such as epilepsy or cerebral palsy have higher rates of hyperkinetic syndrome, though most hyperkinetic children do not show signs or evidence of neurological damage. Goodman & Stevenson (1989) found no relationship between hyperactivity scores and perinatal adversity. EEG investigations have also not produced any consistent results. Finally, Pomeroy et al (1988), in a study of 300 children, found no association between minor physical anomalies and ADHD, the latter being most strongly associated with psychosocial factors.

## Diet

Feingold (1975) maintained that hyperactivity was an allergic response by the child to certain food additives such as tartrazine and salicylates. He therefore proposed a diet which excluded these substances. The subsequent findings appeared to show beneficial results, but the evidence for the general efficacy of these exclusion diets other than as a placebo response is unconvincing. Recently however, Egger et al (1985), using a sophisticated methodological design of food exclusion and challenge, showed that some children with severe hyperactivity and mental retardation did respond to the omission of certain food substances. It is however unclear whether these results would apply to the majority of children with hyperkinetic disorder.

## Lead

While the toxic properties of lead are not in doubt, the relationship between lead intoxication and behaviour, particularly hyperactivity, is still unresolved. A recent study (Thomson et al 1989) of 501 Edinburgh children found a dose-response relationship between high blood lead levels and abnormal hyperactivity scores on the Rutter Scale questionnaires. This study supported earlier reports that high blood lead levels can produce behaviour and cognitive disorders in some children (Needleman et al 1979). The main uncertainty is still the strength and clinical importance of the statistically significant findings found in the various studies.

*Psychosocial factors*

As discussed earlier, poor social circumstances and inadequate parenting can undoubtedly exacerbate the child's problems of impaired attention and overactivity. It is doubtful, though, whether these factors are primarily responsible for the behaviour of most children with ADHD or hyperkinetic syndrome.

## Symptoms

Symptoms vary widely, but some brief additional comments on core symptoms are now discussed. Fig 12.1 shows the ways in which the different symptoms of hyperkinetic disorder can adversely affect the child's development and behaviour. In most circumstances, these factors interact with each other to produce the overall clinical pattern of the disorder.

*Overactivity*

An important component of overactivity is the accompanying sense of restlessness, which is not task-related and has an irritating, disruptive quality that is annoying to other people. Direct observation and recording with actometers confirms this restlessness. By contrast, observation of the child during the initial assessment interview often reveals no overactivity or restlessness, a result probably produced by the child's anxiety about and/or unfamiliarity with the interview situation.

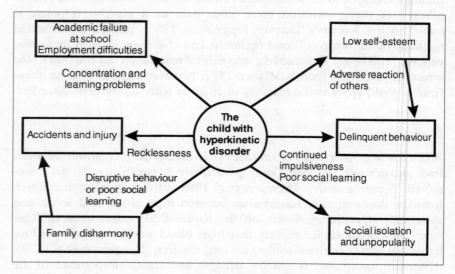

**Fig. 12.1**   Common problems for the child with hyperkinetic disorder

## Poorly sustained attention

This has major adverse effects on the child's performance at school with respect to scholastic progress and relationship with teachers. It also impinges more generally on social relationships as adults are irritated by the child's frequent distractions and inability to stick to the task at hand. The distractible behaviour fluctuates wildly depending on the circumstances and the task. Objective assessment with vigilance tasks shows that hyperactive children make errors of omission (a failure to identify the correct stimulus) and of commission (a response to an incorrect stimulus). Errors of omission indicate poor attention, whereas those of commission imply distractibility.

## Impulsiveness

Impulsivity, that is the inability to delay a response or more overtly intrusive behaviour, is irritating to peers and adults whether it occurs at school, at home or in the community. Objective assessment of impulsivity using measures such as the Matching Familiar Figures Test indicates that hyperactive children have a distinctive response pattern characterised by a short latency of response.

## Secondary problems

**Learning disorders.** Many children with hyperkinetic syndrome or ADHD show evidence of generalised or specific learning disabilities. These probably arise through a combination of factors, including cognitive impairment, direct effects of inattention and distractibility as well as a poor relationship between the child and teachers. These problems are a further burden for the child at school.

**Social relationships.** The irritating and antisocial nature of many symptoms inevitably sours relationship between the child, other children and adults.

**Self-esteem.** Not surprisingly, the child with hyperkinetic disorder often has a poor self-image and low self-esteem because of social rejection from other people and frequent conflict with peers or adults.

## Treatment

The many problems shown by the child with ADHD or hyperkinetic disorder necessitate a diverse range of treatment strategies to resolve the problems (see Table 12.4). The particular combination used depends on the assessment of the individual child and family. The general principles are outlined below; more detailed discussions of the individual strategies are given in Chapter 17.

**Table 12.4**   Symptom management of ADHD/hyperkinetic disorder

| Symptom | Management |
| --- | --- |
| Motor restlessness | Counselling for parents/teachers<br>Behaviour modification<br>Environment manipulation<br>Stimulant drugs<br>Major tranquilliser |
| Inattention | Stimulant drugs<br>Special teaching<br>Training in attentional skills |
| Disruptiveness/aggression | Behaviour modification<br>Conjoint family therapy<br>Individual counselling |
| Academic failure | Special education placement<br>Graded and reward-based instruction<br>Individual counselling |

*Medication*

Bradley (1937) found that Benzedrine, a racemic mixture of dextro- and laevo-amphetamine, produced a dramatic reduction in hyperactivity among a group of disturbed children. Subsequently, many studies (reviewed by Gittelmain-Klein 1987) have confirmed that stimulant drugs are effective in reducing overactivity. Benefits are most clearly established in the short term; long-term effects are less certain.

Three stimulant drugs, amphetamine, pemoline and methylphenidate, have been used most frequently, with methylphenidate the most popular. Their use should be restricted to the small number of children who have severe pervasive hyperactivity, and they should not be prescribed for every child with overactivity. Methylphenidate, in a dosage dependent on age and body weight, should be given in the morning with gradual increments up to a maximum of around 20 mg daily. Higher doses are sometimes necessary for older children or those who are drug-resistant. Beneficial effects are usually immediately apparent, though with pemoline the response may be delayed. If one stimulant drug is ineffective, it may be worthwhile to try another. Most importantly, the drug treatment should be combined with other treatment strategies, particularly behavioural approaches, to increase the likelihood of long-term improvement.

Side-effects of methylphenidate include loss of appetite, insomnia, reduced growth rate and labile mood. Drug 'holidays', when the drug is stopped for periods of time, are very useful, not only to minimise side-effects but also to show whether medication is still necessary. The regular monitoring of growth and weight is essential during treatment.

Other drugs such as chlorpromazine or haloperidol have also been used with some benefits. This appears to be a result of a non-specific sedative response rather than a specific effect on overactivity.

## Dietary measures

Evidence for the role of dietary factors in causing hyperactivity is not convincing, apart from the one study mentioned earlier (Egger et al 1985). Despite justifiable reservations and scepticism, doctors should not be dismissive of requests from parents for information about modification of the child's diet. If nothing else, the change may result in more healthy eating habits with less reliance on 'junk food'. Advice on additive-free and artificial colouring-free products is relatively straightforward and can be easily implemented. Parents should be encouraged to chart behaviour before, during and after the elimination of these items from the child's diet. The increased attention and the accurate recording of behaviour following the alteration of the diet is likely to have a beneficial placebo effect on the child and family.

If the parents wish to pursue a more rigorous approach to the detection of food allergy, referral to an expert dietician is essential to ensure not only that dietary changes are introduced in a rational way but also that an adequate nutritional balance is retained. Some parents can become so preoccupied with the effects of diet on behaviour that it amounts to a Munchausen's syndrome by proxy. Extreme modification of the diet must only be undertaken when the behavioural problem is severe and expert supervision of the programme available. Care should also be taken to ensure that other factors contributing to the disturbed behaviour, such as marital discord or ineffectual parenting, are not ignored.

## Parental counselling

Though no detailed control trials have been carried out, clinical evidence indicates that many parents find this approach useful. Common topics for discussion include:

- counselling about the basis of the child's behaviour
- discussion about the management of behaviour
- the opportunity to talk about parents' own anxieties and concerns.

## Behaviour modification

Application of behaviour modification principles, usually of the operant variety, are useful for target behaviours at home or in school. The main problem is to ensure that the benefits of the programme generalise to other situations and that participants maintain enthusiasm for the programme. As mentioned earlier, a combined behavioural and drug treatment approach is often the best way to proceed. Detailed discussion of behavioural techniques are given in Chapter 17.

*Environmental manipulation*

Advice to teachers or parents about changes in the child's routine or overall environment at home or at school can be useful. Examples include:

- placement of the child in a small, stable teaching group
- time limitation for individual activities
- alterations to classroom layout
- careful control of the number of activities or friends the child has at home after school.

*Remedial education*

Individual remedial programmes for general and specific learning difficulties are necessary for many children.

Finally, Satterfield and colleagues (1987) have described a 'multi-modal' strategy to treat hyperactive children. This is a combined approach involving drug treatment, parents' groups, individual, group and family therapy. Over one-third of 117 children originally included in the study were still in contact at 3 years. A better outcome was obtained with those remaining in contact for this period than with the group who remained in contact for less than 2 years. Unfortunately, the study did not allocate the children and families to the different treatment groups randomly, so that definite conclusions about the relative efficacy of the various treatment strategies cannot be drawn.

## Outcome

Many outcome studies have been carried out, but the poor quality of the original as well as the follow-up data combined with the loss of many patients at follow-up limits the usefulness of the conclusions. Despite these reservations, more recent follow-up studies (Mannuzza et al 1989, Farrington 1990) have shown clearly that the major determinant of long-term adjustment is the co-existence of conduct disorder with the hyperactivity. Children with conduct disorder and hyperactivity have a much worse prognosis, approximately 25% receiving the diagnosis of personality disorder as adults and up to 50% showing criminal behaviour.

Approximately one-third of children continue to show some residual symptoms such as restlessness and aggressive behaviour when reviewed in early adult life. Other problems include educational under-achievement and poor employment records. The presence of learning disabilities also has an adverse effect on outcome. The overall conclusion from follow-up studies is that the prognosis is extremely variable, a finding not unexpected given the heterogeneous nature of hyperkinetic disorder and ADHD.

# 13. Miscellaneous disorders

## INTRODUCTION

This chapter discusses a group of disorders and syndromes that are not easily categorised in terms of aetiology or symptomatology. The group does however have the common feature that most of the psychopathology, usually a mixture of anxiety and behavioural symptoms, arise secondarily to the presenting problem. For example, the antisocial or delinquent behaviour of the child with specific reading disorder usually develops in response to the child's poor academic progress and sense of failure at school. Another common feature of this group of disorders is the wide variation in the severity of the disorder according to the limitations that it imposes on the daily activities of the child and family. This chapter discusses four categories of disorder:

- developmental disorders
- tic and other habit disorders
- sleep disorders
- eating disorders.

## DEVELOPMENTAL DISORDERS

ICD-10 recognises four main categories of disorder:

- disorders of speech and language
- disorders of scholastic skills
- disorder of motor function
- a mixed category of developmental disorder.

This section discusses the three main categories of disorder, that is speech and language, scholastic skills and motor function. As the term suggests, the mixed category involves a combination of the three other categories.

## SPEECH AND LANGUAGE DISORDERS

Language is commonly defined as a system of symbols for the generation of new information that is understandable to someone who knows the

177

symbol system. Language has three essential characteristics. First, it involves the use of symbols. A symbol is commonly defined as something that stands for something else by convention or code rather than just by similarity or resemblance. Second, the symbols are part of a system in which each symbol has a systematic and consistent relationship to the other symbols. Third, as a result of this symbol system, language has the capacity to generate an infinite variety of new or novel messages. Language is characterised by its variety and productivity. By contrast, speech is often defined as the systematised use of vocalisation to express verbal symbols or words. This definition emphasises that speech refers to spoken language as well as to word–sound production, that is the two separate processes of vocalisation and articulation.

Though speech and language disorders are primarily the concern of speech therapists, neurologists and general paediatricians, the child psychiatrist is likely to be involved in the following circumstances:

- where the speech disorder is a reflection of co-existing mental retardation
- where there is an associated psychiatric disorder such as childhood autism
- where there is concern that the family situation is adversely affecting language and speech acquisition
- where there are emotional or behavioural problems secondary to delayed language or speech development.

Many studies (Richman et al 1982, Cantwell & Baker 1985, Rutter & Lord 1987) have shown that children with language disorder are more vulnerable to psychiatric disturbance, mainly because of the associated anxiety and embarrassment caused by the disorder. For instance, Richman et al (1982) found that 25% of 3-year-olds with specific language delay had significant behavioural problems. Consequently, child psychiatrists are likely to see behaviourally disturbed children with language disorders.

## Delayed speech and language disorders

This is a frequent source of parental concern as well as a common reason for specialist paediatric referral. All children without meaningful words by 18 months should be investigated thoroughly. Though it is true that many children do 'grow out of' their delayed speech or language, there should be a sound basis for such professional optimism. Failure to make an adequate assessment at an early age is unhelpful for the following reasons:

- It prevents the initiation of remedial help
- It increases the likelihood of secondary psychological problems
- Parental anxiety will continue
- Parents are not given advice about helping their child's language development.

The important causes of delayed speech or language development are as follows:

- intellectual retardation
- deafness
- childhood autism
- social deprivation
- speech/language disorder.

*Intellectual retardation* is the commonest cause of delayed language or speech, the prevalence rate being approximately 1%. The severity of the language disorder is usually related to the overall delay in development. Consequently, the clinical picture varies widely from mild delay to total failure to acquire meaningful language or speech. Problems with articulation are also common among this group of children.

Similarly, the severity of *deafness* determines its impact on language acquisition, with profound deafness resulting in no meaningful speech production. More commonly, repeated middle ear infection and secretory otitis media or 'glue ear' cause significant delays, particularly with expressive language. Community prevalence studies (MacKeith & Rutter 1972) indicate that 1/1000 have marked language delay due to deafness.

By definition, children with *childhood autism* have delayed language, though the rarity of the condition (prevalence rate 2–4/10 000) makes it an uncommon cause of language delay.

*Social deprivation* is an unsatisfactory term used to describe the situation where inadequate stimulation and interaction at home affects adversely the child's development, including language. It is impossible to quantify the severity or frequency of the psychosocial deprivation, though clinical experience shows that children from deprived backgrounds undoubtedly thrive when they are provided with adequate language exposure and encouragement. It is, however, important to exclude any other more remedial cause of language delay before attributing the delay to poor stimulation. Indeed, the other causes of language delay are quite likely to be found as well among disadvantaged families.

Finally, *specific language or speech disorder*, prevalence rate 1/1000, is an important cause of delayed speech or language (see below).

## Assessment of language and speech skills

Although child psychiatrists are unlikely to be involved in the investigation of language delay, it is nevertheless clinically useful to have some knowledge about the language profile of children with the various types of language disorder. Table 13.1 outlines the important features in the assessment of language and speech skills.

*Imitation* is the child's ability to mimic or engage in imitative games such as 'peek-a-boo' or 'pat-a-cake'. If by the age of 2 years, the child is unable

**Table 13.1**   Assessment scheme for language and speech skills

- Imitation
- 'Inner language'
- Comprehension of language
  - 'Hearing behaviour'
    - hearing
    - listening and attention
    - understanding of spoken language
  - Understanding of gesture
  - Understanding of written language
- Vocalisation and babble
- Language production
  - Mode used (spoken language, gesture, etc)
  - Syntactic complexity
  - Semantic complexity
  - Abnormal qualities of spoken language
  - Social situation in which communication occurs
  - Amount of communication
- Word–sound production
- Phonation
- Rhythm of speech
- Other aspects of development
  - Cognition
  - Socialisation and interpersonal relationships

to take part in such activities, this should be cause for concern and for further investigation. *Inner language* is the child's ability to use a symbolic code in thinking and behaviour. This shows itself in two ways, in the meaningful use of objects and in the ability to engage in pretend or make-believe play. The child should be able by 18 months to use real objects such as a brush or comb in a manner that indicates their function and use. Similarly by the third and fourth year, children should be playing in a make-believe fashion extensively, for instance with dolls. Deficiencies in imitative and inner language skills occur most commonly with childhood autism and to a much lesser extent in severe language comprehension disorders.

*Vocalisation* and *babble* are diagnostically important with deaf children, where these skills are normal until the age of 6 months, and also in childhood autism where the babble is reduced as well as deviant. Disorders of *word–sound production*, for instance dysarthria, are common in several language disorders. Finally, Tables 13.2 and 13.3 summarise the deficits in

**Table 13.2**   Comprehension skills in language and speech delay disorders

| Syndrome | Comprehension skills | | | | | |
|---|---|---|---|---|---|---|
| | 'Inner language' | Hearing | Attention to sounds | Watching face | Spoken language | Gesture |
| Severe deafness | + | − | − | + | − | + |
| Mental retardation | limited | + | ± | + | limited | ± |
| Childhood autism | − | + | − | no | poor | ± |
| Psychosocial retardation | + | + | + | + | + | + |

**Table 13.3**   Expressive skills in language and speech delay disorders

| Syndrome | Expressive skills | | | |
|---|---|---|---|---|
| | Use of gesture | Social conversation | Echolalia | Word–sound production |
| Deafness | +++ | ++ | − | defective |
| Mental retardation | + | + | ++ | poor |
| Childhood autism | − | − | +++ | variable |
| Developmental language disorder | ++ | ++ | ± | variable/poor |

the comprehension and expressive skills of the various language delay syndromes. The analysis of the particular pattern of language skill deficits can be useful in the differential diagnosis of language or speech delay.

## Specific developmental disorders of speech and language

This group of disorders is usually defined as the delayed acquisition of speech or language compared with other aspects of development in the absence of demonstrable physical or neurological disease. Traditionally, there has been a distinction between *comprehension* or *receptive disorders* and *expressive* or *language production disorders*. ICD-10 and DSM-III-R divide the disorders into articulatory, expressive and receptive, though often the clinical picture is mixed. Expressive language disorder, prevalence rate

5/1000, is twice as common in boys as girls, whereas receptive disorder, prevalence rate 1/10 000, has an equal sex incidence.

### Expressive language disorder

Characteristically, there is a family history of slow speech development or reading difficulties. The diagnosis is indicated by the following:

- a language delay which is much greater than other aspects of the child's intellectual development
- no hearing or overt neurological disorder
- the normal social use of language.

Many children are also of below average intelligence and from families with a high rate of psychosocial deprivation, both of which exacerbate the problem(s).

Two principles are important in management, the exclusion of any underlying aetiology and the promotion of normal language development. The latter involves encouraging the parents to stimulate the child's language development, the provision of nursery or other day care facilities and advice from the speech therapist. The parents also require help in the management of the behaviour problems which are also common in this group of children (Richman et al 1982).

The long-term outcome for the language delay is usually good, though the co-existence of low intelligence, behaviour problems and family disharmony means that the child remains at risk of behavioural disturbance.

### Disorders of speech production

These comprise *dyslalia* (speech immaturity), *dysrhythmia* (stuttering/stammering) and *dysarthria* (difficulty with speech or sound production due to structural or neurological dysfunction of tongue, lips or palate).

***Dyslalia.*** This is often a feature of specific language disorder. It commonly involves consonant substitution and lisping. Where necessary, advice and reassurance from a speech therapist is usually the best plan.

***Stuttering or stammering.*** This is an abnormality of speech rhythm consisting of explosive repetitions and hesitations at the beginning of syllables and words. It is a normal, though transitory phenomenon, around the age of 3–4 years. Approximately 3% of children continue to have problems with stuttering. When this occurs, it is often due to parental over-concern leading to further anxiety and low self-esteem in the child. The condition runs in families, though whether this is due to genetic or environmental factors is unclear. Initial management involves advice and reassurance for the parents and the child. Distraction is a useful method to minimise the problem and to promote self-confidence. Persistent and severe stammering requires expert help from a speech therapist. Relaxation exercises and regulated syllabic speech techniques are helpful with many children. Attention to any co-existent emotional or behavioural problems is also important.

*Dysarthria.* This can be divided into *local structural abnormalities* and *neurological abnormalities* of the speech articulation process. Structural abnormalities include cleft lip and palate, disproportion of the jaws, lips and tongue and under-development of the jaw. These anomalies usually produce a characteristic quality to the voice. Neurological abnormalities are many and varied, affecting voluntary and involuntary movements, with cerebral palsy an important cause in many cases.

## Elective mutism

The main feature of this disorder is a persistent refusal to talk in one or more situations despite the ability to comprehend language and to speak normally in other situations. Mild forms of the disorder are common but transitory, usually occurring at the commencement of schooling, while the severe form of the disorder has a prevalence of 1/1000 (Kolvin & Fundudis 1981). Other features include a previous history of speech delay, excessively shy but stubborn temperament and parental over-protectiveness. The latter features are probably important not only in the onset of the disorder but also in its persistence and severity.

### Treatment

A combination of behavioural and family therapy techniques in order to promote communication and the use of speech is most commonly used. Occasionally in-patient psychiatric assessment and treatment are necessary. The prognosis is good for approximately 50% of cases, with failure to improve by the age of 10 years a poor prognostic sign. It is likely that children continue to improve after this age, though definitive follow-up data is not available.

## SPECIFIC SCHOLASTIC DISORDERS

The important disorders are *specific reading disorder, specific arithmetic disorder* and *specific spelling disorder*. The common feature underlying these disorders is that the child's attainments in these subjects are significantly below expectation or prediction on the basis of age and intelligence, hence the word 'specific'. Current ICD and DSM diagnostic guidelines talk in terms of attainments being 'at least two standard errors of prediction below the level expected on the basis of the child's chronological age and general intelligence' to indicate the precise nature of the disability. In practice, this means that the child's attainments are 2 years behind predicted levels.

The key elements in the definition are the inclusion criteria of age and intelligence. For example, a 10-year-old child of average intelligence should have a reading age of 10 years, whereas a child of the same age with superior intelligence or alternatively with mild learning difficulties would be expected to have reading ages of 12 and 8 years respectively. Consequently, if these children were found to have ages of only 10 and 6 years, there would be evidence of specific reading difficulties. Similar concepts are applied to arithmetic and spelling attainments.

These disorders are mainly of educational rather than psychiatric concern, although the child psychiatrist may become involved through the secondary associated emotional or behavioural problems. The latter are particularly common among children with reading disorders, so that the main part of this section concentrates on reading difficulties.

## Reading difficulties

The acquisition of reading is a complex process, requiring visual, auditory and cognitive abilities. Snowling (1991), reviewing contemporary ideas, proposes that children progress successively through three stages:

- logographic
- alphabetic
- orthographic.

In the first or *logographic* stage, the child recognises words according to the first letter or the word length, for instance 'w' for 'water' or 'f' for 'fun', and has no strategy for deciphering unfamiliar words. The subsequent *alphabetic* stage is characterised by the ability to decode words into their constituent syllables or letters and to begin to recognise the correspondence between sounds and words. In the *orthographic* stage, the child's reading strategies become automatic and flexible with the establishment of separate lexical and phonological systems to process familiar and unfamiliar words respectively.

Rutter et al (1970b) popularised the distinction between general reading retardation and specific reading retardation. *General reading retardation* refers to the situation where poor reading attainments parallel the general low level of intelligence, whereas *specific reading retardation* is where reading attainment is significantly below that expected on the basis of age and intelligence, a definition similar to the contemporary term specific reading disorder. Subsequent writers and researchers have followed this distinction, so that these terms have become accepted by educationalists and psychologists. By contrast, the term *dyslexia* has become much less popular. This concept shares many similarities with specific reading disorder, but has been criticised because it implies a single discrete neuropsychological substrate for the disorder, whereas most people believe that several factors, neurological, genetic and social, contribute to the problem in most cases.

*Specific reading disorder*

**Prevalence.** This varies considerably depending on the age group, the test used and the population studied. The most reliable estimates are from the Isle of Wight and London studies carried out by Rutter and colleagues (Rutter et al 1970b, Berger et al 1975). These found prevalence rates of 4% and 10% respectively among 10- and 11-year-olds. The disorder was three times more common among boys and had a strong association with social disadvantage as defined by large family size, overcrowding and low paternal occupational status.

**Aetiology.** This is multifactorial involving genetic, neuropsychological deficits and social factors. Snowling (1991) concluded that children with specific reading disorder had deficits in several neuropsychological processes. These were visual processing, chronological awareness, verbal memory and repetition skills. Social factors probably have a causal as well as a perpetuating role. For example, overcrowding and large family size may not be the ideal circumstances to acquire reading skills with behaviour problems acting as a further impediment.

**Associated features.** An important finding from the Isle of Wight study (Rutter et al 1970b) was the strong association between specific reading disorder and conduct disorder: 25% of children with reading disorder had conduct disorder. Such behavioural difficulties may well be a cause as well as a consequence of the reading disorder. Temperamental characteristics of impulsivity and overactivity may adversely affect the child's chances of acquiring literacy skills, whereas despondency caused by reading difficulties and disillusionment due to school failure may lead to behavioural problems in the older child and adolescent.

**Management.** Detailed psychological assessment of the precise nature of the problem by a clinical or educational psychologist and the initiation of an individually devised remedial programme with a specialist teacher are the best ways to help with these difficulties. Early detection and identification of children at risk, for instance through preschool language screening, are clearly desirable, so that appropriate help can be given right from the outset. Occasionally, paediatric evaluation of visual, auditory or neurological status is useful for the detection and remediation of additional impairments that may be contributing to the problem. Psychiatric involvement is usually confined to those cases where psychiatric disturbance has a major causal role in the reading disorder or is greatly exacerbating the problem. An important goal of all treatments is to prevent the child developing behavioural problems due to disillusionment and despondency. The educational programme for the older child and the adolescent should therefore provide the child with the opportunity to achieve success, for instance with an emphasis on craft or technical subjects where literary skills are less important.

*Outcome.* Despite remedial programmes, many children continue to have major problems with reading and spelling into adolescence and adult life. Hopefully, though, the educational programme will have boosted the child's confidence sufficiently to ensure that secondary behavioural problems are not too serious.

### Other scholastic disorders

Two further conditions, specific arithmetic disorder and specific spelling disorder, have been described. The aetiology, prevalence and prognosis are not well delineated, though it is assumed that they have many similarities to specific reading disorder. Treatment should follow the same general principles as for reading disorder.

## SPECIFIC DEVELOPMENTAL DISORDER OF MOTOR FUNCTION

This is also called *specific motor dyspraxia* or *the clumsy child syndrome* (Gordon & MacKinlay 1986, Henderson 1987) and is characterised by a serious impairment in the development of motor co-ordination involving fine and gross motor skills. Common features are an awkward gait and poor skills in dressing, drawing and constructional tasks.

Neurological assessment reveals neurodevelopmental immaturities such as choreiform movements, 'soft' neurological signs and abnormal reflexes. By definition, there is no diagnosable neurological disorder. The Bruinincks–Oseretsky test of motor proficiency (Bruinincks 1978) is a useful test of balance, agility and dexterity in gross and fine motor movements for children aged between 5 and 14 years of age.

Treatment involves a co-ordinated physiotherapy, occupational therapy and remedial education programme. Psychiatric support and advice may be necessary for the attendant emotional and behavioural problems.

## TICS AND OTHER HABIT DISORDERS

### TIC DISORDERS

Tics are rapid, involuntary repetitive muscular movements, usually involving the face and neck, for instance blinks, grimaces and throat clearing.

### Clinical features

Simple tics occur as a transitory phenomenon in about 10% of the population, with boys outnumbering girls 3 to 1 and with a mean age of onset between 5 and 7 years. They range in severity from simple tics involving the head and neck through to complex tics extending to the limbs and trunk.

The most severe tic disorder is *Gilles de la Tourette syndrome* (also called *Tourette's syndrome*; Gilles de la Tourette 1885). This involves complex tics, coprolalia (uttering obscene words and phrases) and echolalia (repetitions of sounds or words). Like stammering, tics are made worse at times of stress and may be exacerbated by undue parental concern. Other features of tic disorders are positive family history and a previous history of neurodevelopmental delay.

## Differential diagnosis

The main differential diagnosis is from chorea or choreiform movements. The latter can occur in cerebral palsy, Huntington's chorea and the extremely uncommon rheumatic chorea. Choreiform movements differ from tics in that the movements are less co-ordinated and predictable, the pattern is more variable in form and they cannot be suppressed. The other possible differential diagnosis is the shock-like movements of myoclonic epilepsy. These are, however, usually much more discrete and repetitive and involve larger muscle groups. There is also other evidence in support of the diagnosis of epilepsy. Though other habit disorders such as mannerisms and stereotypies can resemble tics, they are usually more purposeful than tics.

## Aetiology

### Genetic factors

Recent genetic studies (Pauls & Leckman 1988) provide evidence for a genetic contribution, particularly for Tourette's syndrome, with a risk of approximately 50% for first-degree male family relatives for some form of the disorder (18% Tourette's syndrome, 31% chronic motor tics and 7% obsessive-compulsive disorder). The most favoured mode of genetic transmission is autosomal dominant.

### Neurochemical and neurological factors

Abnormalities in the basal ganglia of the extrapyramidal system have been proposed but as yet they have not been definitively shown. The proven value of dopamine blockers such as haloperidol in the treatment of Tourette's syndrome is, however, taken to support this hypothesis.

### Individual and family factors

As tics and other movements are made worse by stress, clinicians have traditionally regarded tics as a displacement activity for underlying anxiety in the child or family. Undoubtedly, many children and families show evidence of anxiety when seen in the clinic, though whether this is primary or merely a secondary response to the child's frequent tics is not known. Some evidence for the primary role of individual and family psychopathology is provided by the study by Corbett et al (1969) of children with tics seen at the Maudsley Hospital, London. They found the following features:

- Only 50% initially presented with tics
- One-third of the children had symptoms of tension, aggression or disobedience at home or at school
- Some symptoms, such as speech disorders, encopresis, obsessional and hypochondriacal symptoms, were more common among children with tics than other disturbed children
- Other symptoms, such as aggression, truancy and fighting, were less common among children with tics than other disturbed children.

## Treatment

Many tics resolve spontaneously, or respond to advice, explanation and reassurance to the child and parents. Others, particularly the complex tics associated with Tourette's syndrome, are persistent and difficult to treat.

### Medication

This is effective, but should be reserved for severe cases. Haloperidol (dosage range 0.5–6 mg daily) is the drug of choice for Tourette's syndrome, producing a reduction of approximately 75% in tic frequency (Shapiro & Shapiro 1988). A major drawback with haloperidol usage is the frequent and disabling extrapyramidal side-effects. These include acute dystonic reactions such as torticollis or oculogyric crises, akathisia or motor restlessness and parkinsonian symptoms. The additional prescription of antiparkinsonian medication such as orphenadrine can reduce the severity of such side-effects, but this is nevertheless a decided disadvantage with this form of treatment. Another dopamine blocker, pimozide (dosage 1–10 mg daily) is an alternative to haloperidol, though the side-effects are similar. Clonidine (dosage 0.05–0.25 mg daily), an $alpha_2$ adrenergic receptor agonist, produces an approximately 25% reduction in tic frequency. The main side-effects with clonidine are sedation and hypotension.

### Behaviour modification (see Ch. 17)

Two approaches, the star chart system and massed practice, have been used with good effect. With the star chart technique, the aim is to get an initial baseline frequency record followed by reinforcement with stars or other rewards for tic-free periods. Gradually, the tic-free period is extended, so that the improvement generalises throughout the day. The rationale of massed practice, in which the child is actively encouraged to produce the tics for a 10-minute period twice per day, is that the child learns more effective control of the onset and cessation of tics; it is hoped that this will reduce the daily frequency in the longer term.

### Individual and family counselling

The child and family benefit from explanation and discussion of the factors responsible for the onset and maintenance of the tics. Specific therapy sessions devoted to various aspects of individual or family psychopathology may be useful when these factors have been identified as important in the maintenance of the tic behaviour.

## Outcome

The prognosis for simple and even complex tics is good, while that for Tourette's syndrome is more gloomy, 50% showing persistent symptomatology into adult life. Good prognostic factors are the absence of any additional psychopathology, a stable family background, no history of developmental delay and average intelligence.

## OTHER HABIT DISORDERS

This section discusses the various types of stereotypy as well as masturbation. The latter is discussed in this section rather than in the adolescent chapter (Ch. 14) as it is more likely to be a source of parental concern with the younger child. A stereotypy is defined as an intentional but meaningless pattern of movements carried out in a repetitive manner. The main distinction between a tic and a stereotypy is that the former is not under voluntary control. Stereotypies are usually isolated phenomena, though they may occasionally be a feature of another syndrome, for instance childhood autism. Common stereotypies are rocking and head-banging, hair-pulling and bruxism or tooth-grinding.

### Rocking and head-banging

Many normal and otherwise healthy toddlers indulge in these habits when they are in their cots at night, causing much anxiety and distress to their parents who are also embarrassed by neighbours' complaints about the noise. Most children spontaneously cease this behaviour around their fourth birthday, so that reassurance and support for the parents are usually effective treatment measures. More serious self-injurious behaviours occur among some severely retarded children, some blind children and also children with Lesch–Nyhan syndrome.

### Hair-pulling (trichotillomania)

This uncommon but distressing behaviour produces considerable distress and embarrassment to the child and parents. It is usually an isolated phenomenon, but is sometimes part of a more widespread disturbance. The child repeatedly pulls, twists or tugs his hair, so that a noticeable bald patch appears. The child seems oblivious of the consequences and is unable to refrain from the habit. Occasionally a child, usually mentally handicapped, may swallow sufficient hair to produce a hair-ball or *trichobezoar* in the stomach that may require surgical intervention and removal.

The management depends on assessment. A behavioural strategy is likely to be successful when the hair pulling is the only abnormality, whereas more extensive individual and family interventions are necessary when more widespread disturbance is present.

### Tooth-grinding (bruxism)

Repetitive tooth grinding during sleep occurs commonly in young children after the eruption of the first dentition and may lead to tooth damage and misalignment. Sometimes it may be related to daytime anxiety or stress. Preventative measures such as a night time rubber mouth guard are useful, and occasionally reduction in or treatment of daytime anxiety is necessary.

### Masturbation

This usually attracts attention and concern when it happens excessively. Most infants and toddlers engage in and enjoy touching their genitalia. During middle childhood, this appears less common and/or the child is more discreet. At adolescence, masturbation is probably universal among boys, though less common among girls. Excessive masturbation requires investigation and help. Causes include:

- local skin irritation, particularly among infants
- sexual abuse among older children
- emotional deprivation, where the masturbation represents an attempt by the child to obtain some pleasure from an otherwise unloving environment.

Sexual abuse is a possibility that must be seriously considered.

Some mentally retarded adolescents cause much embarrassment to their parents by masturbation in public. Clear guidelines for the parents about what is acceptable and what is not, for instance masturbation in private is allowable, are the best way to help, together with encouragement to the parents to enforce these rules.

# SLEEP DISORDERS

This section discusses those disorders occurring in older children and adolescents (see Ch. 5 for sleep problems in preschool children). These disorders are common, varied and often misdiagnosed and also a frequent source of concern for the child and parents (Horne 1992).

## Nightmares

These are frightening or unpleasant dreams occurring during REM (rapid eye movement) sleep. The child may or may not wake up, but there will be a clear recollection of the dream if the child does wake up and also in the morning. There is no period of altered consciousness or inaccessibility as with night terrors.

Nightmares are extremely common and not pathological, occurring in most children at some time or another, with a peak frequency around 5–6 years of age. Persistent and recurrent nightmares are, however, extremely distressing for the child and the parents. Daytime anxieties and/or the viewing of frightening television programmes prior to bedtime are contributory factors in many cases. Attention to and correcting these factors is necessary to reduce the frequency of the nightmares.

*Sleep paralysis*, where the child is unable to move or call out for his parents, is a rare but frightening conclusion to a nightmare. It is caused by the persistence of the motor inhibition that is usually present during REM sleep. The child is unable to make any movements apart from breathing, eye movements or possibly moaning. Sustained voluntary eye movement or, if possible, touching by someone else are two effective ways to terminate the sleep paralysis episode. Advice and explanation of these strategies to the parents and child enable them to manage future episodes more successfully and with much less anxiety.

## Night terrors

The usual pattern is for the child to wake up in a frightened, even terrified state, not to respond when spoken to, nor appear to see objects or people. Instead, he appears to be hallucinating, talking to or looking at people or objects not really present. The child may be difficult to comfort during the period of disturbed behaviour, and the state of altered consciousness lasts up to 15 minutes or occasionally even longer. Eventually, the behaviour settles, with or without assistance, and the child goes back to sleep, awakening in the morning with no recollection of the episode. The latter point is invaluable in helping to allay parental anxiety about the episodes. Night terrors arise from stage 4 of deep sleep, so that this explains why the child has no recollection of the episode. The peak incidence of the disorder is between 4 and 7 years with a continuation rate of approximately 2% in older children.

Advice and explanation to the parents and child are the mainstay of management. It is also helpful to identify and ameliorate any identifiable stresses that may occasionally contribute to the problem. Recently, a new behavioural approach which relies on waking the child 15 minutes prior to the expected time of the night terror has been reported with encouraging results (Lask 1988). Occasionally, diazepam 2–5 mg at night is useful, possibly as the drug decreases the amount of stage 4 sleep. The long-term outcome for night terrors is good.

### Sleepwalking (somnambulism)

This often occurs in association with night terrors. The child, usually aged between 8 and 14 years, arises calmly from his bed with a blank facial expression, does not respond to attempts at communication and can only be woken with difficulty. The child is in a state of altered consciousness at the deep level of sleep (stages 3 and 4). The management comprises giving the parents advice about safety and protection of the child during these episodes and also the alleviation of any contributory daytime anxieties.

### Narcolepsy

This is defined as an irresistible urge to sleep, usually during the daytime. The condition is rare before 10 years, becoming more frequent in later adolescence. The onset is usually abrupt and unpredictable and the child falls asleep for between 5 and 30 minutes. Other features are cataplexy (sudden loss of muscle tone resulting in a fall to the floor) and sleep paralysis (inhibition of muscle movement and tone). 10% also have epilepsy. EEG studies show that the individual passes rapidly into stage 4 sleep.

Management involves the exclusion of organic disease such as epilepsy by examination and investigation when necessary. Methylphenidate (5–15 mg in the morning) or clomipramine (10–25 mg three times daily) are effective in reducing the frequency of the episodes. There is a potential danger of drug abuse due to the stimulant effects of these drugs, so that careful supervision of drug intake is essential. Finally, identification and treatment of any associated anxiety is also important.

### EATING DISORDERS (see Chs 5 and 14)

### Obesity

Although there is no universally agreed definition of obesity, a commonly accepted criterion is a weight approximately 20% or more above the expected weight according to age, height and sex. When so defined, community surveys indicate that approximately 10% of children are obese.

Psychological problems may be responsible for the onset of the obesity and/or may arise secondarily to the obesity.

Organic causes are rare and include conditions such as Prader–Willi syndrome and hypothalamic disorders. In such cases, there are usually other features suggestive of the disorder, so that misdiagnosis is unlikely. Obesity is usually caused by several interacting factors. These include genetic, excessive calorie intake, minimal exercise, poor dietary habits and individual or family disturbance.

A collaborative approach involving the paediatrician, the dietician and the psychologist/psychiatrist is most likely to be successful. Education and advice about nutrition and diet, the importance of exercise and the imposition of a calorie-restricted diet are essential. The role of the psychologist/psychiatrist is to identify and to treat the attendant psychological problems and, more importantly, to enlist the co-operation of the child and family in adherence to the dietary regime. Other treatment components include a behavioural programme to modify eating patterns, for instance making the child more aware of the cues associated with excessive eating.

A major problem with treatment programmes is that they do not modify the eating habits sufficiently to ensure that weight loss is maintained when the programme is finished. Consequently, the long-term success rate is not high. Unfortunately, many obese children grow up into obese adults.

## ANOREXIA NERVOSA AND RELATED DISORDERS

Anorexia nervosa occurs in older adolescents and young adults, usually female, but the condition is well recognised and described in prepubertal children (Lask & Bryant-Waugh 1992). The core features of anorexia nervosa are:

- self-induced starvation and weight loss
- a strong desire to be thinner and thinner with a marked fear of weight gain
- a distorted body image (for instance feeling fat when emaciated).

*Bulimia,* defined as periodic bouts of 'binge-eating' or the consumption of high calorific food over a brief period followed by self-induced vomiting, rarely occurs in children.

### Definition

Lask & Bryant-Waugh (1992) have adapted adult criteria for use with prepubertal children (Table 13.4). The key elements are:

- determined food avoidance
- the loss or failure to gain weight in the absence of physical or psychiatric disturbance
- a pattern of eating behaviour designed to prevent weight gain.

**Table 13.4**   Criteria for diagnosing anorexia nervosa in children

---

- Determined food avoidance
- Weight loss or failure to gain weight during a period of preadolescent growth (10–14 years) in the absence of physical or psychiatric illness
- Any two or more of the following:
  - Preoccupation with body-weight
  - Preoccupation with energy intake
  - Distorted body image
  - Intensive exercise
  - Laxative abuse

---

## Prevalence

Crisp et al (1976) found that 1% of 15–19-year-old girls fulfil the criteria for anorexia nervosa. Accurate prevalence figures for younger children are not available, but the illness is much less common. Anecdotal clinical evidence does, however, suggest that it may be becoming more common.

## Clinical features

Table 13.5 lists the common characteristics of anorexia nervosa. The presentation is varied, sometimes mimicking physical illness or the consequences of weight loss and starvation. The core features are:

- weight loss or failure to attain age-related weight gain
- severe dieting
- a distorted body image.

The history is of prolonged self-imposed starvation. Dieting often begins following a chance remark about size or shape, or alternatively as a group

**Table 13.5**   Clinical characteristics of anorexia nervosa

---

- Usually female
- Amenorrhoea (if postpubertal)
- Active maintenance of weight at least 15% below average or failure to gain weight during growth spurt
- Eating behaviour to prevent weight gain
  - avoidance of 'fattening foods'
  - self-induced vomiting
  - self-induced purgation
  - overactivity designed to lose weight
  - excessive use of laxatives
- Distorted body image
- Bulimia (commoner in older adolescents and young adults)

---

exercise with other adolescent girls. Food portions at mealtimes are reduced, some meals such as breakfast or lunch are skipped entirely with the total elimination of high calorific foods such as sweets, puddings or cakes. The individual derives satisfaction from the weight loss which in turn is an incentive for further weight loss. Parents and other adults are often complimentary and pleased at this initial weight loss. More extreme and rigid dieting is then self-imposed to meet the target for further weight reduction. Appetite and hunger pains are prominent, but the prospect of further weight loss is a powerful motivator. Only when the illness is well established does the anorexia and nausea over food become apparent.

Interest and participation in exercise and athletic activities often parallel the dieting in the belief that these activities will enhance weight loss. Later on, excessive laxative use begins in order to reduce weight further.

Despite her increasingly thin physique, the child refuses to accept her emaciated status, still believing and perceiving herself as fat or overweight. This distorted body image is often the first indication to the parents that the child has a serious illness. Increasingly, arguments over food and its consumption combined with the child's implacable refusal to eat convinces the parents that urgent medical help is required. Often, the child is initially referred to a paediatrician or endocrinologist in order to exclude a physical basis for the problem rather than accepting the psychological basis for the weight loss.

## Physical examination

Table 13.6 summarises the main physical findings on examination and investigation. The individual is usually bright and alert despite the evident

**Table 13.6**    Physical findings in anorexia nervosa

**Appearance**
- Bright, alert appearance
- Emaciation
  - prominent cheek bones and sunken eyes
  - bones protruding through skin
  - dry skin and hair
  - blue and cold hands and feet
  - fine downy (lanugo) hair on face, limbs and trunk

**Examination**
- Slow pulse rate
- Low blood pressure
- Hypothermia

**Endocrine changes**
- Low gonadotrophin levels
- High growth hormone and cortisol levels

emaciation. Prominent cheek bones, sunken eyes, bones protruding through the skin, dry skin and hair with blue, cold hands and feet are common features. Severe emaciation is accompanied by the appearance of fine downy hair or *lanugo* on the face, limbs and trunk with a slow pulse rate, low blood pressure and hypothermia. Most biochemical investigations are normal, but low gonadotrophin levels with high growth hormone and cortisol levels are sometimes found.

## Differential diagnosis

Anorexia and weight loss are features of other psychiatric syndromes so that depression, obsessive-compulsive disorder and schizophrenia may need to be excluded. Careful history taking should establish the eating disorder as the primary abnormality in anorexia nervosa, whereas it is secondary or coincidental in the other conditions.

## Aetiology

Almost as many theories have been proposed as the number of people who have researched the condition. Several factors are likely to be responsible, with individual and family factors prominent in most cases. More recently, several investigators have implicated childhood sexual abuse as a factor in the development of anorexia nervosa in adults (Hall et al 1989, Palmer et al 1990), but its relevance to the childhood disorder is unknown.

### Genetic factors

Evidence from twin and family studies suggests that genetic factors may make some contribution, but the strength of the association is unclear (Lask & Bryant-Waugh 1992).

### Neuroendocrine and endocrine changes

Most people believe that the observed changes are secondary or a consequence of the disease rather than a cause. More recently, Craigen et al (1987) have argued that changes in gastric emptying and motility through the release of cholecystokinin (CCK) are important, as they could explain the altered pattern and reduced intake in individuals with anorexia nervosa.

### Individual factors

Review of the premorbid personality characteristics of anorexics often shows them as conformist, conscientious, compliant and high-achieving individuals. Early psychoanalytic writing emphasised that the sexual maturation and the associated conflict posed by adolescence was resolved by the development of anorexia, the 'Peter Pan' solution. Later writers (Bruch 1973) argued that autonomy and independence were the core issues for anorexics with control over food intake the only available means to preserve self-identity and independence. Although these explanations are persuasive and make sound clinical sense, many children with anorexia do not fit these descriptions.

*Family factors*

Family therapists (Minuchin et al 1978, Palazzoli et al 1978) have studied and written extensively about families with an anorexic member. Minuchin et al (1978) argued that anorexia is a psychosomatic disorder produced by a particular family pattern of interaction. 'Psychosomatic' families show four main features:

- enmeshment or over-involvement
- over-protectiveness
- rigidity
- poor conflict resolution.

The ill-defined boundary between the parents and the child causes the parents to over-protect the child and to prevent the development of increasing independence as the child grows older. This in turn is compounded by the family's rigid functioning, so that the parents are unable to meet the child's changing developmental needs. The family's fear of conflict or disagreement means that they are unable to resolve the conflicts that inevitably arise in families with growing up children.

Minuchin and colleagues argue that the child's maladaptive solution to these problems is the development of anorexia nervosa. Similarly, Palazzoli et al (1978) regard anorexia as an indication of the profound conflict within the family. The conflict is so serious and potentially damaging that it cannot be expressed nor discussed, hence the anorexia. The latter, though maladaptive, is seen as less detrimental than the exposure of the family's dysfunctional patterns of interaction.

While many families do show some of the characteristics claimed by family therapists, many do not. Moreover, it is not known whether these family patterns of interaction are merely a response to the child's anorexic behaviour or whether they are specific to anorexia nervosa. Despite these criticisms, the family therapists' models of interactions among families with an anorexic member are clinically useful and do provide a framework within which to assess family functioning.

*Sociological factors*

Society's view of the relationship between female attractiveness and position on the fatness/thinness dimension has veered markedly towards the 'thin end of the spectrum' in the last 40 years. The 'pursuit of thinness' has become a major issue for many women. Inevitably, this is likely to influence the views of younger women and adolescents. It is unclear how important this issue is with younger anorexic patients, but it may be a factor influencing the individual's determination to persist with dieting.

## Management

The severity of the condition varies widely, so that treatment includes out-patient and in-patient management with an emphasis on a 'multimodal' approach. The latter implies that a variety of treatment strategies such as individual, family or cognitive therapies are used, often concurrently but alternatively sequentially depending on individual assessment. Despite the number of treatments, some general principles apply (Table 13.7).

### Recognition and acknowledgement of problem

This is the first crucial step which may necessitate several extended interview(s) with the parents and child. The nature and seriousness of the condition highlighted by avoidance of food and irrational ideas and behaviour about diet and eating habits must be discussed and exposed thoroughly in order to establish a therapeutic alliance with the child and family. Only when the latter has occurred is it possible to commence a specific treatment programme.

### Alteration of eating habits

The two main aims are the restoration of weight loss and the correction of nutritional deficiencies. Advice and collaboration with the dietician are important from the outset, particularly for any nutritional deficiencies. A target weight, usually around the average for the age, height and sex of the child, should be agreed upon, along with the appropriate daily calorific intake to ensure its attainment. Only minimal concessions to food fads or preferences should be allowed, with a standard protocol for regular weight checks.

---

**Table 13.7**  Treatment aims in anorexia nervosa

- Recognition/acknowledgement of the problem
- Alteration of eating habits to ensure
  - restoration of weight loss
  - correction of nutritional deficiencies
- Treatment of individual and family psychopathology
  - individual or cognitive behaviour therapy
  - family therapy
  - drug treatment for any associated conditions, e.g. depression
  - follow-up contact to monitor weight and general progress

---

If the patient is in hospital, the nursing care and support are the most important aspect of management. The nursing staff have to win the co-operation of the child with the treatment plan. They must also be vigilant about food hoarding and surreptitious vomiting. Treatment programmes usually involve a graded series of privileges dependent upon satisfactory weight gain. Once the target weight is attained, the diet should be modified, so that age-appropriate weight gain continues. In-patient programmes often involve nursing staff supervising family meals at home during weekend leave.

## Individual and family therapy

The establishment of a trusting relationship between the child and the individual therapist is important in the early stages of management. Acceptance of the problem and the willingness to discuss attitudes and ideas about body concept and image, growth and development, family and peer relationships are necessary not only to enable the child to modify her eating habits but also to change family and interpersonal relationships. The techniques used may vary according to the style of the therapist, but the underlying aims are the same.

Family therapy, solely or in combination with individual therapy, is now a very popular approach. The theoretical bases of the different schools of family therapy differ, but their aims are common. Minuchin and colleagues (1978) have described in detail the techniques necessary to bring about change in the family's views and attitudes about food and also more general aspects of their interactions (see Ch. 17). Finally, Russell et al (1987), in a randomised intervention study of the comparative effectiveness of family therapy versus individual therapy, found that family therapy was better than individual therapy in the prevention of relapse among anorexics aged less than 18 years of age who had had the illness for less than 3 years. An important limitation of this study was that only 65% of the 80 patients completed the treatment programmes.

## Drug treatment

This was previously used much more extensively to treat the symptoms of anxiety and tension which are frequently present. By contrast, contemporary practice emphasises that there should be a specific indication, for instance the presence of a depressive disorder, before drugs are used as part of the treatment programme.

## Follow-up contact

In many ways, the easiest part of the treatment programme, particularly with in-patients, is the restoration of weight loss. A more challenging and difficult aspect is the restructuring of the child's and family's attitude to food and their pattern of interaction. Regular supervision, support and contact are essential to maintain progress and keep up morale. Very often a compromise has to be made between an ideal resolution of the problem and a realistic appraisal of the child's and family's capacity to change.

## Outcome

Results from follow-up studies vary widely according to inclusion criteria, outcome measures and length of follow-up. Despite these problems, outcome appears to fall into three categories, one-third good, one-third intermediate and one-third poor. Lask & Bryant-Waugh (1992), reporting on the follow-up of 30 cases of childhood anorexia treated at the Hospital for Sick Children, Great Ormond Street, London, found the following features:

- mean age of onset 11.7 years
- mean length of follow-up 7.2 years
- mean age at follow-up 20.8 years (range 14–30 years)
- 67% good physical outcome
- 59% good psychosocial outcome
- 50% good psychosexual outcome
- 35% persistent eating difficulties.

There were two deaths in this sample, though one death was unrelated to the disorder.

The conclusion from other follow-up studies is that mortality is around 10% in the long term, with malnutrition and suicide accounting equally for most deaths. Overall, poor prognostic factors in childhood anorexia are early age of onset, co-existent psychiatric disorders such as depression and poor family functioning.

## OTHER EATING DISORDERS

Two new types of eating disorder have recently been described, *food avoidance emotional disorder* and *pervasive refusal syndrome*. The former, described by Higgs et al (1989), is a disorder of emotions in which food avoidance is a prominent symptom along with other affective symptoms such as depression, anxiety or phobias. There is often a previous history of food fads or food restrictions, but the symptomatology does not meet the criteria for anorexia nervosa. The validity and independence of this syndrome has, however, not yet been established.

Pervasive refusal syndrome (Lask et al 1991) is a severe, life-threatening syndrome characterised by pervasive refusal to eat, drink, talk, walk or engage in self-care skills. Lask et al (1991) describe four children with this syndrome. The children were markedly underweight, with an adamant refusal to eat or drink that ultimately became life-threatening. Although the children fulfilled some criteria for anorexia nervosa, the pervasiveness of the symptomatology made this diagnosis inaccurate. The children required prolonged and extensive in-patient nursing care in order to maintain vital body functions. All children were girls, and there was some suggestion that previous traumatic sexual abuse, often involving violence, might have precipitated the syndrome. The authors also comment that other colleagues have had children with similar symptomatology. The four children eventually made a satisfactory physical recovery, but their long-term psychiatric adjustment is not yet known.

# 14. Adolescent disorders

## INTRODUCTION

This book is mainly concerned with children rather than adolescents and young people. Nevertheless, the clinical practice of child and adolescent psychiatrists involves regular contact with adolescents, so that knowledge about normal and abnormal adolescent development is clearly important. Similarly, other professions caring for children such as paediatricians, teachers or social workers should be familiar with the range and diversity of adolescent problems. Recent British legislation (the Children Act 1989) also enjoins professionals and agencies to provide continuity of care from childhood through adolescence into adult life.

This chapter has two main sections, adolescent psychological development and adolescent psychiatric syndromes.

## ADOLESCENT DEVELOPMENT (TABLE 14.1)

Adolescence is the transition between childhood and adult life. Four maturational tasks must be accomplished successfully to ensure a favourable outcome:

- the attainment of independence
- the establishment of a sexual role and orientation
- the self-control of aggressive and oppositional impulses
- the achievement of self-identity.

Though these tasks are not necessarily complete nor entirely resolved by the end of adolescence, the adolescent should have made substantial progress with them. Three tasks — independence, sex role and orientation, self-control of aggressive and oppositional impulses — refer to specific aspects of psychological development, whereas the fourth — self-identity — is a global term referring to that sense of uniqueness or individuality that distinguishes one person from another. Erikson (1965) believed that the attainment of a stable self-identity during adolescence is the prerequisite for successful adult adjustment. Important components of self-identity for Erikson are *sexual identity* and *career identity*. The Eriksonian unsuccessful

**Table 14.1**   Adolescent psychological development

**Tasks of adolescence**
- Attainment of independence
- Establishment of sexual role and orientation
- Self-control of aggressive and oppositional impulses
- Achievement of identity

**Phases of adolescent development**

| Phase | Age | Characteristics |
|-------|-----|-----------------|
| Pre-adolescence | 11–14 | Onset of biological puberty |
| | | Interest in peers and in teenage pursuits |
| Early adolescence | 13–15 | Questioning attitude towards parents |
| | | Uncritical acceptance of peer group values |
| Mid-adolescence | 14–16 | Sexual experimentation and gender identity issues |
| | | Wider social network outside the family – 'mature dependence' on parents |
| Late adolescence | 17 onwards | Rewarding sexual role/relationships |
| | | Career/vocational choice |

outcome of adolescent conflict is *identity diffusion,* with the person lacking clear goals and direction in the fulfilment of individual ambition.

Adolescent development is commonly divided into four phases:

- the pre-adolescent phase (11–13 years)
- early adolescence (13–16 years)
- mid-adolescence (14–16 years)
- late adolescence (17 years onwards).

The main features of *the pre-adolescent phase* are the onset of biological puberty and an increased interest in peer relationships and teenage pursuits. *Early adolescence* is characterised by the critical questioning of parental values combined with an uncritical acceptance of peer group views.

The establishment of a separate sexual and social identity occurs during *mid-adolescence.* The individual explores and develops his own gender and sexual role. The development of social relationships outside the family enables the individual to have his own social network as well as altering the basis of his relationship with his parents. The latter has been described by Winnicott (1965) as 'mature dependence', implying a healthy balance between the need for increased independence and recognition of the strong attachment between the adolescent and his parents. *Later adolescence* is focused on career or work choice along with expression of the sexual role through more satisfying and enduring relationships.

## DETERMINANTS OF ADOLESCENT ADJUSTMENT

Though the same general factors influence development and adjustment in adolescence as in earlier periods, brief mention will be made of those that are of particular relevance.

### Previous childhood experience(s)

Unsatisfactory earlier experience(s) and relationships, particularly the child–parent(s) relationship, are major factors affecting predisposition to adjustment during adolescence. The individual's capacity to withstand the inevitable stresses of adolescence, and also his resilience, are greatly impaired when the outcome of earlier experiences was unsatisfactory. Adverse childhood experience is an important vulnerability factor in adolescent breakdown.

### Family psychopathology

Parental psychopathology such as marital disharmony or parental psychiatric illness has a powerful influence on children's behaviour throughout childhood, but even more so during adolescence, when conflicts over discipline, control and autonomy are normal and unavoidable. Parental disagreements and disunity on these matters greatly exacerbate the difficulties.

### Schooling

Common problems are:

- academic failure in scholastic subjects
- poor motivation and disillusionment with schooling
- conflicts over authority with teaching staff.

### Peer group

Peer group values and pressure exert enormous influence on the adolescent, so that contact with and membership of a deviant peer group can lead to major problems in school (e.g. truancy) or in the community (e.g. delinquency or vandalism).

### Chronic illness or handicap

The normal adolescent drive for self-appraisal and self-identity leaves the disabled or handicapped adolescent feeling isolated and different from his peers, a most distressing experience. Early childhood feelings of acceptance and tolerance by peers are replaced by feelings of exclusion and separateness and a reluctance or inability to gain peer group acceptance. The adolescent often deals with these feelings of anger and frustration by denial or minimalisation of the seriousness of his condition. This can result in poor compliance with medication or reckless exposure to dangerous situations.

## INTERVIEWING AND ASSESSMENT OF ADOLESCENTS

Though Chapter 4 discussed the general principles of interviewing and assessment, it is helpful to mention some specific points relating to adolescence. Flexibility in approach is essential for successful interviewing. In general, the older the adolescent and the more serious and intimate the problem, the greater the necessity for a separate interview with the adolescent. Usually, this is combined with a family interview in order to complete the assessment.

Many adolescents are reluctant, confused or anxious attenders, so that the clinician must clarify and explain the purpose, sequence and duration of the assessment procedures at the outset. Respect for the adolescent's maturity, right to privacy and confidentiality must be acknowledged clearly. The distinction between 'family business' and 'individual business' must be emphasised to the adolescent and to the parents. Adolescent anxieties about 'seeing the shrink' or 'being treated like a child' must be addressed and talked through. The individual interview may allow the clinician to conduct a thorough assessment of the mental state, though careful phrasing of questions about sexual or psychotic phenomena is essential in order to avoid a dismissive denial and a further increase in anxiety and confusion.

Silence and refusal to talk during the interview are common and often difficult to overcome. The clinician can use three tactics to deal with this problem:

- point out that the silence is just as difficult for the interviewer as it is for the adolescent
- point out that there will be opportunity and time to talk through difficult topics either now or alternatively on another occasion
- terminate the interview if necessary to prevent prolonged or undue tension.

Family interviews are often part not only of the assessment procedure but also of the treatment plan. Details of the various types of family therapy are discussed in Chapter 17. Sometimes, however, it is more appropriate to interview just the parents and the child together rather than the whole family.

## ADOLESCENT PSYCHIATRIC SYNDROMES

These are divided into three categories:

- disorders persisting from earlier childhood

- new disorders arising during adolescence
- disorders with features special to adolescence.

Prior to the discussion of these topics, brief comment will be made about the prevalence of psychiatric disorders in adolescence.

## Prevalence

This varies widely from 10–20% depending upon the population studied, the diagnostic criteria and the age group. Most studies do, however, show a consistent pattern with respect to sex ratio, urban versus rural differences and the range of clinical syndromes. In contrast to earlier childhood, when psychiatric disorder is more common among boys, the adolescent period shows a shift towards an equal sex ratio in early adolescence followed by a subsequent female preponderance in late adolescence and adult life. Prevalence rates in urban populations are at least twice those for rural populations. Schizophrenia, major affective disorder, suicide and attempted suicide, anorexia and substance abuse all begin to appear with some frequency during adolescence, whereas encopresis and enuresis decrease markedly.

## Persistent childhood disorders

Childhood disorders are more likely to continue into adolescence in one or more of the following circumstances:

- when there is a major constitutional factor to the syndrome
- when the adverse circumstances responsible for the onset of the disorder are still present
- when perpetuating or maintaining factors are prominent.

The follow-up study of 10-year-old children in the Isle of Wight study (Rutter et al 1975a, b) showed that 40% of the disorders had persisted into adolescence with a strong continuity for boys with conduct disorder and associated educational problems. This section now discusses the factors responsible for the persistence of some disorders into adolescence from earlier childhood.

### Conduct disorder

The oppositional and defiant character of conduct disorder means that it is very likely to be exacerbated by the rebellious and anti-authoritarian nature of ordinary adolescent behaviour. Studies from the UK (Farrington 1978) and elsewhere have shown that early childhood predictors of persistent conduct disorder are:

- early onset of symptoms

- extensive and varied symptomatology
- severely aggressive behaviour.

Adverse temperamental characteristics, combined with continued exposure to deviant family psychopathology such as deficient and ineffective parenting, marital disharmony or parental psychiatric illness, are thought to be important factors maintaining the conduct disorder. The persistence of the frequently associated learning disorders is another source of frustration and disillusionment for the adolescent, producing conflict with teachers and reluctance to attend school.

## Emotional disorders

Generally, emotional disorders have a good prognosis, often because they arise in response to some identifiable but remedial stress. Consequently, emotional disorder persisting into adolescence implies a more serious underlying cause. School refusal syndrome is the most likely condition to show continuity with early childhood. It may reappear at transfer from primary to secondary school, or early on during secondary schooling. Previous history of separation difficulties, for instance at the start of nursery or primary school, and/or an over-dependent relationship between the child and parent(s) are commonly found. The increased necessity for independence, autonomy and assertiveness at secondary school may prove too much for the vulnerable adolescent.

## Childhood autism

The overt autistic-like behaviour and overactivity prominent in younger children with the disorder often decrease during adolescence, but the majority are still profoundly impaired in social and communication skills, with marked apathy and lack of empathy. Educational and learning disabilities are very evident. Epilepsy also develops in about 15% of individuals (Deykin & McMahon 1979), the risk being greater when severe mental retardation is also present.

## Hyperkinetic syndrome

Overactivity usually decreases during adolescence, but persistent problems with antisocial behaviour, impulsivity, recklessness, distractibility and learning disorders mean that the adolescent with hyperkinetic disorder is likely to remain disturbed. Schacher (1991), reviewing outcome studies, concluded that the following were associated with poor outcome:

- pervasive hyperactivity
- additional conduct disorder symptoms

- inattentiveness and distractibility
- language delay and educational problems.

## New disorders arising during adolescence

These can be divided into two categories, those related to the stress of adolescence and major adult-like disorders arising in adolescence.

### Stress-related adolescent disorders

During adolescence, the distinction between normal and abnormal behaviour is often imprecise, so that it is more important to understand why the adolescent's behaviour is such a cause of concern than whether the behaviour fulfils the criteria for the disorder in a diagnostic classification system.

In many cases, conflict arises between the adolescent and his parents over independence and control issues. Allied with pressure from peers, this often leads the adolescent to engage in antisocial or conduct-disordered behaviour. Delinquency, vandalism and out of control behaviour are common, sometimes mixed with a pattern of alcohol or drug abuse. Persistent antisocial disorder often culminates in criminal behaviour and arrest by the police. Coexistent family problems and limited capacity to resolve issues also contribute to the severity of the disorder.

Eventually, it may be necessary for the adolescent to leave the family home and to be provided with alternative care arrangements, for instance with foster parents or community carers. Another solution sometimes adopted by the adolescent is to run away from home. Although the majority of runaways eventually return home, a minority stay away and become involved with the homeless subculture found in large cities.

The common neurotic or emotional responses to adolescent stress are affective symptoms such as irritability, lability of mood and anxiety symptoms, particularly related to social situations or mixing with peers. The latter may sometimes lead to marked social withdrawal.

*School refusal* may sometimes present during early adolescence, when it represents a combination of adolescent stress and the revival of an earlier over-dependent parent–child relationship. The increased need for independence and autonomy posed by the demands of secondary school precipitates an avoidance response to school attendance by the adolescent. Anxiety symptoms often masquerade as physical complaints such as headaches or abdominal pain. The prompt exclusion of organic pathology with the minimum amount of investigation is essential in order to prevent the secondary elaboration of physical symptomatology. Delay in the recognition of the underlying psychological basis for the problem greatly exacerbates the difficulties. The prognosis is not good for a significant minority of adolescents, up to one-third failing to maintain regular school attendance (Hersov & Berg 1980). Poor prognosis is usually a sign of more serious underlying family psychopathology. Follow-up studies into adult life have shown that anxiety or agoraphobic symptoms are present in about 20% (Berg 1982).

*Obsessive-compulsive disorder* sometimes begins during adolescence, when its occurrence can be seen as a maladaptive response to the stress of adolescence. There is often a previous history of earlier childhood obsessional and anxiety traits. The key element in the maintenance and exacerbation of the disorder is usually the willingness of the family to participate in the ritualistic behaviour. Flament et al (1985) reported considerable improvement among 19 adolescent patients treated with clomipramine, though the follow-up showed continued symptoms and disability in two-thirds of patients (Flament et al 1990). More recently, 5-hydroxytryptamine uptake inhibitors such as fluoxetine have been tried with some success, but the long-term benefits have not been established.

### Major adult-like disorders arising in adolescence

Two categories of disorder, schizophrenia and affective disorder, begin to occur with increasing frequency during adolescence (see also Chs. 7 and 8 respectively).

*Schizophrenia* may cause some diagnostic problems, as first-rank Schneiderian symptoms are not prominent at the outset. The usual presentation is insidious rather than florid, with gradual social withdrawal and increased internal preoccupation. Dysphoric symptoms are common, so that a diagnosis of affective disorder is sometimes made. The adolescent is often able to conceal his bizarre ideas from parents and peers. It is the presence of increasingly unpredictable and erratic behaviour that indicates that something more serious is occurring. The possibility of drug abuse is an important alternative diagnostic possibility.

*Depression* is much less of a diagnostic problem, though hypomanic episodes may be initially confused with drug-induced states or with schizophrenia. The assessment of the suicidal risk (see Ch. 8) is an essential feature in the management of adolescents with depressive disorder or with adolescents after they have attempted suicide.

*Anorexia nervosa* is another disorder likely to occur with increasing frequency during adolescence (see Ch. 13).

## SPECIAL TOPICS

### Substance abuse

This ranges from readily available and legal substances such as tobacco or alcohol to more uncommon and illegal substances such as heroin or cocaine. Though the latter give rise to more public concern, there is little doubt that cigarette smoking and excess alcohol consumption have a far more deleterious effect on the health of the population as a whole. A recent survey (Dunnell 1990) found that 14% of girls and 12% of boys were regular or occasional smokers, with strong continuity between adolescent and adult smoking habits. Similarly, Plant et al (1982) in a survey of 15- and 16-year-olds in Scotland found that the average alcohol consumption for males and females was 18 and 19 units per week respectively, with approximately 25% having experienced at least one hangover in the previous 6 months. Adolescents are, however, only rarely referred to psychiatric services because of their smoking or alcohol habits.

*Solvent abuse ('glue sniffing')*

Ashton (1990), reviewing the available literature, estimated that 5–10% of adolescents have at some time inhaled solvents and that 0.5–1% were regular users. Since 1971, the death rate from solvent abuse overdose has risen from 2 per annum to over 100 per annum. Solvent abusers tend to show the following characteristics:

- male sex
- peak age 13–15 years
- more commonly from lower socioeconomic groupings, minority ethnic groups and disrupted families.

Inhaled substances include many everyday items such as adhesives, aerosols, dry cleaning fluids and cigarette lighter fuel. The substances are inhaled by using paper bags, saturated rags or direct inhalation. Sniffing often occurs as a group activity in the socioeconomically disadvantaged areas of large cities, and regular solitary sniffing is a cause for more serious concern.

The immediate effect is euphoria followed by confusion, perceptual distortion, hallucinations and delusions. The regular user is often able to titrate the 'sniffs', so that a pleasantly euphoric state is maintained for several hours. The characteristic appearance of red spots around the mouth is highly suggestive of solvent abuse.

Sudden death during inhalation can occur from anoxia, respiratory depression, trauma or cardiac arrhythmia. The latter accounts for over half such deaths, while anoxia, usually from the inhalation of vomit, is responsible for over 10%. Accidents or suicide attempts while intoxicated are another cause of death, particularly with toluene adhesives. Long-term effects include neurological damage (peripheral neuropathy, encephalopathy, dementia and fits) as well as renal and liver damage.

Most solvent abusers do not come into contact with psychiatric services, unless they are referred following hospital admission with acute intoxication.

School-based educational programmes and community-resource initiatives are more likely to be beneficial in the long-term. The encouragement of retailers and shop owners to enforce the restrictions on the sale of solvents is also useful. A number of solvent abusers are referred for psychiatric assessment, usually when the abuse is seen as part of more widespread individual or family psychopathology. Finally, most adolescents do not persist with the habit, but a minority progress to more addictive drugs such as heroin or cocaine.

*Abuse of other substances*

These include 'soft' drugs such as cannabis (marijuana) or 'hard' drugs such as amphetamines, cocaine, heroin, lysergic acid diethylamide (LSD) and the recently available designer drugs such as Ecstasy. Up to one-third of older adolescents and young people have occasionally smoked cannabis, although a much smaller proportion are regular recreational users. The effects are euphoric and relaxing in the short term, but apathy and inertia set in with chronic use. Most individuals do not progress from cannabis to other more seriously addictive drugs, and its consumption is not indicative of underlying psychological disturbance.

Hard drug consumption is a far more serious problem, having deleterious effects on physical and psychological well-being as well as the risk of physical or psychological dependence. In addition to euphoric and pleasurable effects, most such drugs can produce acutely distressing symptoms such as panic, fright or hallucinations. This can result in suicidal behaviour or an increased risk of accidents. Long-term use of, for example, amphetamines or cocaine can precipitate a florid psychotic episode with hallucinations, often visual, and paranoid delusions. Psychological withdrawal symptoms such as an unbearable craving for a 'fix' and physical withdrawal symptoms such as nausea, vomiting and diarrhoea make giving up the drug extremely difficult. Physical neglect and malnutrition are also common and exacerbate the problems. The necessity for a regular supply of the drug means that the individual frequently resorts to crime to support his addiction. The practice of needle-sharing is a major health hazard, with HIV infection a strong possibility. Referral of the adolescent to a specialist treatment centre and support for the parents are essential to prevent the serious social and psychological problems that are inevitable with long-term drug abuse.

## Sexual problems

Three topics are discussed:

- sexual abuse and sexual offenders in adolescence

- gender identity disorders
- teenage pregnancy.

*Sexual abuse and sexual offenders in adolescence*

Sexual abuse can present in two ways, direct disclosure of abuse and indirect manifestations of abuse. The same principles of practice and management apply with adolescents as with younger children (see Ch. 5), but some special features are important. Open disclosure by the adolescent is often accompanied by the plea for complete confidentiality and no further action. Clearly this guarantee cannot be given and the adolescent must be counselled about the necessity for open investigation and the convening of a child protection conference.

Indirect manifestations of abuse occur in two forms, sexually-related behaviour and psychiatric symptomatology. Sexually-related manifestations include pregnancy, venereal disease and promiscuity. This last often arises because the adolescent relates readily to adults in a sexual manner as a result of his/her earlier experience of sexual abuse by an adult. Paradoxically, the promiscuous behaviour may also lead some adults not to believe the adolescent's claims of abuse or that the adolescent was not responsible for the initiation of sexual contact. The psychological presentations of abuse are numerous, with distress a prominent feature. Common presentations include depression, deteriorating school performance or attendance, suicidal behaviour and running away from home.

Help for the sexually abused adolescent has two aims, the protection of the adolescent and the provision of therapy to lessen the psychological consequences of the abuse. The first aim is usually achieved by ensuring that the perpetrator is either no longer living at home and/or does not have contact with the adolescent. A wide range of therapies is used including individual counselling and support, family therapy and group therapy.

Group therapy for adolescents who have been sexually abused has become extremely popular recently. This approach has several advantages: the adolescent realises that others have had a similar experience; he/she has the opportunity to discuss and share feelings with other adolescents who are in a similar predicament; and he/she may feel less stigmatised. The group approach is probably less successful when the predominant feeling of the adolescent is betrayal. In this instance, it is more useful to offer individual psychotherapy to enable the adolescent to establish trust with the therapist, so that disclosure and discussion can occur in a confidential setting.

A more recent development has been the provision of treatment strategies for adolescents who have perpetrated sexual offences. The latter include exhibitionism or indecent exposure as well as sexual abuse of other, usually younger, children. The treatment programme(s) involve(s) an assessment of the offender's sexual knowledge and attitudes as well as his social skills and relationships (Salter 1988). Treatment programmes use a variety of approaches, often in combination, including social skills training, sex education and cognitive–behavioural approaches.

### Gender identity disorders

Society's attitudes towards sexuality have been changing in recent years, so that more open discussion of sexual values and behaviour is possible, along with greater tolerance of and less stigma associated with homosexuality, whether in males or females. Homosexual behaviour in some form is quite common during the pre-adolescent and adolescent years, occurring in approximately 20% of boys and 10% of girls. It is clearly a transitory pattern of behaviour, as estimates of adult male and female homosexuality are 3% and 1.5% respectively. While homosexuality per se is most unlikely to be a reason for psychiatric referral, anxiety and depression associated with doubts about the homosexual role are occasionally sufficiently severe to warrant referral.

A core distinction is made between individuals who display anomalous gender role behaviour and those with gender identity disorder, and clinicians are more likely to be involved with the latter.

*Anomalous gender role behaviour* is the individual's preference for interests, activities and clothes normally associated with the opposite sex. For example, effeminate boys prefer girls' style of clothing and like to play with dolls, while 'tomboy' girls like aggressive contact games and boys' style of clothing.

By contrast, the essential feature of *gender identity disorder* is the persistent wish to be of the opposite sex. This is confirmed by the frequent expression of this wish and by extensive anomalous gender role behaviour such as cross-dressing. Zuker & Green (1991), quoting figures derived from the Achenbach Childhood Behaviour Checklist (Achenbach & Edelbrock 1983), state that positive response to the questions 'behaves likes the opposite sex' and 'wishes to be of the opposite sex' were more likely with girls than with boys. This finding is in contrast to most clinical studies (Zuker & Green 1991) which show that boys are more likely than girls to be referred with gender identity disorder problems. During adolescence, referral is often sought for problems associated with cross-dressing, homosexual behaviour and social ostracism by peers. Trans-sexualism, the wish for permanent change of gender assignment, can also become an issue.

The search for aetiological factors in gender identity disorder has not been fruitful, with no convincing evidence for chromosomal, physiological or endocrine abnormalities. Most clinicians believe that several psychosocial factors acting in combination are responsible. Initial parental tolerance of the anomalous sexual behaviour followed by subsequent acceptance and reinforcement is a common finding in referred children, together with an over-dependent mother–child relationship.

Treatment strategies for gender identity disorder include individual and family therapy, parental counselling and behaviour therapy. The most important aspect of treatment is to define and agree goals with the parents and the child. Clinic studies (Zuker & Green 1991) indicate that the earlier treatment is commenced the better the prognosis. Behavioural programmes with attainable short-term goals are much more likely to be successful than more ambitious plans. Minimising anomalous gender behaviour such as cross-dressing and the promotion of gender appropriate behaviour is the basis of intervention strategies. Treatment of co-existing individual and family psychopathology is also beneficial. Finally, the long-term follow-up of 66 effeminate boys (Zuker & Green 1991) found that three quarters were bisexual or homosexual as adults.

*Teenage pregnancy*

Recent articles (Black 1986, Rosenberg & McEwan 1991) have reviewed the trends and problems associated with teenage pregnancy. The UK pregnancy rate for 15–19-year-olds in 1980 was 44/1000 compared with 96/1000 in the US and 14/1000 in the Netherlands. Approximately 1500 girls under 16 become mothers each year in the UK. The other major trend in the past 15 years has been that the abortion rate has doubled, so that 70% of teenage pregnancies now end in termination. The obstetrics risks compared with older women are small and relate probably to social factors rather than to the youthful age of the mother. There is, however, a slightly higher rate of preterm delivery, low birth weight and later presentation for antenatal care among teenage expectant mothers.

Most pregnancies occur in girls who are in a stable relationship, usually with a boy of the same age. The options for the girl, termination or continuation of the pregnancy, are fraught with complications. Expert counselling should be available to the girl and family to arrive at an informed decision and the girl's wishes should be paramount. Schooling is likely to be seriously disrupted and many girls are embarrassed to attend antenatal clinics with older mothers so that special antenatal clinics and the provision of social and educational help, including postnatal contraceptive counselling, are not only desirable but essential. Clearly, better education about sexual relationships and contraception is the best way to prevent this upsetting and disruptive event happening to the adolescent.

## TREATMENT

Often, the most difficult aspect of providing help is getting the co-operation and agreement of the adolescent and family that treatment is necessary. The principles of treatment approaches are outlined in the chapters on the individual syndromes, while detailed discussion of treatment techniques is provided in Chapter 17.

# 15. Psychiatric aspects of mental retardation in childhood

## INTRODUCTION

Child psychiatrists are likely to become involved with children who have mental retardation in several different ways. Sometimes, they are responsible for the provision of the specialist medical care for these children, but more commonly they are asked for advice from other professionals about the emotional and behavioural problems that are quite frequent in this group of children. This chapter discusses first the clinical features of mental retardation in childhood and secondly the psychiatric disorders of children with mental retardation.

## CLINICAL FEATURES OF MENTAL RETARDATION IN CHILDHOOD

### Terminology (Table 15.1)

As discussed in Chapter 3, many terms, such as *mental subnormality* and/or *mental handicap*, have been used in the past. ICD and DSM use IQ (intelligence quotient) or mental age as the basis for classification. As discussed in Chapter 3, IQ is defined as mental age/chronological age x 100. The mean or average IQ is therefore 100, with a standard deviation (s.d.) of 15 (Fig. 15.1). The normal or Gaussian distribution of intelligence means that approximately 2.5% of individuals are 2 s.d. below the mean, corresponding to an IQ of 70. This is usually taken as the dividing point between the normal range of intelligence and mental retardation.

ICD and DSM have four categories of mental retardation:

- mild (IQ 50–69 approximately)
- moderate (IQ 35–49 approximately)
- severe (IQ 20–34 approximately)
- profound (IQ less than 20).

The other important defining criterion is that there should be evidence of social impairment and limitation in the individual's daily activities and self-care skills. The latter is usually the way in which the mental retardation manifests itself. The Vineland Adaptive Behavior

217

**Table 15.1**   Classification of mental retardation

| Term (ICD/DSM categories) | Approximate IQ range |
| --- | --- |
| Mild | 50–69 |
| Moderate | 35–49 |
| Severe | 20–34 |
| Profound | Below 20 |

**Note**: Educationalists use other terms:
- Mild learning difficulties (comparable to IQ 50–70)
- Severe learning difficulties (comparable to IQ 50 or below)

Scales (Sparrow et al 1984) are a useful means of assessing the child's independence and self-help skills from birth to adolescence. The assessment is carried out by means of a semi-structured interview conducted by a specially trained interviewer with a person who is familiar with the individual child. In practice, the interview is normally carried out with the mother. Four functional domains or dimensions are assessed:

- communication
- daily living skills
- socialisation
- motor skills.

These scores are then collated to produce an *adaptive behaviour composite* which provides an accurate assessment of the child's level of independence and self-care skills.

Another source of confusion with terminology is that educationalists and teachers dislike terms such as mental retardation or handicap which they feel are pejorative. Instead, they prefer to use the terms *mild learning difficulties* (comparable to IQ range 50–70) and *severe learning difficulties* (comparable IQ range 50 and below). This terminology has been adopted in the UK in the Education Act 1981.

This Act produced major changes in philosophy and the provision of services for children with special educational needs. It recognised that up to 20% of children met the criteria for special educational need. It also made the following recommendations. First, there should be a clear statement or document of the educational needs of every child with special educational problems. This statement should be drawn up as soon as practical and also provide the basis for decisions about the provision of specialist educational resources for the child. Second, parents should be actively involved in this process of decision-making about their child's educational needs. Finally, children with special educational needs should be integrated into mainstream schooling whenever possible rather than remaining at a special school.

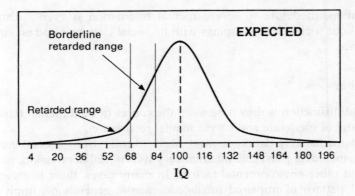

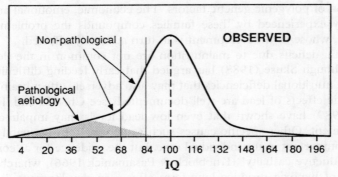

**Fig. 15.1** Population distribution of intelligence.  **a.** Distribution of Stanford–Binet IQs expected from the normal curve.  **b.** Approximate distribution of IQs actually found: individuals with pathological aetiology separated from those without pathological aetiology.

## Prevalence (Fig. 15.1)

The normal distribution of intelligence throughout the population implies that by definition 2–3% of the population are in the mildly retarded range (IQ 50–70). This prevalence figure does not, however, provide any meaningful indication of the range and severity of the learning difficulties experienced by this group of children. In practice, they vary very widely. Children in the mildly retarded range tend to come from families in the lower socioeconomic groupings and have parents of similar intellectual ability. They often experience psychosocial deprivation in varying degrees of severity which further impairs their developmental progress.

The rate of moderate to profound mental retardation (IQ 50 or below) is 3/1000. This is greater than would be expected because of the occurrence of several specific syndromes associated with mental retardation, for instance Down's syndrome, which are responsible for the 'hump' on the downward tail of the IQ distribution curve (Fig. 15.1). Unlike mild mental retardation, moderate to severe mental retardation is evenly distributed throughout social class groupings with no social class bias and an equal sex incidence.

## Aetiology

A broad distinction is drawn between the causes of mild mental retardation and those of moderate and severe mental retardation.

Mild mental retardation is most likely to arise from a combination of factors, including polygenic inheritance, psychosocial deprivation, malnutrition and other environmental factors. In many cases, there is a consistent familial pattern of impaired intelligence across generations, implying the operation of polygenic genetic factors. The economic, emotional and social adversity experienced by these families compounds the problem for the children, whose own development is in turn adversely affected.

Specific deficits due to malnutrition are not common in the developed world, though Skuse (1988) has argued that early feeding difficulties may produce nutritional deficiencies that may also adversely affect brain growth. The toxic effects of lead are well documented (see Ch. 12) and Thomson et al (1989) have shown that even low lead levels may impair cognitive development. Other specific causes such as anoxia from perinatal damage may be important in the individual case, but the evidence for a 'continuum of reproductive casualty' (Knobloch & Pasamanick 1966), whereby minor degrees of hypoxia produce long-term effects on development, is unconvincing.

By contrast, aetiological factors in moderate to profound retardation are more clearly defined (Table 15.2):

- chromosome factors 40%
- genetic factors 15%
- pre- and perinatal factors 10%
- postnatal factors 10%
- unknown 25%.

### Chromosome factors

**Down's syndrome (trisomy 21).** This is the most common abnormality, accounting for 75% of chromosome abnormalities, that is, nearly one-third of all cases of mental retardation. 95% of cases are caused by the addition of an extra chromosome 21 (non-disjunction type), whereas in the remaining 5% the extra chromosome is displaced from one site to another with no increase in chromosome number (translocation type). The non-disjunction type risk increases with maternal age, whereas the translocation type risk depends on whether the translocation is new or whether one parent is a carrier.

**Table 15.2**  Common causes of mental retardation

| Syndrome | Aetiology | Features |
|---|---|---|
| Down's syndrome (trisomy 21) | Non-disjunction/translocation types | Upslanting eyes with epicanthic folds, short nose with flat nasal bridge and large tongue |
| | | Fingers are short with incurved little finger and single palmar crease |
| | | Short stature |
| | | Hypotonia (reduced muscle tone) |
| | | Cardiac abnormalities |
| Fragile X syndrome | Long arm X chromosome breakage on exposure to low folic acid | High forehead with prominent supra-orbital ridges |
| | | Low-set, protruding ears with prominent jaw |
| | | Autistic features such as hand flapping and poor eye contact |
| Cri du chat | Deletion of chromosome 5 | Microcephaly (small head size) |
| | | Hyperteleorism (widely spaced eyes) |
| | | Cat-like cry |
| | | Failure to thrive |
| Prader–Willi syndrome | Short arm deletion chromosome 15 | Severe language and speech delay |
| | | Hypotonia (reduced muscle tone) |
| | | Hypogonadism (small genitalia) |
| Phenylketonuria | Autosomal recessive | Fair hair and blue eyes with retarded growth |
| | | Other features include epilepsy, microcephaly and hyperactivity |
| Tuberous sclerosis | Autosomal dominant with variable penetrance | Epilepsy, butterfly rash on face, white skin patches and multiple 'tuber' tumours in kidney and lungs |
| Rubella | Viral infection in first trimester | Blindness and cataract |
| | | Deafness |
| | | Microcephaly |
| | | Congenital heart disease |
| Toxoplasmosis | Infection during pregnancy | Hydrocephaly (large head size) |
| | | Retinal damage |
| | | Enlarged liver and spleen with jaundice |
| | | Epilepsy |
| Lesch–Nyhan syndrome | X-linked recessive | Normal at birth |
| | Defect in purine metabolism | |
| | | Progressive extrapyramidal movement disorder |
| | | Increasing self mutilation involving fingers, lips and other parts of body |
| | | Aggressive behaviour |

*Fragile X syndrome.* This is so called because of the breakage that occurs on the X chromosome when the cells are cultured in a medium deficient in folic acid. An X chromosome breakage rate greater than 2% is regarded as diagnostic. The syndrome is the second most common cause of mental retardation after Down's syndrome, accounting for 10% of moderate to profound retardation in boys. Inheritance is complicated, and 10% of affected males and 70% of female carriers are within the normal intelligence range. Affected individuals often show some autistic features, for instance hand-twirling and poor eye-contact, but it is unclear whether these factors are more common in the fragile X syndrome than among other individuals with similar degrees of mental retardation. It is important to exclude the syndrome as a cause of mental retardation, though the results of diagnostic tests are often inconclusive.

*Cri du chat syndrome (partial deletion of chromosome 5)* and *Edward's syndrome (trisomy 18)* are rare causes of mental retardation.

*Prader–Willi syndrome* is associated with mental retardation, marked obesity, hypotonia and hypogonadism. There is usually a history of marked speech and language delay, though the mental retardation may only be mild. A major problem for the parents is controlling the child's voracious appetite in order to minimise obesity.

Finally, sex chromosome abnormalities such as *Klinefelter's syndrome (XXY genotype)* or *Turner's syndrome (XO genotype)* are usually associated with only mild degrees of mental retardation.

### Genetically-determined metabolic abnormalities

These account for 15% of cases and include phenylketonuria and a large number of other metabolic 'storage' disorders. In most cases, the enzyme deficiency results in the accumulation of substances in excessive amounts or in a deficiency of substances essential for the control of body metabolism.

### Pre- and perinatal causes

These include infections during pregnancy such as rubella, toxoplasmosis and, more recently, HIV virus as well as perinatal abnormalities such as birth trauma or anoxia. These causes are responsible for approximately 10% of mental retardation.

### Postnatal causes

These include head injury or trauma, severe central nervous system infection and cardiac or respiratory arrest.

**Table 15.3** Psychiatric disorder in children with mental retardation

- Approximately 40% have signs of significant psychological disturbance
- Range of disorders is similar to children of average ability except that the following occur much more frequently:
  - Pervasive developmental disorders
  - Pervasive hyperkinetic syndrome
  - Severe stereotyped movement disorder
  - Self-injurious behaviour and pica more common

*Unknown causes*

These account for the remaining 25% of cases where no clearly defined pathology can be identified. Many of these children do, however, have some other abnormality such as epilepsy or a developmental anomaly so that an as yet unidentified cause is likely to be responsible.

## PSYCHIATRIC DISORDER IN CHILDREN WITH MENTAL RETARDATION

### Prevalence (Table 15.3)

The Isle of Wight study (Rutter et al 1970b) found that approximately one-third of children with mental retardation showed signs of disturbance, the rate rising to 50% among moderate to severely retarded children. A more recent epidemiologically based survey of severely mentally retarded children aged 5–15 years in South London (Corbett 1979) found that 43% had significant psychiatric disorder. The children exhibited the same range of disturbance as children of normal ability but in addition three disorders were much more frequent:

- childhood autism
- pervasive hyperkinetic disorder
- severe stereotyped movement disorder.

Finally, self-injurious behaviour and pica were also more frequent.

### Aetiology (Table 15.4)

It is important, to distinguish between the factors responsible for disorders occurring in mildly mentally retarded children and in those with moderate to severe retardation. Children with mild mental retardation probably have the same risk factors as children of average ability, but to a greater extent, that is adverse temperamental characteristics, specific learning disorders and family psychopathology. The last is particularly important as parents of children with mild mental retardation are also likely to be within the lower range of intellectual ability. Consequently, their parenting capacity may be

**Table 15.4**   Causes of psychiatric disorder in children
with moderate to severe mental retardation

- Brain damage leading to:
  - loss of specific functions or skills
  - active disruption of normal brain activity
  - increased risk of epilepsy

- Specific learning difficulties

- Adverse temperamental characteristics:
  - impulsivity
  - overactivity
  - distractibility

- Psychosocial consequences of handicap:
  - Child – social isolation and low self-esteem
  - Parents – overprotection/rejection

limited, with inconsistent discipline and control prominent features. In addition, this may be combined with marital disharmony and socioeconomic disadvantage, so that this group of children is considerably more vulnerable to psychiatric disturbance.

Another important causative factor in many children with severe mental retardation is the presence of brain damage. Several studies (Crome 1960, Rutter et al 1970a,b) have found that half of children with moderate to severe mental retardation have demonstrable brain damage. This increases the risk of psychiatric disturbance in several ways: loss of specific functions or skills; active disruption or dysfunction of normal brain activity; and increased risk of epilepsy. Children with moderate to severe mental retardation are also more likely to have specific learning difficulties which further increases vulnerability. Adverse temperamental characteristics such as impulsivity, distractibility or overactivity are more common among children with severe mental retardation. The psychosocial consequences of handicap for the child and the family also make a contribution in some cases, though the relative contribution is difficult to estimate. The child's feelings of social isolation and low self-esteem, combined with inappropriate parental attitudes such as over-protection or rejection, are important factors in some cases.

## Psychiatric syndromes specifically associated with moderate to severe retardation

Although most types of disorder are found among children with moderate to severe mental retardation, certain syndromes which are generally uncommon are found much more frequently.

## Childhood autism

80% of children with childhood autism have an IQ of less than 70. Corbett (1979) found that childhood autism accounted for up to 17% of psychiatric disturbance in a community survey of severely mentally retarded children living in south London. Many clinicians distinguish between those individuals who have childhood autism and those who have severe mental retardation with some autistic features. Such features include stereotypies, mannerisms and deficits in comprehension and expressive language. These symptoms, which are quite common among retarded children, tend to occur in isolation, so that the individual does not fulfil the diagnostic criteria for childhood autism. Clinical practice and research findings do not, however, provide clear-cut criteria for deciding the dividing line between childhood autism and severe mental retardation with autistic features. Consequently, clinicians tend to have their own personal preferences in terminology and classification.

Autistic behaviours are also features of some syndromes associated with mental retardation such as tuberous sclerosis, rubella, fragile X syndrome and infantile spasms. In some cases, for instance with rubella, the autistic behaviour seems to be a response to the coexisting sensory deficit rather than the separate occurrence of childhood autism. Finally, individuals with some extremely uncommon neurodegenerative diseases such as subacute sclerosing panencephalitis or disintegrative disorder often show autistic-like stereotypic behaviour.

## Hyperkinetic syndrome

Like autistic behaviour, overactive or hyperkinetic behaviour is common among children with severe mental retardation. In most cases, the overactivity occurs in some situations but not others and reflects an immaturity in behaviour and language skills. A much smaller but nevertheless significant number of children with severe mental retardation do show pervasive hyperactivity with other features of that syndrome, including distractibility, impulsivity and aggressive behaviour.

## Stereotypic and self-injurious behaviour

Stereotypic movements such as body-rocking or hand-flapping have been reported as frequently as 40% in mild to severely mentally retarded children (Corbett 1979). Self-injurious behaviour such as head-banging, biting of limbs or eye-gouging is much less common but more potentially harmful and also difficult to eradicate. The Lesch–Nyhan syndrome is particularly associated with the development of self-mutilating behaviour. The self-destructive behaviour is usually a reflection of the poverty of the individual's skills and abilities and/or the lack of stimulation provided by his surroundings and immediate environment.

Murphy (1985) reviewed the treatment methods for these intractable and destructive behaviours. Protective devices such as helmets, treatment with major tranquillisers such as haloperidol and behavioural approaches have all been used with some success. A real danger with drug treatment is that once started, it is difficult to stop, so that the individual can remain on drug for several years, often with increasing dosage over time. A behavioural approach is more likely to produce long-lasting benefits, but it is more time-consuming to carry out and more demanding of staff co-operation.

*Pica*

The ingestion of substances not normally regarded as edible is a transitory phenomenon in normal toddlers and is even more common in children with severe mental retardation. The main adverse consequence of this behaviour is possible lead intoxication from the licking of painted objects. Faecal smearing and ingestion occur among some severely retarded children, particularly those with an additional sensory handicap such as blindness.

## Mental retardation syndromes associated with specific behavioural characteristics

Traditionally, children with certain mental retardation syndromes have been said to show a characteristic behavioural or personality profile, though contemporary opinion is more sceptical about such associations.

*Down's syndrome*

Children with this syndrome are often described as sociable, musical, contented and easy-going, features they share with their siblings. Overall, these children have a slightly increased rate of disturbance, a minority showing aggressive and oppositional behaviour, usually associated with the translocation trisomy.

*Phenylketonuria*

Untreated, these children develop severe mental retardation with autistic and hyperkinetic behaviour prominent. Successful dietary treatment usually results in normal growth and development, but treated children have a greater risk of psychiatric disturbance, with overactivity, distractibility and restlessness common.

*Lesch-Nyhan syndrome*

This sex-linked disorder of purine metabolism, occurring only in boys, is associated with an extrapyramidal movement disorder including chorea and

**Table 15.5**  Management of mental retardation in childhood

Key elements are:

- Breaking the news
- Promotion of normal development
- Treatment of medical and behavioural problems
- Educational provision
- Genetic counselling
- Long-term case work support

athetosis, severe mental retardation and self-injurious behaviour. This last is extremely difficult to treat and eliminate.

## Prader–Willi syndrome

The main behavioural feature associated with this syndrome is the explosive outbursts associated with the dietary restriction frequently imposed to control voracious appetite and accompanying obesity.

## Hydrocephalus

Children with hydrocephalus were previously described as showing the 'cocktail party' syndrome. This is characterised by verbosity in the form and superficiality or shallowness in the content of their conversation. The early detection and treatment of hydrocephalus has now produced a reduction in morbidity, so that these features are less commonly seen.

## Management (Table 15.5)

Many professionals, including paediatricians, teachers and psychologists, are likely to be involved in the provision of care for children with mental handicap and their families. A multidisciplinary approach to assessment and treatment is vital. Different aspects of management are important at various stages during the child's life.

### Breaking the news

This topic is discussed more fully in Chapter 16, so that only brief comments are made here. The ability to communicate bad news in a sensitive manner is a skill rarely taught to medical students or junior doctors. Many parents complain justifiably that their initial interview with the doctor was unsatisfactory and distressing. Tact, sympathy and time are essential to enable the parent(s) to begin to grasp and understand the implications of the situation. Honest discussion, combined with an emphasis on the hopeful aspects, are the important prerequisites for a satisfactory interview.

### Promotion of normal development

Parents should be encouraged from the outset to develop the skills of their child in the social, self-care and educational aspects of development to the maximum. A 'normalisation' and 'optimalisation' strategy is the basis to the approach. Specific treatment packages, for example the Portage scheme, are helpful in enabling the parents to set realistic targets for their child.

### Treatment of medical and behavioural problems

Advice from neurologists, physiotherapists and occupational therapists is important in the management of the neurological deficits frequently present in this group of children. Behavioural problems are managed in a variety of ways including medication (for instance with major tranquillisers), protective devices (e.g. for excessive head-banging) and operant or time-out procedures (e.g. for maladaptive behaviour). Treatment approaches are discussed more fully in Chapter 17.

### Educational provision

Parents need advice from an early stage about the most appropriate educational provision. The recent changes in the UK education legislation are designed to ensure that a comprehensive assessment of needs and available resources is undertaken for every child with special educational needs. Specialised preschool nursery provision is beneficial, along with the consideration of later special educational placement. Some children with mental retardation may be helped by attendance at schools which specialise in the education of children with communication or autistic-like disorders.

### Genetic counselling

This is clearly essential for all parents, especially when a specific syndrome is identified.

### Long-term casework and support

Clinical experience and practice suggest that many families find this type of help invaluable in the long term. The identification of a key professional worker who co-ordinates the care plan for the child is very useful. A social worker or a professional from a voluntary organisation with counselling skills is often the person best placed to fulfil this role.

Recently, Byrne & Cunningham (1985) have provided a useful conceptualisation of the ways in which mental retardation affects the family. They identified three factors as crucial in determining outcome:

- the stressful effects of handicap on family life
- the material and practical consequences of the handicap for the family
- on the positive side, the increased resourcefulness and coping skills developed by the family as a result of their experience.

The authors believe that the outcome, favourable or otherwise, is determined by the relative balance of costs and benefits for the family. They conclude that a gloomy outcome is not necessarily inevitable.

## Outcome

Treatment programmes, with their emphasis on maximising potential, minimising adverse effects and integration into the community, are successful for many children with mental retardation and their families. Despite cognitive impairment, behaviour problems are reduced by treatment programmes and families learn to adapt satisfactorily. The policy of the UK government to close institutions for individuals with mental retardation and to integrate them into the community is also likely to promote better adjustment in the long term.

# 16. Psychological aspects of illness and disability

## INTRODUCTION

The recent revolution in the treatment of acute illness in children and the dramatic improvement in survival rates for children with many serious illnesses mean that the management of chronic illness and disability is an important component of contemporary paediatric practice. The psychosocial adjustment of the child and family to these conditions varies widely depending upon the illness, the child, the family and the effects of treatment. This chapter discusses the psychosocial aspects of chronic illness or handicap in three sections:

- general features
- specific syndromes
- miscellaneous aspects of illness and handicap.

Before discussing these aspects, it is useful to define the terminology more precisely as the terms are often used in a confusing and interchangeable fashion. Recently, the World Health Organization (WHO 1980) has proposed the following definitions:

- An *impairment* is an anatomical defect, or the absence or loss of a specific psychological or physiological function, that can arise from a disease or from an intrinsic pathological state
- A *disability* is a restriction in the ability to perform a task or activity within the range normally expected of someone of the same age or level of maturity
- A *handicap* is a social disadvantage preventing the fulfilment of a normal social role.

Thus a disfiguring facial deformity can be seen as an impairment not producing disability but associated with handicap, probably from social rejection.

## GENERAL FEATURES

Approximately 15% of children have some form of disability from either a chronic illness (5%), cognitive or educational impairment (5%) or

231

**Table 16.1**  Adjustment to illness and disability

**Predisposing factors**
- Temperamental characteristics
- Physiological and psychological response to stress
- Family influences
- Societal and cultural attitudes

**Precipitating factors**
- Acute or insidious onset
- Severity of stressful response

**Perpetuating factors**
- Continuation of stressful response
- Management of attendant anxiety
- Social reinforcement of illness role
- Family and societal attitudes

**Protective factors**
- Adaptable temperamental characteristics
- Harmonious family relationships
- Peer group support

behavioural abnormality (5%) (Rutter et al 1970b). The Isle of Wight study (Rutter et al 1970a) showed clearly that children with chronic illness were on average twice as likely to be disturbed as healthy children, rates varying from 33% for children with central nervous disease to 12% for children with asthma or diabetes. The Isle of Wight study also showed that children with chronic illness had the same range of disorders as other disturbed children. This implies that in most cases the mechanisms involved in the increased morbidity associated with chronic illness are probably indirect and non-specific rather than direct or specific to each illness or disability.

Illness and disability impose psychological stress on the child and family not only at the time of diagnosis but also in the long term. Although these two stages are discussed separately, there is clearly a gradual transition from one phase to the other. Table 16.1 lists the four types of factor that determine the individual's adjustment to illness or disability.

## The initial impact of diagnosis

The initial emotional response of the parents and the child, depending on age, has similarities to the grief reaction associated with a major loss such as a bereavement. Four phases are recognised: shock, denial, anger and sadness, and adjustment. The four phases usually follow one another in a sequential manner, though at any one time a mixture of the various components may be experienced.

*Shock* describes the brief period of intense emotional arousal immediately following the disclosure of the diagnosis. It lasts for only a short period and is succeeded by *denial*, inability or reluctance to accept the seriousness or likely outcome of the illness. Initially, the response is adaptive, as it enables the parents and child to realise gradually the implications of the disease. Prolonged or excessive use of denial becomes maladaptive when it results in poor treatment compliance and reluctance to accept the limitations or restrictions imposed by the illness. This pattern of behaviour is a more frequent feature of the long-term adjustment of older children and adolescents who have illnesses that necessitate adherence to a strict treatment regime.

*Sadness and anger* begin to emerge when the child or parents start to appreciate the long-term implications of the disease. As such, these emotions are not pathological, but represent an understandable response to the predicament imposed by the illness. Sadness usually elicits a supportive response from professionals, other family members and friends. Anger is usually expressed through the 'why me?' or 'why us?' question, often manifest as a critical attitude by the parents towards doctors and other care staff, or as unprovoked outbursts of temper or frustration in the child.

## Long-term effects

As stated earlier, children with chronic illness or disability and their families are more at risk for developing disturbance. There is, however, a wide variation in outcome, with the majority of children and their families making a reasonable adjustment. Traditionally, research interest has focused on the adverse impact on the child and family. By contrast, a recent review (Byrne & Cunningham 1985) emphasised the potential benefits and enrichment that may occur when the child and family adapt successfully. The increased competence and sense of mastery, combined with an enlarged repertoire of coping mechanisms, can be a considerable asset to the child and family. Table 16.2 summarises the various ways in which chronic illness or disability can adversely affect the child and family.

### Effects on the child

Illness or disability can adversely affect the child's development in three ways:

- the acquisition of skills and of outside interests
- the development of the self-concept
- the development of adaptive coping behaviour.

Many illnesses or disabilities inevitably limit and restrict the child's ability and opportunity to acquire everyday skills and to develop interests and hobbies. For example, the child with cerebral palsy has a significant motor impairment that makes the skilful execution of movement more difficult; the exercise limitations imposed by asthma can preclude participation in gymnastic or other sporting activities; the unpredictable occurrence of seizures can make cycling or swimming a hazardous pursuit for children with epilepsy. Additionally, educational problems are common among this

**Table 16.2**    Impact of chronic illness or disability on child and family

**Prevalence**
- 15% have chronic illness/impairment/disability

**Rate of disturbance**
- General population: 7%
- Chronic illness not affecting CNS: 12%
- Chronic illness affecting CNS: 33%

**Effects on child**
- Reduced ability/opportunity to develop skills and interests
  - Physical – cerebral palsy
  - Dietary – diabetes
  - Exercise – asthma
  - Some activities – epilepsy
- Educational problems are common
  - School absence
  - Specific learning difficulties
  - Low expectations of teachers and parents
- Poor self-concept
- Body image – distorted
- Self-esteem – pessimistic opinion of abilities and of the future

**Effects on family**
- Parents
  - Rejection (uncommon)
  - Over-protection
  - Inability to discipline and control
  - Marital disharmony
- Siblings
  - Excessive responsibility
  - Loss of friendships
  - Neglect of own needs

group of children for a variety of reasons including increased absence from school, specific learning difficulties, especially among children with epilepsy, and the low expectations of parents and teachers.

Illness and disability can adversely affect the child's self-concept through the effect on his body image and self-esteem. Many children with chronic illness have a distorted view of their bodies, believing their disability to be very prominent or disfiguring. These ideas are often reinforced by adverse comments from parents and peers. Self-esteem can also be impaired by a faulty cognitive appraisal of themselves combined with a pessimistic and despondent response to that evaluation. This leads the child to have low self-esteem along with a gloomy view about his illness and the prospects for the future. This is particularly likely to occur in older children and adolescents and may have a very disabling and deleterious effect on their development.

Successful adaptation to chronic illness or disability depends upon the acquisition of a range of coping behaviours and the use of defence mechanisms to lessen anxiety to an acceptable level. Effective coping strategies include:

- regulating the amount of stress into manageable amounts, for example 'taking one thing at a time'
- obtaining information from several sources
- rehearsing the various outcomes of treatment, including adverse consequences
- assessing the situation from several viewpoints.

Parents, nursing staff and paediatricians have an important role in promoting this repertoire of skills in children with chronic illness or disability. Defence mechanisms such as denial, rationalisation or displacement can be helpful for the child during the transition phase from the initial to the long-term adaptation to the illness or disability.

The other important factor influencing the child's adaptation is his concept of the causation of the illness or disability. Children below the age of 6 years often regard their illness as a punishment for some misdemeanour, while during middle childhood the child commonly thinks that he or she has 'caught' the illness or disability from someone or something. It is only from around 10 years onwards that the child begins to acquire adult-like concepts of the causation of illness and disability.

*Effect on the parents*

Most parents eventually arrive at some degree of adaptation, though for a minority maladaptive behaviour patterns emerge and are prominent. Surprisingly perhaps, the rate of psychiatric disturbance or marital disharmony is not significantly different among this group of parents compared with the general population (Byrne & Cunningham 1985). Though some parents seem to respond to the child's illness or disability with friction and disharmony, this group is counterbalanced by another group who are united by the adversity caused by their child's illness or disability.

The common reaction is over-protection – the parent(s) is unable to allow the child to experience the normal disappointments and upsets inevitable during childhood, so that the child leads a 'cotton-wool' existence. Less frequently, the parent(s) are rejecting and indifferent to the child because the disability is so damaging to the parents' self-esteem or because it exacerbates an already precarious parent–child relationship. Over-protection and rejection are sometimes combined. Finally, the parents may also find it difficult to provide appropriate discipline and control as they irrationally fear that such control may exacerbate the child's illness. For example, the parents of children with epilepsy may think that thwarting the child's wishes may induce a seizure.

*Effects on siblings*

This can manifest itself in several ways: the oldest sibling may be given excessive responsibility for the care of the child with the illness or disability; the siblings may lose friendships because they are reluctant to bring their friends home in case the ill or disabled child is an embarrassment; and finally, the siblings' own development needs may be neglected, with consequent resentment and frustration.

## SPECIFIC SYNDROMES

## CHILDHOOD MALIGNANCIES

Cancer is an important cause of death in childhood and adolescence, brain tumours and acute lymphoblastic leukaemia (ALL) accounting for 40% of cases. ALL is most common between the ages of 2 and 4 years. The rapid improvement in survival rates over the past 30 years (up to 60% and rising with ALL) have been achieved through the development of rigorous treatment regimes involving chemotherapy, irradiation, surgery and bone marrow transplantation. These procedures are also likely to increase the risk of psychological morbidity not only because of their stressful and painful nature but also because some treatments, for instance cranial radiation in leukaemia treatment, has a direct effect on brain function. The heroic nature of the treatment regime allied with the improved survival time means that the quality of life for survivors is an increasingly important component in the evaluation of treatment outcome (Mulhearn et al 1989).

### Psychological morbidity

It is probably not helpful to conceptualise the child's adjustment to malignancy in terms of conventional diagnostic categories such as anxiety or depression, but rather as a response to a major stressful event, so that the notion of *post-traumatic stress syndrome* is most useful. Consequently, assessment of adaptation and coping strategies is as important as the measurement of psychological morbidity.

Three stages in the illness are likely to be associated with psychological distress:

- the initial diagnosis
- the active treatment phase
- the post-treatment survival period.

*Initial diagnosis*

Clearly, the impact of the diagnosis is distressing to the child and family, anxiety in the child and shock and bewilderment among the parents being extremely common and understandable. The family's capacity to adapt and to begin to develop coping strategies during this initial phase is an important predictor of subsequent long-term adjustment. Koocher & O'Malley (1981) coined the term 'Damocles syndrome' to describe the predicament posed for the child and family by the diagnosis of leukaemia. (In classical mythology, Dionysus ordered a sword to be suspended on a single hair above the head of Damocles during a banquet to emphasise the precarious nature of power, life and death.) The association between the response to diagnosis and the long-term adjustment is probably a reflection of the premorbid characteristics of the child and family.

*Treatment phase*

The necessity for repeated courses of treatment, painful procedures such as bone marrow aspiration and the adverse side-effects of treatment such as hair loss and susceptibility to infection inevitably lead to considerable morbidity for the child and family. The child commonly displays symptoms such as anxiety, sadness, withdrawal and excessive clinging behaviour, with rates of disturbance of around 30% on formal assessment by questionnaire or interview measures (Maguire 1982). Interestingly, Maguire found that mothers were extremely reluctant to disclose their distress as they were fearful that this would upset the child or expose their own failure to be stoical in adversity. This study also found considerable morbidity among the siblings.

*Long-term survival*

The improved survival rates for childhood malignancies have been achieved at considerable cost to other aspects of development and residual defects include short stature, major organ failure or even secondary malignancy. Koocher & O'Malley (1981), reviewing 114 survivors of childhood cancer on several measures of psychosocial adjustment, found that 40% had some residual symptomatology with 26% rated mild, 10% moderate and 11% severe. The survivors were also less well-adjusted than individuals with other long-term chronic illnesses. Interestingly, the authors reported that favourable outcome was associated with the adaptive use of denial mechanisms during treatment. A more recent study of 52 survivors (Fritz et al 1988) found that successful adaptation was associated with open communication between the child, parents, clinicians and other professionals along with an effective peer group support. Finally, despite the consensus from studies about factors associated with successful adaptation, it would be wrong to be prescriptive about the best way to cope satisfactorily. Clinical experience supports the view that generalisations are invalid and that an idiosyncratic response style suitable for the individual is often the best determinant of outcome.

## Special clinical problems

### School problems

These include school refusal, learning difficulties and school-based behaviour problems. Refusal or reluctance to attend school sometimes occurs when the child has had a relapse or when there is a high risk from intercurrent infections. Realistic appraisal of the risk and a firm insistence on regular attendance are the best strategies.

Learning difficulties are common — several factors are responsible, including frequent absence from school and the direct consequences of the brain lesions associated with the disease or with cranial irradiation treatment. Short-term memory loss and poor concentration are also frequently found (Cousens et al 1988). Finally, behavioural problems in school can arise from the understandable reluctance of teachers to impose firm discipline on children with such a serious condition.

The necessity for strict adherence to the treatment regime and the unpleasantness of some procedures mean that non-compliance can be a problem with some children, particularly the older child and adolescent, and also with some families, particularly those who are already disharmonious or disorganised.

### Stressful medical procedures and chemotherapy

Distress is an almost inevitable consequence of current treatment regimes, which require repeated lumbar punctures, bone marrow aspirations and the administration of drugs with strong nausea- and vomit-inducing properties. Many strategies, including pharmacological, cognitive-behavioural and hypnotic techniques, have been used to alleviate the discomfort, with some considerable success (Redd et al 1987, Zeltzer et al 1989).

## Treatment approaches

The wide range of psychosocial problems shown by children with malignant disorders means that most treatment approaches have been used with some children for some problems at some stage during the illness (Holland & Roland 1989). Drug therapy with antidepressants or major tranquillisers is useful for depressive and anxiety or confusional symptoms respectively, while individual psychotherapy and parental counselling programmes have also been used extensively. The overall results from intervention parental counselling programmes have been mixed: some studies showed clear-cut benefits (Stein & Jessop 1984) while others did not (Nolan et al 1987).

Despite the inconclusiveness of these studies, there is no doubt that children and parents require considerable support throughout the child's illness.

Finally, more specialised psychopharmacological approaches for pain relief, confusional states and the management of the terminally ill child are also necessary in some cases (Holland & Roland 1989).

## NEUROLOGICAL DISORDERS

### Epilepsy

*Clinical features*

Epilepsy is the most common serious, chronic neurological condition in childhood, with an approximate prevalence rate of 4/1000 (Dreifuss 1989). Moreover, 75% of individuals who develop epilepsy begin to have seizures before their 18th birthday. Childhood epilepsy is characterised by a wide range of seizure patterns including generalised or tonic/clonic seizures, complex partial seizures or temporal lobe seizures, with a mixed seizure pattern a common feature.

Additionally, several epilepsy syndromes such as infantile spasms or West's syndrome and Lennox–Gastaut syndrome arise only in childhood and have considerable morbidity and some mortality. These syndromes are associated with severe intractable seizures, often of a mixed motor pattern, as well as mental retardation. The latter may be a primary feature of the syndrome or arise secondary to the prolonged epileptic status that frequently occurs. Co-existent cognitive and learning disabilities are also common among children with epilepsy, so that educational problems are often a source of concern.

*Psychiatric disturbance*

Many studies (Rutter et al 1970a, Hoare 1984), Hoare & Kerley 1991) have shown that children with epilepsy have an increased risk of psychiatric disturbance compared with children who have illnesses not affecting the central nervous system and healthy children. Until recently, disturbed children with epilepsy were regarded as an example of the 'brain-damaged child' syndrome with a stereotyped pattern of disturbance characterised by overactivity, impulsivity, aggression and distractibility (Strauss & Lehtinen 1947). Subsequent research (Rutter et al 1970a, Stores 1978, Hoare 1984a) has, however, found that most disturbed children with epilepsy have the same range and type of psychopathology as other disturbed children. The concept of the 'epileptic personality' or the 'epileptic child' has therefore been abandoned.

A recent study (Hoare & Kerley 1991) involving children with chronic epilepsy attending a seizure clinic at a children's hospital has confirmed that

**Table 16.3**   Causative factors of psychiatric disturbance in children with epilepsy

**Neurological factors**
- High fit frequency
- Complex partial seizures (temporal lobe epilepsy)
- Bilateral active brain abnormality

**Individual characteristics of the child**
- Adverse temperamental factors
- Cognitive and learning difficulties

**Stressful effects of chronic illness**
- Marital disharmony
- Parental psychiatric illness
- Stigma/prejudice

**Anticonvulsant medication (usually older anticonvulsants)**
- Overactivity
- Depression
- Poor concentration
- Distractibility

disturbed children with epilepsy have a similar range of disturbance to other children. This study also found that emotional or neurotic disturbance was the commonest diagnostic category with similar rates of disturbance in boys and girls, findings not reported in earlier studies.

Several factors, acting directly and/or indirectly, are important in the development of disturbance in children with epilepsy. Table 16.3 lists the main factors involved with this increased vulnerability.

Children with frequent seizures, complex partial seizures or evidence of neurological damage on examination or investigation are more likely to develop psychiatric disturbance. Adverse temperamental characteristics such as impulsivity or distractibility and the presence of cognitive and learning disabilities are also risk factors. The Isle of Wight study (Rutter et al 1970b) found that learning difficulties, known to be a general risk factor for childhood disturbance, are more common among children with epilepsy.

Factors stemming from the stressful effects of epilepsy on family life such as marital disharmony or parental psychiatric disorder further increase the child's vulnerability. The promotion of increasing independence and responsibility during childhood are two of the more important maturational tasks that parents have to do for their children. These skills are often deficient in the parents of children with epilepsy, who understandably find it difficult to allow their child to become independent in an age-appropriate fashion and also to exert effective control over the child's behaviour.

While it is difficult to quantify the importance of stigma or prejudice as a risk factor, epilepsy does have certain features that make such a possibility more likely. First, it is paroxysmal, so that it is not possible to predict and/or prevent the occurrence of a seizure, thereby undermining the child's self-esteem and confidence. Second, seizures often occur in public and are frightening and demeaning as well as frequently dangerous. These factors can combine to engender a sense of low self-esteem and poor self-image in the child. The unpredictable and often bizarre behaviour sometimes associated with seizures is a further reminder to the child that he is not the same as his peers. The child's own experience, allied with inappropriate parental attitudes, can reinforce dependent and immature behaviour. This may lead to further restrictions on the activities of the child and family, to their mutual detriment.

Epilepsy also imposes on the child and the family the necessity for continued and prolonged treatment with anticonvulsant drugs. The latter not only reduce the tendency to seizures but also have marked effects on behaviour and mood. The older anticonvulsants, particularly pheno-barbitone, are likely to cause depressed mood, overactivity and irritability, while even the newer anticonvulsants such carbamazepine or sodium valproate can adversely affect alertness, concentration and attention.

## Impact of epilepsy on the child and the family (Table 16.4)

The following factors are important in determining the impact of epilepsy on the individual child and family:

- the type and severity of epilepsy
- the presence of additional handicaps
- the maladaptive responses of the family to chronic illness
- the disruption and distortion of the child's normal developmental progress.

As discussed earlier, childhood epilepsy varies markedly in frequency and severity. The intractable epilepsies such as Lennox–Gastaut syndrome or

**Table 16.4**   Factors affecting impact of epilepsy on the child and family

**Type and severity of epilepsy**
- Lennox–Gastaut syndrome
- Severe complex partial seizure disorder

**Presence of additional handicaps**
- Cerebral palsy
- Mental retardation

**Maladaptive responses of the family to chronic illness**
- Parental over-protectiveness
- Unrealistic fears about seizures, for instance death or serious injury
- Neglect of the needs of the other siblings

**Disruption and distortion on the child's normal developmental progress**
- Preschool child – over-protectiveness and lack of effective control and discipline
- School-age child – social isolation and low self-esteem
- Adolescent – lack of independence, peer relationships and career choice

severe complex partial seizures impose considerable restrictions and limitations on the child's daily life, numerous seizures and prolonged status epilepticus being common occurrences. Again, 10–20% of children with epilepsy have additional disabilities such as mental retardation or cerebral palsy which place a further burden on the child and family (Hoare & Kerley 1991).

In common with other chronic illnesses, epilepsy can provoke maladaptive responses in the family at various stages during the illness. For instance, the fear of death or risk to life is very common among parents at the onset of the child's seizures. Similarly, the prospect of injury or permanent physical damage is a realistic fear for parents of some children who suffer repeated trauma from fits. Siblings are also likely to be affected by neglect of their own needs and sometimes the assumption of excessive responsibility for the welfare of their epileptic sibling. Hoare (1984b) found that the rate of psychiatric disturbance was significantly greater among the siblings of children with chronic epilepsy than among the siblings of children with newly diagnosed epilepsy, implying that continued treatment for epilepsy adversely affects the health of siblings.

Finally, epilepsy can impede the child's developmental progress in various ways throughout childhood. During the preschool period, excessive parental anxiety can produce over-protectiveness and a lack of effective discipline and control over the child. With the school age child, social isolation and low self-esteem become apparent, whereas with the adolescent, anxiety over lack of independence, peer relationships and career choice assume increased importance.

## Management of the child with epilepsy

The best management strategy for the child with epilepsy is based upon a collaborative model involving hospital and community resources. The hospital paediatrician should be responsible for the choice of anticonvulsant, which depends upon the accurate diagnosis of the seizure type, as well as for ensuring the regular monitoring of serum anticonvulsant levels. Treatment with the chosen anticonvulsant at the correct dosage is essential not only for the successful management of the medical aspects of epilepsy but also in the promotion of healthy psychosocial adjustment. Key elements of the latter include:

- the continuity of medical care by a specialist multidisciplinary out-patient service
- the provision of a clinic-based counselling service, particularly at the onset of treatment
- the detection and treatment of learning difficulties
- close liaison with schools and general practitioners.

Finally, referral to child psychiatric services can be useful sometimes for the more intractable behavioural or family problems associated with childhood epilepsy.

## Cerebral palsy

### Clinical features

This is a non-progressive, permanent motor disability involving paralysis or loss of movement (for instance hemiplegia), impairment of balance (for instance ataxic cerebral palsy) or involuntary movements (for instance choreo-athetoid cerebral palsy). The prevalence rate is approximately 2/1000. Aetiologically, pre-, peri- or postnatal factors are responsible, prematurity and low birth weight being of major importance in many cases.

The severity of the disability varies widely, ranging from a mild weakness affecting one limb to profound handicap involving all four limbs and associated with severe mental retardation. Problems usually arise in the first year of life when feeding difficulties, floppy or stiff limbs and delayed motor milestones become apparent. 50% of children with cerebral palsy have an IQ less than 70, though some children, particularly those with choreo-athetoid cerebral palsy, are of normal or above average intelligence. Cognitive development is adversely affected for two reasons. First, the brain damage causing the cerebral palsy also affects other areas of the brain responsible for cognitive function. Second, the physical restrictions and limitations imposed by the cerebral palsy may reduce the child's activities and opportunities for exploration and learning.

Children with cerebral palsy frequently have problems with language, perceptual and motor co-ordination skills. The language deficits involve not only articulatory problems caused by the cerebral palsy but also other aspects of language such as comprehension and expression. The perceptual problems may be visual, auditory or tactile, while the motor co-ordination problems involve the execution of skilled movements. A major consequence of these problems is that the child finds it difficult to perform everyday activities such as dressing, feeding or writing in a skilful manner.

### Psychiatric disturbance

The Isle of Wight study (Rutter et al 1970a) showed clearly that children with cerebral palsy were at least five times more likely to be disturbed than healthy children. The study also found that disturbed children with cerebral palsy showed the same range of disorders as other disturbed children, but that overactivity and autistic features were more common among the group of children who had mental retardation as well. Important contributing factors to the increased risk of disturbance are :

• underlying brain dysfunction

- rejection by peers and siblings
- poor self-image and low self-esteem
- the family disturbance which is frequently present
- learning difficulties.

Children with cerebral palsy are frequently teased and ridiculed by other children, which in turn further reduces the child's self-esteem. During adolescence, the sense of peer rejection and social isolation are likely to become more evident and disabling.

## Management

A comprehensive and co-ordinated multidisciplinary assessment, involving medical, physiotherapy, speech therapy, education and social work professionals, is clearly needed from the outset to meet the child's and family's varied needs. Regular review and reassessment of needs are also indicated. The promotion of the child's normal social development and long-term support for the family are an integral part of the treatment plan for the child and family. Specialist referral to psychiatric services may be necessary to meet the more intractable and complex emotional and behavioural problems.

## Cerebral tumours

### Clinical features

Cerebral tumours are the second most common childhood malignancies after the leukaemias. Unlike in adults, the tumours arise in deep structures of the brain such as the midbrain or cerebellum, so that the pressure symptoms caused by the growth of the tumour in a confined space dominate the clinical picture. The symptoms are often non-specific, for instance headache, irritability or aggression, while common signs are unsteadiness in walking or paralysis of the eye muscles, producing squints. The steady progression of the symptoms means that diagnosis is not usually in doubt.

### Psychiatric aspects

Treatment by surgical removal and/or brain irradiation causes considerable disability as well as increasing the risk of psychiatric disturbance. Post-treatment morbidity is high, with up to 50% showing signs of disturbance (Kun et al 1983). Educational problems such as general or specific learning difficulties are common and special schooling is necessary in many cases. Long-term survival is associated with considerable disability in many cases (Lannering et al 1990). This is more likely with an early age of presentation and also following cranial irradiation treatment.

## Head injury

### Clinical features

Trauma, particularly from road traffic accidents, is a major source of mortality and morbidity throughout childhood and young adult life, approximately 15% of children attending a hospital casualty department at least once a year. Though most injuries are minor with subsequent complete recovery, a significant minority are associated with long-term sequelae, most commonly severe head injury. Epidemiological studies of children involved in road traffic accidents have shown that they are not a random group of children, but rather have the following features:

- They are boys rather than girls
- They have adverse temperamental characteristics such as impulsivity, aggression, overactivity and distractibility
- They are associated with psychosocial disadvantage, for instance single or divorced parents, poor supervision or control and parents in manual or unskilled occupations.

### Cognitive and psychiatric outcome (Table 16.5)

Rutter and colleagues (Brown et al 1981, Chadwick et al 1981) conducted an influential prospective study into the psychiatric and cognitive sequelae of serious head injury in children. They found that the best predictor of outcome was the duration of the PTA (Post-traumatic amnesia) period, that is, the length of time between the accident and the subsequent re-emergence of continuous memory. They also found two other findings of general importance, a threshold effect and a dose–response relationship. For the subsequent development of cognitive or psychiatric sequelae, the minimum necessary period of PTA was 2 weeks or 1 week respectively. There was also a clear dose–response relationship between the PTA period and the severity

---

**Table 16.5** Cognitive and psychiatric sequelae of head injury in children

**Cognitive impairments**
- PTA greater than 2 weeks
- Dose-response relationship between severity of injury and cognitive impairment
- Recovery mainly in first year following injury
- Visuospatial or visuomotor deficits more common than verbal deficits

**Psychiatric outcome**
- Disturbance more likely when PTA greater than 1 week
- Disturbance occurs independently of any residual cognitive or neurological impairment
- Usual range of disorder, except that socially disinhibited behaviour more common
- Site of lesion unrelated to symptomatology, except depression is more common with right-sided frontal and left-sided posterior lesions

of the cognitive deficit, with definite effects more likely when the PTA period lasted longer than 3 weeks.

Cognitive impairments were more likely to involve visuospatial or visuomotor skills rather than verbal deficits and there was little evidence of an association between site of injury and the type of cognitive deficit. Follow-up of the children showed that most cognitive recovery and improvement occurred in the first year, though there was some evidence for continuing improvement into the second year, especially when the head injury was severe.

Chadwick et al (1981) found that psychiatric disorder was more likely to develop when the PTA period was greater than 1 week, though a dose–response relationship between adjustment and severity of injury was not so evident. The occurrence of disorder was independent of any residual neurological deficit or cognitive impairment. Generally, children had the usual range of disorders, but socially disinhibited behaviour was more common in children with severe head injury. Finally, most studies have not found a consistent relationship between the site of injury and the type of symptomatology, except that depression has been linked with right frontal and left posterior lesions (Shaffer 1985).

### Management

A comprehensive rehabilitation programme involving medical, physiotherapy, psychology and educational staff is required for many children with severe head injury. Clinical experience (Silver et al 1987) suggests that carbamazepine and propranolol can have a useful role in the management of the disinhibited and aggressive outbursts commonly found in this group of children.

## Spina bifida

### Clinical features

This condition, caused by failure of fusion of the vertebral arches of the spinal column, varies widely in severity from a simple anatomical defect to a major disability producing motor and sensory deficits, bowel and bladder dysfunction and hydrocephalus. Paediatric surgical practice has altered over the years, so that operative procedures are now only undertaken when the subsequent quality of life is likely to be reasonable. Despite this selective approach to treatment, many children with spina bifida still have considerable disabilities affecting bowel and bladder function as well as intermittent problems associated with the drainage shunts inserted to treat the hydrocephalus. Intellectually, the children are delayed and many are in the below average to mildly retarded range.

*Psychiatric aspects*

In common with other children who have chronic neurological problems, these children are at greater risk for psychiatric disturbance because of the associated neurological damage, cognitive deficits and maladaptive family responses. Adolescents seem particularly at risk, with a high rate of depressive symptoms, social isolation and low self-esteem together with embarrassment over bowel and bladder dysfunction and anxieties over sexual function and interests (Dorner 1976).

*Management*

Careful, co-ordinated and sensitive long-term support from the multidisciplinary team, including advice about education, is essential for satisfactory adjustment. Voluntary agencies and local support groups can be particularly useful in providing sensible help and advice for the parents and child with spina bifida. Referral for more specialist psychiatric advice is sometimes useful.

## PERCEPTUAL IMPAIRMENTS

The two major categories are deafness and blindness, or rarely both together.

### Deafness

*Clinical feature*

Deafness can be classified in various ways according to onset, severity or absolute amount of hearing loss.

The onset category is divided into two groups:

- prelingual (before onset of spoken language)
- postlingual (after onset of spoken speech).

The severity dimension comprises two categories:

- hard of hearing (able to use some communication skills)
- profoundly deaf (unable to use communication skills).

Absolute hearing loss is categorised according to the loss of hearing as measured in decibels (dB) :

- mild (25–40 dB)
- moderate (41–65 dB)
- severe (66–95 dB)
- profound (96+ dB).

Mild to moderate hearing loss is commonly due to disease of the middle ear such as secretory otitis media, whereas severe and profound deafness is often the result of sensorineural deafness associated with some genetically determined syndromes or following infection with rubella or cytomegalovirus. Currently available hearing aids enable many children with mild to moderate hearing loss to communicate effectively, so that deleterious effects on communication and social interaction are thereby reduced.

*Psychiatric aspects*

The two major determinants of long-term adjustment are the presence of additional handicaps and the severity of the deafness. Cerebral palsy, visual impairment and cognitive delay are more common among deaf children, so that developmental progress is frequently adversely affected. The severity of the deafness determines the child's ability not only to develop language but more crucially to acquire other communication and interpersonal skills along with the development of social relationships.

Freeman et al (1975) found that 20% of deaf children had significant behaviour problems, with restlessness, dependency and aggression prominent features. An important factor determining the psychological adjustment was the presence or absence of communication difficulties in the deaf child.

*Management*

Skilled intervention and support from knowledgeable professionals are essential in the promotion of the normal development of the deaf child. A major but unresolved dilemma for many parents and professionals is the best means to develop communication skills, that is, whether to rely on aural methods alone, whether to promote the acquisition of sign language or whether to use a combination of both. A clear-cut decision is often not possible, so that the best policy is to choose the method(s) on the basis of individual assessment and to review progress regularly.

Psychiatric assessment and intervention often require the assistance of an interpreter or other experienced professional in order to understand the problem accurately and also to be able to communicate helpful and realistic suggestions about management.

## Blindness

*Clinical features*

Visual impairment has many causes such as the rare genetic syndromes, retinal fibroplasia of prematurity and prenatal rubella infection. The majority of severe cases usually become evident around birth or soon thereafter. Despite this, clinical experience shows that professionals are sometimes initially reluctant to accept parental concern about the child's visual abilities, a factor that greatly increases parental anguish and anxiety when the condition is subsequently correctly identified. Severe visual impairment requiring special schooling has a prevalence rate of 4/10 000 with additional disabilities such as cerebral palsy or learning difficulties quite common. Developmental delay, present in up to 70% of visually impaired children, is the other important factor determining outcome and adjustment.

Blindness affects the child's development in two main ways, interaction with the environment and development of the self concept. Visual impairment radically limits the child's ability to explore and investigate his immediate surroundings, so that his concepts of the external world are slow to develop. This is further exacerbated by the restriction on mobility imposed by the visual impairment. The child's rate of progress is therefore much slower. For the parents, these problems can be compounded by the child's failure to respond to and be interested in the visual world.

These handicaps increase further the child's difficulty in developing a sense of himself as a distinct and separate individual who relates to but is separate from other aspects of the environment. Concepts of time, continuity, separation and distance are extremely difficult for the blind child to comprehend.

## Psychiatric disorder

Freeman (1977), reviewing the available research findings, found that approximately 40% of blind children showed moderate to severe signs of disturbance. Feeding and sleep disorders are common in the younger child, while social isolation and stereotypies are prominent in older children. The stereotypies include hand-flapping, rocking and eye-pressing. These were previously known by the special term blindisms. This term is not useful, as the stereotypies in blind children probably arise for the same reasons as in other children, that is sensory deprivation, boredom, self-stimulation and sometimes anxiety.

During adolescence, social relationships and anxiety about sexual interests are common.

## Management

Parents require expert advice and guidance from the outset to enable them to maximise their child's developmental potential. Toys with strong tactile or auditory features are extremely useful. Special school provision is essential for children with marked visual impairment. The promotion of language skills and the acquisition of Braille are important not only in their own right but also as an aid to cognition and in the development of concepts about the outside world and its functioning. Residential schooling is often beneficial for the older child and adolescent, as it provides them with social activities and the opportunity to develop social relationships. Teachers and other staff members are able to give sensible advice about future career prospects and job opportunities.

## MISCELLANEOUS DISORDERS AND CONDITIONS

### The burned child

Burns are second only to road traffic accidents as a cause of accidental death in childhood (Campbell & McIntosh 1992). Severe burns are physically, psychologically and socially catastrophic, requiring prolonged hospitalisation and long-term rehabilitation (Sawyer et al 1983, Stoddard et al 1989). Four phases can be recognised:

- pre-injury predisposing factors
- the acute injury stage
- the reparative and rehabilitation phase
- long-term adjustment.

*Pre-injury predisposing factors*

Preschool children from overcrowded, poorly supervised home backgrounds and those with certain temperamental characteristics such as impulsivity, recklessness or overactivity are particularly vulnerable. Preschool children are also at risk of non-accidental injury from their parents, for instance by cigarette burns or from scalding with hot water.

*Acute injury phase*

The psychological aspects of this phase include:

- management of severe pain and distress
- the acute stressful response to the hospital admission and to the necessity for frightening and/or painful procedures
- sometimes an acute confusional state produced by the severity of the injury and/or the medication to reduce the distress.

The acute confusional state may include acute anxiety symptoms, disorientation in time and place as well as hallucinations, illusions or delusions.

*Reparative and rehabilitation phase*

A serious burn injury requires frequent and often painful procedures to ensure satisfactory healing followed by numerous plastic surgery operations to tackle the subsequent cosmetic and functional disabilities. Debridement, the application and removal of antibacterial dressings, and bed linen changes are routine procedures that can become sources of anxiety and tension between child and staff. Children's responses vary markedly, from overt opposition to passive compliance. Dependent and regressive behaviour, as well as attention-seeking and defiant behaviour, are also common. Specific psychological techniques such as relaxation training and hypnosis have been used successfully for the many distressing treatment procedures often necessary with burned children.

The involvement of the parents during this stage is vital. The parental sense of guilt and responsibility for the injury, whether realistic or not, is a prominent feature, so that the opportunity for counselling about this topic is important. The participation of the child's parents in the treatment programme is not only helpful for the child but also of assistance to the staff.

### Long-term adjustment

Discharge from hospital and re-integration into the community, particularly re-entry to school, are stressful stages that require careful planning and consideration. Anticipation of problems and the proposed subsequent response are important aspects of the discussions between the staff and the child and family prior to discharge. A planned school visit by the child with a hospital staff member is a useful preliminary to school return.

Finally, the child may also benefit at this stage from skilled individual psychotherapeutic help to enable him to adjust to the marked changes in his appearance and physique consequent on the injury. In many cases, the child and family may require long-term support following discharge from hospital.

## Diabetes

### Clinical features

Diabetes in childhood (prevalence rate 2/1000) usually presents acutely, with marked symptoms such as abdominal pain, excessive thirst, increased urine production and weight loss, or even more dramatically as diabetic coma from ketoacidosis. There is a total or near total failure of insulin production by the pancreas, so that the child requires life-long injection of insulin and strict dietary control.

The medical management of childhood diabetes has two main phases, the initial institution of the insulin and dietary regime and the long-term supervision of diabetic control. The introduction of the treatment regime is usually carried out in hospital, where the child and parents are taught the principles of insulin injection, dietary management and urine testing for diabetic control. Subsequently, the child and parents attend the diabetic clinic where the multidisciplinary team of doctors, nurses and dieticians review regularly the various aspects of diabetic management.

*Psychiatric aspects*

Though many studies have been carried out into the psychiatric morbidity of diabetic children, the results have been conflicting, usually because of the wide variation in the age range of children in the various studies and also because of the use of non-standardised measures of psychiatric assessment. Despite this confusion, the consensus view is that children with diabetes are more at risk for psychiatric disorder than healthy children (Johnson 1988). Most studies have shown that children with diabetes have the same range of disorders as other disturbed children with no evidence of any specific type of psychopathology.

Disturbance commonly arises through two mechanisms operating separately or sometimes in combination. First, the limitations and restrictions imposed by diabetes result directly in the child developing symptoms such as anxiety, depression or low self-esteem. Second, the burden of diabetic management compromises a precariously functioning family where inadequate parental care and control and family conflict are already present.

A particularly important problem is the management of the adolescent with diabetes, as successful management depends upon the resolution of the normal adolescent conflicts surrounding control and autonomy against the need for a well-regulated life style.

*Management*

The multidisciplinary diabetic team is usually able to manage most of the emotional and behavioural problems shown by the children and their families through a combination of advice, counselling and individual support. A recent evaluation of the diabetic service at a children's hospital (Bloomfield et al 1990) found, surprisingly, that the presence of an additional specialist counselling and support service did not have any long-term effect on adjustment. There are however several features of the study that may explain this unexpected result:

- the overall rate of disturbance among the children was low
- the routine service provided by the clinic was comprehensive and thorough
- the children in the study were mainly prepubertal, with a mean age of 9 years.

Consequently, it would be unwise to generalise from the findings of this study.

Sometimes, however, referral to psychiatric services is necessary. Behavioural techniques, family therapy and group therapy, particularly for adolescents, are frequently used. Minuchin and colleagues (1975) have proposed that children with diabetes and their families are an example of the so-called psychosomatic family which shows a distinct type of psychopathology (see Ch. 17 for more detailed discussion). This group also believed that structural family therapy was especially useful in resolving such maladaptive patterns of interaction, though the available evidence for this is not conclusive.

Finally, admission to hospital for a combined paediatric and psychiatric approach is sometimes necessary to treat the more intractable problems of compliance and poor diabetic control. Very occasionally, the admission may reveal that the poor control is caused by Munchausen syndrome by proxy (Meadow 1982), usually involving the mother.

## Asthma

### Clinical features

Asthma is a disease characterised by the episodic and recurrent increase in resistance to air entry into the lungs. It is a common condition affecting approximately 5% of children depending upon diagnostic criteria. The onset is usually in the preschool period with a favourable long-term outcome in most cases.

Traditionally, the disease is regarded as the classical psychosomatic illness, psychological factors having a role not only in the onset of the illness but also in determining its course. By contrast, contemporary views emphasise the importance of genetic and allergic factors in the predisposition to the disorder, while psychological factors are involved in the precipitation and severity of individual attacks. The cornerstone of medical management is the correct usage of bronchodilators, prompt treatment of respiratory infection and the judicious usage of steroids. The promotion of a normal lifestyle with minimal restrictions is also important.

### Psychiatric aspects

Rutter et al (1970b), in the Isle of Wight study, found that children with asthma were twice as likely to be disturbed as healthy children. Paediatricians are usually able in most cases to successfully manage any emotional or behavioural problems in asthmatic children. Specialist referral to psychiatric services is sometimes necessary for specific treatment(s) such as a behavioural relaxation programme to reduce anxiety over asthmatic attacks or family therapy for intractable family dysfunction. Lask & Matthew (1979) showed that brief, focused family therapy to improve communication within the family was not only successful in that regard but also produced an objective improvement in respiratory function as well.

## Congenital malformations

Cleft lip and palate — prevalence rate 3/2000 — and hypospadias (the opening of the external urethral orifice on the underside of the penis rather than at the tip) — prevalence rate 1/350 male births — are the two congenital malformations most likely to be associated with psychiatric disturbance.

### Cleft lip and palate

Parents of the child with cleft lip or palate are understandably shocked and dismayed initially at the sight of their child's disfigurement. Current paediatric practice involves early surgical intervention to correct the deformity. Parents require advice about feeding problems and also information about the likely outcome, usually very favourable in most cases. Pictures of other similarly affected children pre- and postoperatively are often very reassuring to parents in the early stages. Advice from an audiologist or a speech therapist may also be useful in promoting language development.

Older children with some residual disfigurement are often teased by their peers, so that counselling and social skills training are necessary to encourage satisfactory adjustment.

### Hypospadias

Early and repeated surgical operations are necessary to correct this anatomical deformity. Follow-up studies of treated children (Schultz 1983) show that this group of children are likely to have anxieties about their sexual attractiveness and competence and also lower self-esteem than their peers.

## Congenital heart disease

Congenital heart disease — prevalence rate 1/150 children — is the most common congenital malformation, with a wide range of severity from relatively benign conditions to those with a fatal or inoperable outcome. There is a genetic component to many lesions, which are often part of another syndrome such as Down's.

Children with serious heart lesions and their families clearly require long-term support and commitment from the paediatric medical and surgical teams. Careful preparation for and explanation of the procedures are essential not only for the parents but also for the child, depending on his age and cognitive development. Psychological disturbance is twice as common among this group of children, with over-protectiveness and decreased independence common problems (Kramer et al 1989). Cognitive development and educational attainments are usually within the normal range for most children, though as a group their IQ tends to be lower than their siblings. Finally, expert counselling and support are necessary for those parents whose child has an inoperable lesion or when the cardiac operation has had a fatal outcome.

## HIV-spectrum disease

### Clinical features

Infection with human immune deficiency virus (HIV) and the development of AIDS (acquired immune deficiency syndrome) is an increasingly important aspect of contemporary paediatric practice. The virus can be transmitted in several ways:

- by contamination with transfused blood products, previously commonly in boys with haemophilia
- through contaminated blood products from the syringes of drug-abusing adolescents
- though sexual molestation of children by HIV-positive adults
- by vertical transmission from HIV-positive mothers to their offspring during the perinatal period.

The latter currently accounts for approximately 80% of paediatric cases. Follow-up studies of children HIV-positive at birth indicate that approximately 20% are still positive at 18 months.

The central nervous system is a major site for HIV infection, so that widespread neurological and cognitive impairment is likely with the development of AIDS (Krenner & Millar 1989). Indeed, an AIDS dementia complex (ADC) has been reported in older children and adolescents with established AIDS. Features include impaired concentration and attention, memory loss, mild frontal lobe dysfunction and difficulty with complex sequential cognitive tasks. Magnetic resonance imaging (MRI) shows that the white matter of the brain is affected more than the grey matter.

### Psychiatric aspects

The psychiatric skills involved with the treatment of HIV-spectrum disease are multiple and include the assessment and identification of developmental, neuropsychiatric and affective symptomatology as well as the management of life-threatening illness. An important practical decision in many cases is whether the HIV-positive infant should remain with the drug-abusing mother or whether alternative long-term care arrangements are necessary. Finally, a sad but increasingly common clinical situation is the predicament posed by the death of the drug-abusing mother from AIDS, often leaving the child an orphan. Skilled counselling and support are vital for the mother and child in this aspect of management.

## MISCELLANEOUS TOPICS

### Hospitalisation

Admission to hospital is unfortunately a common experience during childhood, approximately 25% of children having been admitted on at least one occasion by the age of 4 years. For most children, this is a short admission for a brief, treatable illness, while a minority, approximately 4%, remain in hospital for at least a month. While most parents and children cope successfully with the admission, children who are repeatedly admitted with minor illnesses often show evidence of disturbance that may have been the reason for admitting the child to hospital in the first place (Quinton & Rutter 1976).

Admission to hospital can have adverse effects in the short term as well as in the long term. Bowlby (1969) wrote extensively about the immediate and distressing effects upon the preschool child of short-term separation from the mother. He described the sequence of the separation reaction in terms of protest, despair and detachment (see Ch. 2). At the time that Bowlby observed these reactions in young children, it was the usual hospital practice to restrict contact between parents and child during hospitalisation in the belief that this reduced the likelihood of the child being exposed to infection. Contemporary paediatric medical and nursing practice recognises the importance of continued contact between the parents and the child during hospitalisation, so that open-access visiting is strongly encouraged and the parents are active participants in many of the procedures involved in the care of the ill child.

Table 16.6 summarises the main factors determining the child's response to hospitalisation. The contributory factors can be grouped under three headings:

- child and family factors
- the nature of the illness
- the policy and practices of the hospital and its staff.

*Child and family factors* include the child's age and temperament, any previous experience of hospital, the quality of the parent–child relationship and the current family circumstances. Children between the ages of 1 and 4 years are particularly affected by separation from familiar figures. Consequently, parents should be actively encouraged to maintain contact with the child and to visit regularly throughout. Children with adverse temperamental characteristics such as poor adaptability or irregularity of habits are more likely to be adversely affected by admission than other children.

Children also vary in their repertoire of coping strategies. An active rather than a passive response-style to stressful situations is more likely to be adaptive and to facilitate adjustment to hospitalisation (Petersen 1989). The child's previous experience of hospital, if any, will also influence the

**Table 16.6**    Factors affecting the child's adjustment to hospitalisation

**Child and Family**
• Age
• Temperament
• Child's coping strategies
• Previous experience of hospital
• Parent–child relationship
• Current family circumstances

**Nature of illness**
• Emergency/routine admission
• Type of illness
• Associated pain
• Necessity for painful procedures

**Policy and practices of hospital and its staff**
• Rooming-in facilities
• Organisation of ward routine
• Visiting arrangements
• Adequate provision of play staff and teachers
• Preparation of child for painful procedures
• Training of the nursing and medical staff to minimise the child's distress and to respond appropriately to the child's anxiety

**Note:** Short-and long-term effects are possible

response to the current admission. For instance, if previous contact was favourable, then subsequent admissions are likely to be less stressful. If the parent–child relationship was unsatisfactory prior to admission, hospitalisation is likely to exacerbate this problem because of the additional stress associated with admission. Adverse family circumstances such as marital disharmony or financial hardship may also be exacerbated by the child's admission to hospital.

*The nature of the illness* also influences the response to hospitalisation. Some illnesses, for instance burns, are more frightening and distressing than others, and there is a wide variation in the amount of associated pain. Again, painful procedures such as debridement for burns or bone marrow aspirations are more likely with some illnesses than with others. Finally, an acute or emergency admission to hospital is likely to be more stressful than an elective or routine admission.

*The policy and the practices of the hospital and its staff* can considerably reduce the distress associated with hospitalisation (Table 16.7). Whenever possible, the parents and child should visit the ward prior to admission. The hospital should provide the parents and the child with a booklet explaining the unfamiliar aspects of hospital practice such as admission procedures or ward routines. With young children, the parents should be encouraged to read the child a story book explaining about hospital and what happens there. Good rooming-in facilities for parents and active encouragement of visiting by parents and siblings are also beneficial.

**Table 16.7**   Principles of good practice to lessen the distress of hospitalisation

---

- Preparation for admission whenever possible
- Opportunity for parents and child to visit ward prior to admission
- Parents and child to read story book about hospital
- Good rooming-in facilities for parents
- Active encouragement of visiting by parents and siblings
- Child-centred approach to the organisation of the ward routine
  - Flexible approach to meal/bedtimes
  - Allocation of individual nurses to each child
  - Training of nursing/medical staff to minimise distress
  - Adequate preparation for unpleasant clinical procedures
  - Ward play staff and teachers to provide play and teaching materials
- Ready availability of social work, psychology and psychiatric support services
- Opportunity for ward staff to discuss psychosocial problems
  - Joint liaison meetings between paediatric and psychiatric teams
  - Staff support group

---

The organisation of the ward routine should be centred around the needs of the child rather than the staff. For instance, there should be a flexible approach to meal and bedtimes in order to encourage a less institutionalised atmosphere on the ward. Additionally, the daily shift routine of the ward should ensure that each child has a designated nurse who is primarily responsible for his care. The senior nursing and medical personnel should ensure that their junior staff receive adequate training in the more sensitive aspects of paediatric practice, including management of the child's distress, the ability to console and comfort the distressed child and preparation for painful procedures. Play leaders and teachers should also be readily available on the ward, so that the children have the opportunity to engage in play activities and also to receive education when appropriate. The play staff are often an important source of emotional support for the child, as their more informal and relaxed approach may facilitate the child's expression of concerns and anxieties.

The paediatric medical and nursing staff should also have access to social work, psychological and psychiatric services in order to meet the social and emotional needs of the children. A common and useful practice is to have a regular joint 'psychosocial ward round' involving paediatric social work and psychiatric staff. The success of this approach is, however, crucially dependent on the involvement and encouragement from the senior staff of the participating professions. Finally, many specialised paediatric services such as neonatal intensive care or burns units have established staff support groups to enable the staff to discuss their own anxieties about working in such a stressful environment. The child psychiatrist or any other similarly

**Table 16.8**   Breaking bad news to parents: principles of good practice

- Most senior doctor should see the parents
- Interview both parents together
- Privacy for interview is essential
- Begin the interview by asking parents about their knowledge of the problem
- Tell parents frankly and honestly using simple and non-technical language
  - nature of the problem
  - explanation for investigations
  - basis for the diagnosis
- Encourage parents to ask questions
- Emphasise the positive as well as the negative aspects of the diagnosis, e.g.
  - child able to have physiotherapy and special equipment
  - child able to go to school
  - effective control of pain possible
- Facilitate the expression of emotions by the parents
- Offer further opportunity to talk about the problem
- Many parents find it helpful to continue the discussion with nurse or social worker after the interview

trained professional can often perform a useful role in the organisation and supervision of the staff support group.

## Breaking bad news to parents

This distressing but inevitable aspect of paediatric care comes in various guises, for instance, the birth of a child with Down's syndrome or the diagnosis of cystic fibrosis. Unfortunately, most undergraduate and postgraduate training includes very little teaching about this important topic.

While the details vary with each case, Table 16.8 summarises the important general principles. There are several reasons why the most senior clinician involved with the child's care should be responsible for meeting the parents to discuss the child's problems. First, the parents are more likely to respect his/her knowledge and experience. Second, the senior clinician is more likely to be able to answer the parents' questions in a more authoritative and knowledge manner. Third, the presence of the senior clinician is an acknowledgement to the parents of the seriousness of the problem and the importance that is attached to the discussion.

It is essential to make every effort to ensure that both parents are seen together. This not only reduces the misinformation that may arise between the parents but also allows them to be mutually supportive from the outset. The clinician should also set aside an adequate length of time for the interview, so that the parents are aware that they have the undivided attention of the clinician. It is wrong to arrange the interview at the end of a ward round or of an out-patient session when only a brief period is available. The interview should also take place in complete privacy, not only as a matter of courtesy and dignity to the parents but also because this will allow them to express their emotions more freely.

After the initial introductions, it is often useful to begin by asking the parents about their knowledge of the child's problems. This provides the clinician not only with invaluable information about their views but also with the opportunity to assess their appreciation of the seriousness of the problem as well as whether there is any discrepancy in their view of the problem.

The next stage involves the clinician telling the parents frankly and honestly the nature of the problem, the explanation for the investigations and the basis for the diagnosis. Clearly, simple and non-technical language must be used in this discussion. The clinician should then encourage the parents to ask questions about the situation. The use of open-ended questions, for instance asking the parents to elaborate on their understanding of the diagnosis, is helpful. The clinician should also emphasise the positive as well as the negative aspects of the diagnosis. For instance, the child will be able to have physiotherapy and will also be provided with special equipment to increase mobility, the child should be able to continue to attend school and effective pain relief will be available when necessary.

The clinician should facilitate expression of emotion by the parents through a sensitive and sympathetic response to their distress and crying. The interview should conclude with a definite offer from the clinician of a further appointment to talk things over again. Finally, many parents find it helpful to continue the discussion with a nurse or social worker after the interview with the clinician has finished.

The importance of these guidelines has been confirmed in a recent study by Wooley et al (1989). This retrospective study involved interviewing the parents of 70 children who had life-threatening illnesses. The parents appreciated greatly the opportunity to discuss the implications of the illness at an open, sympathetic, direct and uninterrupted interview at the time of diagnosis. They disliked evasive, unsympathetic or brief interviews. Perhaps surprisingly, the degree of satisfaction or dissatisfaction with the interview was not influenced by the current psychiatric morbidity of the parents, though the assessment measures used to assess the latter were not necessarily the most sensitive or appropriate.

## Care of the dying child

Death in childhood is an uncommon event in developed countries. There are nearly 11 000 childhood deaths in the UK each year, 4000 in the neonatal period, 50% acute and unexpected and about 1600 from degenerative disorders and malignancies.

Sudden or unexpected death is often the most difficult for families and health professionals to manage as by definition there has been little preparation for the event. Hospital staff have usually no previous contact with the child or family, so that knowledge about their personalities and domestic circumstances is lacking. The burden of follow-up and subsequent support is the responsibility of the primary health care and community resources. That response may be fragmentary and uncoordinated, so that families often feel that their needs have not been adequately met.

By contrast, the care of the child with terminal illness and his family is usually the focus of considerable concern and attention from hospital and community resources. Goldman et al (1990) have reviewed the options available, including the relative merits of hospital, hospice or home care. Parents usually undergo two periods of grief response when the child enters the terminal phase of the illness, firstly, at the onset of this phase (the *initial phase*) and then at the approach of death (the *terminal phase*). These phases show the features of the normal grief response, that is shock and numbness, denial, the development of somatic symptoms and/or affective features such as anger, anxiety or depression. This is usually followed by some degree of acceptance. Parents often feel guilty that they may be relieved at the approach of death in their child and need encouragement to be able to express these thoughts.

Concern is often expressed about what to tell the child. This is clearly influenced by the child's age and intelligence. Below the age of 5 years, children have little realistic appreciation of the permanence of death and its irreversibility. Subsequently, they begin to acquire more adult-like concepts of death. The child's conceptualisation of death is also facilitated if he has had first hand experience of it, for instance the death of a member of the family or of a family pet. Dying teenagers often present the most difficulty. The full realisation of the permanence of death frequently leads to regression, anger and aggressive outbursts.

Generally speaking, current paediatric practice is to facilitate discussion with the child about his illness and its implications. Parental wishes should, however, be respected, while nevertheless indicating to the parents the advantages of a more open attitude. Consequently, there are no absolute rules but a sensitive and flexible approach is most likely to be beneficial. Recent research (Wooley et al 1991) has emphasised the value of a 'key worker' in helping the child and family make a more satisfactory adjustment to the implications of the disease and its outcome. All families should be offered the opportunity of bereavement counselling following the death of the child in order to facilitate their subsequent adjustment. Predictors of poor long-term adjustment include:

• premature changes in life-style in response to the child's death, for instance a rapid change of job or occupation
• retention of the child's possessions for more than a year after the death

- a too early new pregnancy
- prolonged and extensive involvement with charitable organisations related to the child's disease.

## Stillbirth and neonatal death

The stillbirth rate (the number of infants born after the 28th week of gestation who do not breathe or show other signs of life per 1000 total births) and the neonatal mortality rate (the number of deaths in the first 27 days of life per 1000 live births) are currently 5 and 4.5 respectively in the UK. Placental abnormalities and congenital malformations are the common causes of stillbirths, while respiratory distress syndrome, congenital malformations and birth complications are the main causes of neonatal death.

Recently, several authors (Forrest et al 1981, 1982, Bourne & Lewis 1991) have reviewed the psychological impact of these conditions as well as proposing ways to alleviate the associated distress. Parental responses vary considerably, though most couples are profoundly shocked initially. This is then followed by a bereavement response for the loss of the child. Hospital staff should be sensitive and responsive to the parents' feelings and wishes.

The issue of a certificate of stillbirth or a death certificate and the arrangements for the funeral are particularly distressing for the parents. Mourning is facilitated by providing the parents with the opportunity to see and hold their dead child as well as having a photograph to remember the child. The results of investigations, including post-mortem examination should be communicated to the parents to allay their anxiety and also to advise them about future pregnancies. Grief counselling does seem to facilitate the mourning process (Forrest et al 1982).

Oglethorpe (1989), reviewing the evidence about subsequent parenting following perinatal bereavement, argues cogently for the adoption of the above principles in order to assist the parents to make a satisfactory adjustment. The author also suggests that these procedures also reduce the risk of the 'replacement child syndrome' in future pregnancies.

## Sudden infant death syndrome (SIDS)

This is the commonest cause of death in infants between 1 month and the end of the first year, with a prevalence rate of 2–3/1000 live births. The peak instance is between the fourth and sixth months. The sudden and unexpected nature of the event produces a profound effect on parents with shock, disbelief and numbness followed by a bereavement response. The mourning may continue for several months.

The family doctor and the health visitor usually have important roles for the family during this period. Skilled counselling is essential, as most parents inevitably feel responsible for the child's death and are over-critical of themselves in consequence. Several charitable support groups such as the Foundation for the Study of Infant Deaths provide a useful source of support for some parents.

The provision of home monitoring facilities to alert the parents if a child develops respiratory difficulties requires careful consideration. False alarms are frequent, thereby increasing parental tension and anxiety. Understandably, there is considerable stress within the family in the months subsequent to the child's death, with a likely exacerbation of any pre-existing difficulties in the marital relationship.

# 17. Treatment in child and adolescent psychiatry

## INTRODUCTION (TABLE 17.1)

Several factors are usually responsible for the development of psychiatric disturbance in children, so that it is unlikely that a single treatment method will resolve the problem(s). All treatment approaches rely on common elements that are not only desirable but also essential for a successful outcome. These elements include:

- active co-operation between the therapist, the child and the family
- general agreement about the aims of treatment
- a mutual trust to enable the achievement of the aims.

As the relative efficacy of different treatment approaches is not clearly established for many disorders, the choice of treatment is often based on the therapist's training and experience rather than an absolute indication for a particular approach in many instances. In clinical practice, several approaches are often used simultaneously or sequentially in order to help resolve the different aspects of the problem(s) for the child and family.

Two other notable features characteristic of contemporary child psychiatry practice in the UK are first, active therapeutic collaboration between the different professional disciplines and second, the use of co-therapy or joint therapeutic work in many clinics and departments. The collaborative

**Table 17.1** Treatment principles in child and adolescent psychiatry

- Several factors are usually responsible for the development of disturbance
- All treatments share common elements that are necessary and essential for successful outcome
    - active co-operation between therapist, the child and the family
    - agreement between the therapist, the child and the family on the aims of treatment
    - mutual trust to enable the achievement of the aims
- Choice of treatment approach often a reflection of therapist's training and experience
- Few absolute indications for one particular approach rather than another in many cases
- Several treatment approaches may be used simultaneously or sequentially to help resolve the different aspects of the problems for the child and family

participation of psychiatrists, social workers and clinical psychologists is thought to be beneficial as this enables varying professional skills to be used in the treatment of different aspects of the clinical problem(s).

Joint or co-therapy is practised particularly when family therapy is the treatment method. This is usually carried out in one of two ways. First, the therapists interview and see the family together each time they attend the clinic. Second, one therapist interviews the family, while the other therapist(s) observes the interview. The latter approach is often carried out through the use of a one-way screen or closed-circuit television system to enable 'live' observation and supervision of the family therapy session. This approach is particularly useful for trainee child psychiatrists who have thereby an unrivalled opportunity for supervision of their clinical work. The approach does, however, make considerable demands upon staff resources in the clinic, so that it is probably only justified in specialised training or teaching centres.

Irrespective of the treatment approach adopted, the formulation of the clinical problem undertaken during the initial diagnostic assessment interview(s) should provide the basis for the treatment plan (see Ch. 4). Four dimensions are critically important in determining the components of this. These are:

● the individual features of the problem
● the current level and stage of family functioning
● school factors
● community factors (Table 17.2).

The range, duration and severity of symptomatology influence the treatment method chosen. For instance, circumscribed problems such as sleep disorder in the preschool child should respond effectively to a behavioural approach, whereas extensive early emotional deprivation combined with a current failure in interpersonal relationships may require prolonged individual psychotherapy. The age and ability of the child also affect the treatment options: for instance, cognitive strategies are not possible with younger children. Finally, the co-existence of physical illness or handicap may not only impose limitations or restrictions on the child's abilities but also act as an additional burden which further affects the child's long-term adjustment and self-esteem.

Three aspects of the family's functioning affect the choice of treatment:

● the developmental stage of the family's life cycle
● the parents' capabilities and relationships
● the family's interactional patterns.

Like the individual, the family undergoes a series of changes or developmental stages during its life span (McGoldrick & Carter 1982). For some families, certain stages are more problematic or difficult than

**Table 17.2**   Factors determining the choice of treatment programme(s)

Careful analysis of the following elements is necessary to devise a treatment programme

- Individual characteristics
    - range, severity and duration of symptomatology
    - age and cognitive ability
    - physical illness or handicap
- Family
    - developmental stage, for instance a family with preschool children or one with adolescents
    - psychiatric health of parents
    - marital relationship
    - parenting qualities
    - communication within the family
    - ability to resolve conflict
    - support network, for instance availability of extended family
- School
    - scholastic attainments
    - attitude of child and parent(s) to authority or school
    - peer relationships
- Community
    - quality of peer relationships and of role models
    - neighbourhood and community resources

others. For instance, the prominent role of nurtural and control tasks in the family with preschool children is in marked contrast to the conflicts over autonomy and independence so characteristic of the family with adolescent children.

The parents' current psychiatric adjustment and marital relationship may be so impaired that they require treatment in their own right before attending to the needs of the child. Again, the competence of the parents to fulfil the parental role affects the treatment options available.

The quality of the family's communication patterns and its skills in conflict resolution and problem solving are important factors determining whether a family therapy approach is suitable or appropriate. Finally, the availability of additional support from the extended family or from other community resources may be extremely useful to families whose coping capacity is likely to remain precarious on a long-term basis.

Information about the child's academic progress at school as well as his relationships with teachers and other pupils is essential not only because this may indicate the need for specialist help but also because schooling may be a source of satisfaction and enhanced self-esteem for a child in an otherwise unsatisfactory situation. Similarly, information about the child's own neighbourhood and community may enable the mobilisation of local resources to improve the facilities and opportunities available to the child and the family.

This chapter is mainly concerned with the description of current treatment methods in child psychiatry, while the last section reviews the evidence for the efficacy of psychotherapeutic treatments, the most commonly used form of treatment.

## TREATMENT METHODS

Psychiatric treatments can be divided into two broad groups, physical and psychological. Physical methods include drugs, ECT and psychosurgery. The last two methods are so rarely used in child psychiatry that they will not be discussed further (see Kendell & Zealley 1993 for further details). Psychological treatments (the psychotherapies) are treatments that use psychological methods to relieve distress and produce improvement. A wide range of methods are used including individual therapy, behaviour therapy, family therapy and group therapy as well as counselling and advice for parents.

The last part of this section discusses other treatment approaches such as residential treatment programmes and liaison/consultation work. In the latter the child psychiatrist or a member of the child psychiatric team works with the professionals directly involved with the disturbed child rather than with the child himself in order to enable them to manage the child more effectively. This approach is popular for paediatric problems and also as a way of helping staff to manage disturbed children in residential institutions such as children's homes or schools.

## DRUG TREATMENT

Recent reviews (Campbell & Spencer 1988, Gadow 1992) indicate that the absence of clear syndrome definitions for many child psychiatric disorders combined with the failure to conduct adequately designed double-blind trials has limited the use of drugs as a method of treatment in child psychiatry. Concern has also been expressed about the use of powerful psychotropic drugs in children whose growth and development may be adversely affected. Consequently, drugs are mainly used on an empirical and individual basis in situations where their clinical value has already been established. They are most effective in the treatment of specific symptoms, producing symptomatic relief rather than a curative effect in most cases. They should therefore only be used for a defined period of time, and with the additional proviso that the necessity for continued usage is reviewed regularly. Table 17.3 summarises the main indications for drug treatment in child psychiatry.

**Table 17.3** Drug treatment in child psychiatry

| Drug | Usage | Comment |
| --- | --- | --- |
| **Anxiolytics** | Anxiety/phobic conditions | Short-term adjunct to behaviour treatment |
| **Neuroleptics** | | |
| Phenothiazines, e.g. chlorpromazine | Schizophrenia/hyperkinetic syndrome | Extrapyramidal side effects common |
| Butyrophenones, e.g. Haloperidol | Complex tics/Tourette's syndrome | Extrapyramidal side effects common |
| **Tricyclic antidepressants** | | |
| Imipramine/amitriptyline | Enuresis | Effective, but high relapse rate |
| Clomipramine | Major affective disorder | Most useful with persistent and sustained mood disturbance |
| **Stimulants** | | |
| Methylphenidate | Hyperkinetic syndrome | Effective in the short term |
| | | Long-term effects on growth, sleep and appetite |
| Fenfluramine | Pervasive developmental disorder | Effectiveness not established |
| | | Side effects include irritability, anorexia and weight loss |
| **Hypnotics,** e.g. trimeprazine/promethazine | Persistent sleep disorder in pre-school children | Only short-term |
| **Lithium** | Recurrent bipolar affective disorder | Close supervision of blood level for signs of toxicity |
| **Laxatives,** e.g. bulk-forming (methylcellulose), stimulants (senna), softener (dioctyl) | Encopresis with constipation | Facilitates formation and passage of faeces |
| **Central alpha-agonist,** e.g. clonidine | Unresponsive Tourette's syndrome | Sedation and rebound hypertension |

## Anxiolytics

*Indications.* Benzodiazepines such as diazepam or chlordiazepoxide are not used very much in the treatment of childhood anxiety states. Their most common use is as part of a combined treatment programme for severe school refusal. In this instance, the drug is usually taken prior to the child leaving home to go to school. Diazepam has also been used in some sleep disorders such as night terrors. Recently, propranolol, a beta-adrenergic blocker, has been used to treat the somatic symptoms of anxiety and also in acute anxiety states associated with post-traumatic stress disorder.

*Dosage.* Diazepam up to 15 mg daily in divided doses.

*Side effects.* Drowsiness and dry mouth.

*Comment.* Dependency problem with long-term usage. Prescription in short-term only.

## Neuroleptics/major tranquillisers

### Phenothiazines

*Indications.* Phenothiazines such as chlorpromazine are used to treat acute psychotic symptoms associated with schizophrenia or hypomania. Previously, the sedative properties of chlorpromazine were used to treat the overactive behaviour of the hyperkinetic syndrome. Regular fortnightly intramuscular injections of depot phenothiazines such as fluphenazine decanoate are used as a maintenance treatment in the prevention of relapses in chronic schizophrenia.

*Dosage.* Wide variation, depending upon the symptomatology, some-times up to 300 mg daily in adolescents.

*Side effects.* The parkinsonian symptoms of tremor, rigidity and bradykinesia (difficulty in initiating movements) are more likely with higher dosage. Other symptoms include dry mouth and hypotension. More serious long-term side-effects may include tardive dyskinesia — repetitive, stereo-typed movements involving the face and tongue — as well as choreo-athetoid movements (slow writhing movements) of the upper limbs.

*Comment.* Sedation is common with high dosage, along with risk of parkinsonian side effects. The latter can be reduced by the addition of anticholinergic drugs such as orphenadrine. Other phenothiazines such as trifluoperazine are less sedating, but have a greater risk of parkinsonian side-effects.

### Butyrophenones

*Indications.* The most popular drug of this group is haloperidol. It is useful in the treatment of acute psychotic episodes, particularly hypomania, as well as being the drug of choice for treatment of complex tics and Tourette's syndrome. It is also used for behavioural abnormalities in pervasive development disorders such as stereotypies and overactivity and to reduce the unpredictable aggressive outbursts that occur in severely mentally retarded adolescents.

*Dosage.* Up to 5 mg daily in divided doses in adolescents.

*Side effects.* Sedation and parkinsonian symptoms are frequent with high dosage. Acute dystonic reactions (muscle spasms) involving facial and eye muscles are common, particularly when treatment is first begun.

*Comments.* Orphenadrine is often necessary to counteract the parkinsonian side-effects. Haloperidol is a very useful drug, but requires close and continual supervision to avoid distressing side-effects.

## Tricyclics

### Imipramine/amitriptyline

*Indications.* Useful as part of treatment package for persistent nocturnal enuresis in children over 6 years of age.

In depressive disorder(s), it is most likely to be useful when sustained and prolonged mood disturbance occurs in association with other symptoms such as apathy or agitation. Amitriptyline is more useful when agitation is a marked feature, whereas imipramine is better when there is marked apathy.

*Dosage.* Up to 50 mg at night for nocturnal enuresis. In depressive disorder, gradual increase in dosage up to 150 mg daily, depending upon age.

*Side effects.* Dry mouth, blurred vision and hypotension are common.

*Comment.* Relapse is frequent when the tricyclic drug is discontinued in the treatment of nocturnal enuresis. The therapeutic benefit in depressive disorder should become apparent after 3–4 weeks. A major risk associated with tricyclic usage is drug overdose, either intentionally or accidentally. More recently, some case reports of unexplained death in children prescribed the tricyclic desipramine have been described, so that ECG monitoring prior to and during treatment with tricyclics may be indicated.

### Clomipramine

*Indications.* Several studies have shown that clomipramine can be effective in the reduction of obsessional thoughts and rituals in children with obsessive-compulsive disorder. The beneficial action may be related to its effect on serotonin metabolism.

*Dosage.* Up to 150 mg daily in divided dosage (depending on age).

*Side effects.* Drowsiness, tremor and dizziness are common. There is an increased risk of epileptic seizures.

*Comments.* Symptoms may be exacerbated when treatment is discontinued. It is essential to combine its use with the other approaches in the treatment of obsessional disorders.

## Stimulants

### Methylphenidate

*Indications.* This drug is of proven value in the treatment of overactivity associated with the pervasive hyperkinetic syndrome. It has also been used successfully in the treatment of narcolepsy. The mechanism of action is unknown, though complex effects on central neurotransmitters are probable. Depending on age and severity, the maximum dosage is around 20 mg daily. It is essential to give methylphenidate in a divided dosage in the morning and at lunchtime.

*Side-effects.* Marked reduction in appetite and sleep requirements as well as in growth rate. Excitability in high dosage.

*Comment.* This drug is now only available on a named patient basis from the pharmaceutical company. It is essential to monitor growth, appetite and weight during treatment and advisable to have 'drug holidays' periodically. Drug treatment must be combined with other treatment approaches such as behaviour modification. Close supervision of drug treatment is essential, along with regular review of necessity for continued treatment. Dextro-amphetamine is preferable to methylphenidate when there is a history of seizure disorder. Similar precautions apply with dextro-amphetamine.

### Fenfluramine

*Indications.* Some recent studies have found that the drug can decrease the stereotypies and hyperactivity as well as improve the social responsiveness of children with childhood autism. The drug is known to produce a reduction in serotonin levels.

*Dosage.* Mean daily dosage of 1.5 mg/kg in divided dosage.

*Side-effects.* Similar to other stimulants. Common side-effects include anorexia, weight loss, decreased growth rate and drowsiness.

*Comment.* Definite benefits in treatment of childhood autism have not been clearly established. In common with other stimulants, caution is necessary in its use.

### Hypnotics

This category covers a variety of drugs, including antihistamines such as trimeprazine and benzodiazepines such as nitrazepam.

*Indication.* Short-term relief of sleep disorder in the preschool or older child.

*Dosage.* Trimeprazine 30–60 mg at night. Nitrazepam 5 mg at night.

*Side-effects.* Early morning drowsiness and irritability.

*Comment.* Only justified as a means of providing brief relief for the child and a respite for the parents before they embark on more effective behavioural methods to improve the sleep disorder.

### Lithium

The use of this drug in child and adolescent psychiatry is extremely limited. Its main value is as a prophylactic measure to prevent further relapses in manic-depressive disorder. Prior to treatment, careful screening of cardiac, thyroid and renal function is necessary. During treatment, regular monitoring of serum levels of the drug is essential in order to prevent toxicity. Adult psychiatric text books (Kendell & Zealley 1993) provide more details about treatment.

*Laxatives (see Ch. 11)*

These include bulk-forming agents such as methylcellulose, bowel stimulants such as senna and stool-softeners such as dioctyl. Their main indication is in the treatment of encopresis associated with constipation.

*Other drugs*

*Clonidine.* This drug, a central alpha-agonist for the treatment of hypertension, has been used recently in Tourette's syndrome with a beneficial reduction in tic frequency. The dosage is gradually built up to approximately 0.25–0.45 mg daily. Until the results from double-blind controlled trials are available, it is probably sensible to restrict the use of this drug to those individuals who have failed to respond to standard treatment for Tourette's syndrome. The drug should be discontinued slowly to avoid a rebound hypertensive reaction.

*Naltrexone.* This is a long-acting opiate antagonist that has recently been used to treat self-injurious behaviour in children with pervasive developmental disorders. The rationale is that the drug will reduce the elevated levels of endorphin thought to be present in this group of children. Further studies are, however, required in order to confirm the preliminary beneficial findings.

*Fluoxetine.* This drug, a serotonin re-uptake inhibitor, has been found to be effective in adults with depressive disorder and also obsessive-compulsive disorder. There are some recent case reports available of similar studies in children. Further studies are clearly needed to define the role of the drug in the treatment of affective disorder in childhood.

## PSYCHOTHERAPIES

Psychological treatments are the commonest therapeutic approach in contemporary child psychiatric practice. They encompass a wide range of treatments linked to a diverse set of theoretical explanations for the abnormal behaviour(s). The psychotherapies can be categorised along three separate dimensions:

- their explanatory theories
- their treatment methods
- their approach to problem solving.

These differences will be highlighted during the following sections devoted to the various psychotherapies. Despite this diversity, all psychotherapies share common features that are essential for their successful implementation. As mentioned earlier, these are:

- the establishment of a trusting relationship between the therapist and the patient(s)
- the close supervision of the treatment programme
- usually, the active involvement of other key individuals such as parents or teachers.

## BEHAVIOURAL PSYCHOTHERAPY (MCAULEY & MCAULEY 1977, HERBERT 1981)

This approach is based on the application of findings from experimental psychology, particularly learning theory, to a wide range of problems such as enuresis, encopresis, temper tantrums and aggression. Originally, the term *behaviour modification* was used to describe this approach, as the focus of treatment was on the modification or alteration of overt behaviour using conditioning or operant methods. More recently, the range of techniques subsumed under this approach has increased considerably, so that even covert processes such as cognitions or thoughts are regarded as suitable for a behavioural approach, hence the newer term *cognitive–behavioural methods*. For clarity, however, the latter techniques are discussed separately in the next section. This section now discusses behavioural approaches under three headings: principles, techniques and applications.

### Principles

The behavioural model categorises deviant or maladaptive behaviour into three groups:

- insufficient desirable behaviour
- excessive undesirable behaviour
- avoidant behaviour (Table 17.4).

*Insufficient desirable behaviour* is the failure to acquire the wide range of social and interpersonal skills necessary for adaptive daily living. Parents and children devote a lot of time during childhood to the acquisition of such skills, for instance, self-care skills, communication and language skills and social behaviour. Failure to acquire these skills results in age-inappropriate behaviour that is distressing to the parents or the child and also further impedes developmental progress. Systematic exposure to the desired behaviour through modelling and/or reinforcement of desired behaviour through shaping and operant methods are common approaches to remedy the deficiencies.

**Table 17.4**    Behavioural conceptualisation of deviant or maladaptive behaviour

| Categories | Example | Techniques to modify behaviour |
|---|---|---|
| Insufficient desirable behaviour | Self-care skills | Operant methods<br>Shaping<br>Modelling |
| Excessive undesirable behaviour | Temper tantrums<br>Aggression | Operant methods (extinction, time-out, punishment)<br>Stimulus control<br>Self-monitoring |
| Avoidant behaviour | Social/school phobia | Desensitisation<br>Graded exposure<br>Flooding<br>Modelling |

*Excessive undesirable behaviours* are usually antisocial in nature and include aggression, tantrums and acting-out behaviour. The reduction of these behaviours can be achieved through operant methods or with methods to increase the individual's awareness of the stimuli that trigger the undesirable behaviour. Stimulus control and self-monitoring are examples of the latter approach.

*Avoidant behaviour* such as separation anxiety or school phobia is maladaptive as it impedes the child's development and socialisation. Remedial behavioural techniques for avoidant behaviour are desensitisation, grade exposure, flooding and modelling.

Despite the diverse nature of the techniques used and the varied theoretical basis, all behavioural psychotherapies have a common approach that is distinctive from other psychotherapies in the ways shown in Table 17.5.

**Table 17.5**    Characteristics of behavioural approach

- Define problem(s) objectively with reference to the Antecedents, the Behaviour itself and the Consequences (the ABC approach)
- Emphasis on current behaviour rather than past events
- Construct hypothesis to account for the behaviour
- Pre-treatment baseline to determine the frequency and severity of the problem
- Devise behavioural programme on an individual basis to test the validity of the explanatory hypothesis
- Evaluate outcome of treatment programmes
- Tackle one problem at a time

*Problem definition*

People, including parents, vary markedly in their description and labelling of individual items of behaviour. For example, one parent may describe a child taking some food from the refrigerator as stealing, whereas many parents would regard this behaviour as unremarkable. Similarly, arguments between siblings can be seen as healthy sibling rivalry or alternatively as indicative of serious underlying jealousy.

The ABC (Antecedents, Behaviour, Consequences) approach is a useful way to analyse behaviour. Important aspects of the Antecedent question are the circumstances immediately prior to the occurrence of behaviour, with reference to place, time of day, persons present etc. Accurate description of the Behaviour with respect to frequency, severity, duration and persistence is also essential. The Consequences of the behaviour, particularly in terms of positive reinforcement such as increased parental attention, are important in determining whether the behaviour persists and is maintained.

*Emphasis on current behaviour rather than past events*

Unlike psychodynamic psychotherapies, which emphasise the importance of early experiences in determining current behaviour, behavioural approaches regard contemporary circumstances and contingencies as the main factors influencing behaviour. Though individual predisposition is acknowledged, over-riding importance is attached to the ABC sequence or stimulus–response model. The term *functional analysis* is applied to this process of exhaustive analysis of the circumstances surrounding the occurrence of the maladaptive behaviour.

*Construction of explanatory hypotheses*

The functional analysis of the problem provides the basis for setting up a hypothesis to explain the maladaptive behaviour. For example, the preschool child has a tantrum at the supermarket check-out because similar behaviour has previously been followed by the mother giving the child some sweets. Again, the child who wakes up during the night begins to cry and scream because this behaviour has usually caused the parents to come into the child's bedroom. The sweets and the increased attention from parents are seen as positive reinforcers that increase the likelihood that tantrums and night-time screaming will persist. In both instances, positive reinforcement is hypothesised as the basis for the persistence of the maladaptive behaviour.

*Creation of a pretreatment baseline record*

This is a core feature of the behavioural approach. It comes in many guises such as star charts, record sheets or diaries (Fig. 17.1). The baseline record

| Day of the week | First week | Second week | Third week | Fourth week | Fifth week |
|---|---|---|---|---|---|
| Monday a.m. | | | | | |
| Monday p.m. | | | | | |
| Tuesday a.m. | | | | | |
| Tuesday p.m. | | | | | |
| Wednesday a.m. | | | | | |
| Wednesday p.m. | | | | | |
| Thursday a.m. | | | | | |
| Thursday p.m. | | | | | |
| Friday a.m. | | | | | |
| Friday p.m. | | | | | |
| Saturday a.m. | | | | | |
| Saturday p.m. | | | | | |
| Sunday a.m. | | | | | |
| Sunday p.m. | | | | | |

**Fig. 17.1**  Record/diary/star chart sheets

has two main functions. First, it provides an accurate description of the frequency and severity of the problem prior to treatment, thereby allowing a pre- and postintervention comparison. In most instances, it is the occurrence of the positive or desired behaviour that is recorded on the chart, as this provides the basis for the assessment of improvement during treatment. The second purpose is to assess the child's and the parents' motivation or commitment to the treatment programme. Clearly, if the child and parents are unable to keep an accurate record of therapy, they are even less likely to be able to carry through successfully a demanding behavioural intervention programme.

*Devising an individual treatment programme*

Three factors determine the choice of the intervention programme:

- the explanatory hypothesis
- the symptomatology
- the age and capabilities of the child and the competence of the parents.

The identification and isolation of the contingencies that provide positive reinforcement for the maladaptive behaviour are of crucial importance in elaborating *the explanatory hypothesis*. For instance, increased parental attention from acting-out behaviour or the reduction in separation anxiety produced by non-attendance at school are likely to influence the choice of intervention strategies. Two aspects are usually tackled simultaneously: first, the elimination of reinforcement for the maladaptive behaviour; and second, the promotion of the desired behaviour through positive reinforcement.

*Symptomatology* also influences the content of the treatment programme. Generally, operant methods are successful with excessive or insufficient desirable behaviour, whereas exposure methods such as desensitisation or flooding are preferable for avoidant behaviour.

*The age and capabilities of the child and the competence of the parents* affect the repertoire of treatment possibilities. The older, more mature child is usually more likely to take an active part in planning and participation in the programme than a younger more immature child. Similarly, the competence and enthusiasm of the parents are essential to ensure that the programme is completed satisfactorily. Indeed, the most important clinical skill for successful behavioural treatment is the ability of the therapist to devise a treatment programme that not only accomplishes its aims satisfactorily but also is within the capabilities of the child and parents.

A feature of good programmes is that the maladaptive behaviours are broken down into their constituent parts, so that beneficial change, though on a small scale, is more likely to occur. The establishment of realistic targets and of obtainable goals are the signs of a good behavioural programme. Success breeds success, whereas failure begets despondency and pessimism.

### Evaluation of outcome

The systematic assessment of the outcome of the intervention programme is the hallmark of the behavioural approach. The records provided by sheets or diaries enable the therapist to decide whether the intervention programme has produced a reduction in the maladaptive behaviour and an increase in the desired behaviour. A major feature of the approach is close supervision of the programme to ensure that misunderstandings with parents and child are minimised and the chances of success enhanced. Supervision of the programme through telephone and/or regular clinical contact is a major reason why behavioural approaches make so much demand upon the clinician's time.

If the intervention has failed despite good compliance and adherence from the parents and the child, two explanations are likely. First, the original hypothesis for the maladaptive behaviour was incorrect. Second, the intervention was too complex or ambitious, so that the child and parents were unable to change behaviour adaptively. In both instances, the clinician must modify the programme accordingly. The early detection of failure and subsequent amendments to the programme when necessary are character-istic of successful programmes.

## Tackle one problem at a time

Parents usually describe a wide range of problem behaviours with their child. The assessment phase of treatment should establish a clear definition of the problem and also a priority ranking or hierarchy for the various maladaptive behaviours. This should enable the therapist and the parents to agree upon a sequence or order in which to deal with the problems. The focus on a single problem increases the chances of initial success, so that the child's and the parents' enthusiasm and commitment for the approach are enhanced.

## Techniques

As discussed earlier, behavioural approaches rely upon the application of learning theory principles to the modification of behaviour. The fundamental idea underlying learning theory is the close link between the stimulus, the response and the reinforcement. Reinforcement, positive or negative, is the means by which the strength of the association between the stimulus and the response is increased or decreased. As mentioned earlier, the child's temper tantrum at the supermarket check-out is positively reinforced or rewarded by the mother giving the child some sweets. The strength of the association between the stimulus (the supermarket check-out) and the response (the temper tantrum) is thereby increased.

Broadly speaking, behavioural techniques can be grouped into two main categories, exposure or stimulus modification techniques and operant or

**Table 17.6**  Behavioural techniques

- Exposure techniques
  - Desensitisation
  - Flooding
  - Modelling
  - Response prevention
- Operant techniques
  - Reinforcement
    - positive
    - negative
  - Extinction
  - Punishment
    - application of aversive stimuli
    - removal of reinforcer
- Shaping, prompting and fading

response modification techniques (Table 17.6). The table also lists punishment as a means of behaviour modification. This is included for two reasons. First, parents frequently use 'punishment' as a means to modify behaviour. Second, psychologists make an important theoretical distinction between negative reinforcement and punishment, so that the difference should be made clear. However, punishment is a technique that has ethical implications for professionals who recommend it, so that the indications for its use should be clearly demonstrated.

## Exposure techniques

### Desensitisation

Desensitisation is useful in the treatment of clinically incapacitating phobias. These include fear of animals, especially dogs, the dark, examinations, medical procedures and school phobia or refusal. The technique involves the graded and gradual exposure to the feared object or situation while the individual is simultaneously in a relaxed state. The rationale is that exposure to the previously fearful object while relaxed loosens the association between the anxiety and the feared situation.

The technique has two components, the construction of a fear hierarchy and relaxation training. The fear hierarchy consists of about ten situations that the child finds frightening. They range in severity from the least fearful to the most fearful. For instance, in a child with school phobia, the least noticeable anxiety may be experienced when packing the school bag the night before school and the maximum panic while playing in the playground prior to the start of school. Between these two extremes, there is a series of intermediate situations. A frequent problem with children is their inability to construct a satisfactory hierarchy or series of graded fearful situations. The therapist often requires considerable ingenuity in order to devise a useful and workable hierarchy.

Relaxation training can be taught in several ways. In the formal procedure, the therapist teaches the child to tense and relax his muscles in sequence, so that the child is able to recognise the level of muscle tension. Additionally, the child is taught ways to reduce the level of muscle tension, often by simultaneously imaging a calm or peaceful scene such as lying on the beach or in a grassy meadow on a summer's day. More usually, however, the relaxation component is provided by an adult, often the parent, who accompanies the child while graded exposure is carried out.

The key element in successful desensitisation treatment is the pace or rate of graded exposure: too fast brings no anxiety reduction while too slow decreases motivation. Traditionally, exposure can be achieved in two ways, in vitro or in vivo. In vitro desensitisation involves the patient imagining or visualising the feared situation during the therapy session at the clinic, while in vivo desensitisation confronts the individual with the real live feared object or situation in a controlled and graded manner. In vivo desensitisation is much more preferable with children as not only do they find imagining feared situations more difficult but the presence of a reassuring adult during the in vivo desensitisation also facilitates greatly the anxiety reduction.

The results from clinical practice suggest that desensitisation is most effective for discrete and isolated phobic objects or situations, but less effective when there is additional evidence of more widespread disturbance.

## Flooding

This approach reduces the anxiety by 'jumping in at the deep end of the swimming pool' rather than by 'putting your toes in at the shallow end', as with desensitisation. Flooding, known also as *implosion*, consists of exposing the individual to the most feared object or situation with the individual remaining there until the anxiety decreases and the patient is able to tolerate the situation. Clearly, complete co-operation and explanation are essential for this method to be successful. Sometimes it can succeed when desensitisation has failed. Most studies have been carried out with adults, though some case reports of dramatic success with school and animal phobias have been described with children. Flooding is probably not the method of choice for children, but may be considered when the situation is severe and other exposure methods have been unsuccessful.

## Modelling (imitation)

This comprises exposing the child to the skilled performance of the desired behaviour, so that the child has the opportunity to observe the necessary skills in action. For instance, watching someone playing in a relaxed manner with a large dog shows the child how to tolerate the dog's boisterousness, limit excessive physical contact and control the dog's behaviour. Modelling techniques are often combined with other operant techniques such as shaping. For instance, the child with dog phobia is initially introduced to a small puppy followed by a series of larger and more threatening animals, so that successive shaping or approximation to the desired goal is gradually attained.

## Response-prevention techniques

These have been applied most frequently in obsessive-compulsive disorder in adults and older adolescents. The behavioural formulation of obsessive-compulsive disorder proposes that the compulsions and the rituals are an attempt to reduce the anxiety induced by the obsessional thoughts. As they produce a temporary reduction in anxiety, these behaviours are reinforced and maintained.

Response prevention involves the identification of the stimulus or trigger that produces the urge to engage in the rituals or compulsions. When the stimulus arises, the patient is actively encouraged to resist the compulsive behaviour, often by performing some distracting behaviour such as tapping the table or twanging the wrist with an elastic band, thereby making the performance of the ritual impossible. The gradual abatement of the anxiety without the necessity for the compulsions reduces the association between obsessional thoughts and compulsive behaviour. Bolton et al (1983) have described the use of these techniques with adolescents who have severe obsessive-compulsive disorder requiring hospitalisation. In addition to the use of response prevention techniques, this study also found that successful treatment depended on active co-operation from the adolescents' families, as they were often directly or indirectly involved in the performance of the rituals.

## Operant methods

These rely on altering the contingencies or consequences of the behaviour, so that the frequency of the behaviour is changed with either an increase or a decrease. Reinforcement is the main concept underlying this approach to behaviour modification. A positive reinforcer or reward is something that increases the likelihood that the preceding behaviour will occur again in the future. For example, if a child is given pocket money for completing household chores, then he is more likely to finish these chores again in the future. A negative reinforcer is usually a stimulus, often aversive or distasteful, that increases the probability that the behaviour that resulted in its removal or termination will recur. For instance, an electric shock applied to a barbed wire fence increases the likelihood that the individual will avoid touching the wire again. Commonly, aversive stimuli lead to the development of escape or avoidance behaviour.

Punishment occurs when a stimulus or event leads to the cessation of a particular behaviour. It can happen in two ways, by the application of an aversive stimulus or by the loss or removal of all reinforcers. For example, application of an electric shock to a wire causes the individual to refrain from touching the wire. The aversive stimulus has therefore two properties, a punishing role by suppressing behaviour and a negatively reinforcing role by developing escape and avoidance behaviour. The second method, the loss or removal of all reinforcers, includes the loss of attention or privileges and the implementation of time-out. Time-out or 'time-out from positive reinforcement' implies the loss of all available reinforcers, usually for a brief period of time. This often involves the child being removed to his bedroom or to a corner of the room where all reinforcers such as adults' attention, toys or television are unavailable.

## Positive reinforcement

This is the most common and useful means of promoting the development of desirable behaviour. It is the principle underlying the use of star charts, contracts etc. The essential feature is that the occurrence of the target behaviour is followed by a positive reinforcer or the reward. The close temporal relationship between the desired behaviour and the positive reinforcer is crucial to a successful programme. For example, the occurrence of a dry bed at night or a defined period without aggression should be clearly followed by a reward or positive reinforcer. Diaries or star charts provide a simple and effective means to record the occurrence of the desired behaviour.

Rewards can be categorised into three groups:

- material rewards
- social rewards
- additional privileges.

Material rewards include tokens, stars, sweets and money. Selection depends on the problem, the child and the family. Visually attractive charts such as star charts or the smiley faces style of chart are particularly useful with young children. Tokens can be exchanged or converted into money or small gifts as appropriate.

*Social rewards* such as praise from parents and teachers should be an integral feature of any programme, and are usually the mainstay of the programme on a long-term basis.

The acquisition of *additional privileges* such as an extra half hour of dedicated time with one parent is often a useful adjunct to some programmes, depending on the child and the problem.

Commitment and motivation from the child and parents together with close supervision from the therapist are the essential ingredients of successful programmes.

## Extinction

When positive reinforcers for a behaviour are removed, the behaviour will gradually decrease in frequency and eventually disappear or become extinguished. The initial period after the removal of the positive reinforcer may see a temporary increase in the behaviour followed by a gradual and continued reduction in frequency. For example, if temper tantrums have led previously to increased parental attention, the parents are instructed to ensure that they avoid giving any attention to such behaviour. In everyday terms, the parents are instructed to ignore the deviant behaviour.

Clearly, many parents find such a strategy difficult to enforce and in some circumstances it may not be possible. They should also be warned that there may be this temporary increase in the frequency of the behaviour when the programme is initially started. Providing the parents can be consistent and also ensure that the child is not exposed to risk, this strategy can be effective. It is, however, much more likely to be successful when it is used in combination with another programme designed to promote desirable behaviour. The motto should be: promote the good, ignore the bad.

### Time-out procedures

As discussed earlier, this type of punishment involves the removal of all reinforcers. It can be extremely effective provided that the procedure is thought through prior to the commencement of the programme. It is often extremely useful with the more severe behaviour problems and also when implemented by more psychologically sophisticated personnel such as nursing or care staff.

Two important practical considerations are the location and the duration of the time-out procedures. Many parents think that banishing the child to the bedroom or bathroom is the best option. Usually, however, there are major disadvantages with this choice. For instance, the room may contain toys that provide unwanted stimulation or has hazards such as hot water that are dangerous unless closely supervised. A much better choice, depending upon individual assessment, is the corner of the room or the hallway where there is little stimulation or the risk of causing danger. The duration of the time-out procedure should be approximately 5–15 minutes depending upon the age of child, the nature of the problem and the local circumstances. It is not suitable nor worthwhile to continue for a longer period. The crucial factor is to ensure that there is strict adherence to the no-stimulation rule during the procedure itself. This may inevitably result in the time-out procedure lasting much longer.

*Implementation of time-out.* McAuley & McAuley (1977) advocate a three-stage procedure (Fig. 17.2). First, the child is clearly asked to do something or to stop doing something. If the child complies, he is rewarded. Non-compliance invokes the next stage when the child is asked again to complete the task, coupled with the warning about the time-out procedure unless there is compliance. If compliance now occurs, the child is again rewarded. Further non-compliance is followed by the imposition of the time-out procedure. An important factor in the successful implementation of the time-out procedure is the clear verbal and non-verbal instructions that the adult gives the child about compliance. Simple, unequivocal statements are the best.

Despite the simplicity of the procedure, parents or other adults often experience major problems with implementation. Three difficulties are common:

- the child refuses to go to the time-out location
- the child refuses to remain there
- the child refuses to leave the location at the end of the procedure.

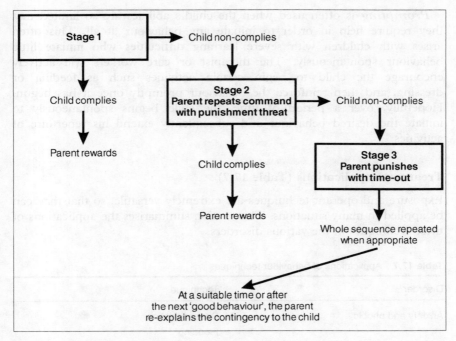

**Fig. 17.2**    Three-stage procedure for the implementation of time-out

Close supervision and guidance from professional staff, including direct observation at home is often necessary in order to help parents manage this procedure effectively. The necessity for the direct supervision of the procedure is a major limitation to its application on a widespread basis. Often it is necessary for parents or teachers to spend some time at the day or in-patient child psychiatric unit in order to receive training in the techniques.

*Shaping, fading and prompting*

**Shaping** involves a series of operant procedures involving positive reinforcement whereby the behaviour increasingly approximates to the desired goal. For instance, a child with a short attention span or overactivity is rewarded initially by the teacher for remaining still and concentrating for a 5 minute period in the classroom. Gradually, this time period is extended until the child is able to cope with a whole lesson. Subsequently, this may be extended for longer periods of the school day.

**Fading** is the procedure whereby the initial positive reinforcers of certain operant behaviours are gradually reduced and eliminated. They are then replaced by other, less overt rewards. For instance, initially the parent remains in the bedroom with the child who has woken up during the night for approximately 5 minutes. Gradually, this time period is reduced until the parent leaves the room as soon as the child has been settled.

*Prompting* is often used when the child's abilities are so limited that they require help in order to initiate any behaviour at all. This often arises with children with severe learning difficulties who initiate little behaviour spontaneously. The therapist or care workers will actively encourage the child to begin certain activities such as feeding or dressing, and then reinforce the behaviour promptly once it has begun. Hopefully, over a period of time, the child begins spontaneously to initiate the desired behaviour and subsequently extend his repertoire of activities.

## Treatment applications (Table 17.7)

Exposure and operant techniques are extremely versatile, so that they can be applied in many situations. This section summarises the applications of these techniques in the various disorders.

**Table 17.7**   Applications of behaviour techniques

| Disorder | Technique |
| --- | --- |
| Anxiety and phobic | Desensitisation |
| | Flooding |
| | Relaxation |
| Obsessive-compulsive | Relaxation |
| | Response-prevention |
| Depressive disorders | Cognitive–behavioural |
| | Relaxation |
| Conduct disorders | Positive reinforcement |
| | Extinction |
| | Time-out |
| Hyperactivity syndromes | Positive reinforcement |
| | Extinction |
| | Time-out |
| Pervasive developmental disorders | Positive reinforcement |
| | Extinction |
| | Time-out |
| | Aversive techniques |
| Encopresis/enuresis | Positive reinforcement |
| Mental retardation | Positive reinforcement |
| | Extinction and time-out |
| | Prompting and shaping |
| | Aversive techniques |
| Tics | Massed practice |

*Anxiety and phobic states*

General anxiety states and specific phobic disorders are readily managed through exposure procedures such as desensitisation and flooding. In vivo rather than in vitro exposure is the usual practice, with the relaxation and support component provided by the parent or other professional actively involved in the programme.

*Obsessive-compulsive disorder*

Anxiety is regarded as central to the development of this disorder, so that relaxation training and anxiety management are components in most treatment packages. Usually, however, response-prevention techniques are used as they provide a more specific strategy to reduce the obsessional thoughts and compulsive rituals found in this disorder.

*Depressive disorders*

Cognitive–behavioural techniques (see next section) are now an important non-pharmacological treatment approach. Relaxation and anxiety management techniques are also useful in some circumstances when anxiety is a prominent feature of the disorder.

*Conduct disorder*

Behavioural approaches have two main applications, the promotion of desirable behaviour and the elimination of undesirable behaviour. Prosocial behaviour can be developed through operant techniques, while extinction and time-out procedures are most useful for undesirable behaviour.

Patterson and colleagues (1982) have developed a wide ranging behavioural training programme for parents to modify their child's behaviour. The parents are taught the principles of behavioural management such as reinforcement or time-out, followed by systematic training with training manuals and weekly sessions in order to observe, rate and record deviant as well as desirable behaviour. Subsequently, specific behaviours for promotion or elimination are targeted as part of the intervention programme. Evaluation of the outcome results indicates substantial improvements which are maintained at follow-up. Major limitations with this approach are, however, the commitment required by the family to complete the programme and difficulties presented by the presence of other family problems that frequently compromise compliance and motivation.

*Hyperactivity syndromes*

Behavioural techniques are frequently used as part of the treatment package to complement the beneficial effects produced by stimulant drug treatment.

The operant techniques of positive reinforcement, extinction and time-out are used to promote prosocial behaviour and to eliminate undesirable behaviour. The goals of school-based programmes are often to improve attention and concentration span and to decrease distractibility by the application of operant techniques such as positive reinforcement. Finally, extinction and time-out schedules are used for the antisocial behaviour problems frequently present at home and at school.

### Childhood autism

The promotion of language and social skills through operant techniques is an important goal in the treatment of children with childhood autism (Rutter 1985b). Active participation of parents and teachers in these programmes is desirable in order to increase the likelihood of long-term improvement in behaviour and social development. Aversive techniques for self-injurious behaviour are sometimes considered necessary when other methods have failed.

### Enuresis and encopresis

The use of positive reinforcement techniques such as star charts is the treatment of choice for these disorders in many cases. The behavioural strategy is usually a part of a more comprehensive treatment package involving other methods, for example, the buzzer alarm in enuresis or laxative drug treatment in encopresis.

### Mental retardation

The behavioural approach is used extensively in the treatment of behaviour disorders in children with severe learning disability. Positive reinforcement is used to develop new skills and behaviours, while extinction and time-out are used to reduce the frequency of deviant or damaging behaviour. Prompting and shaping techniques are common features of many behavioural programmes, as it is important to increase the child's repertoire of skills, particularly for self-care and independence.

Self-injurious behaviour, sometimes a problem with the severely retarded child who has additional sensory or motor disabilities, can be extremely difficult to eliminate, so that aversive or punishment techniques may require serious consideration, especially when other methods such as time-out or protective devices have failed.

### Tic disorders

*Massed practice*, in which the individual performs a behaviour repeatedly and continuously over a period of time, has been shown to reduce the frequency of tics in Tourette's syndrome. The rationale with this approach is that the positive reinforcement previously associated with the performance of the tic is reduced and finally eliminated. Unfortunately, the tics can re-occur when the massed practice is discontinued.

## COGNITIVE BEHAVIOURAL TECHNIQUES

### Cognitive theory of depression and anxiety

Beck (1970, 1976) has elaborated a general theory to explain the origins of neurotic disorders, particularly depression and anxiety. The main premise of this theory is that *cognitions* or thoughts are primarily responsible for the development of symptoms, other manifestations of disturbed mood or behaviour being regarded as secondary phenomena. Thus, depressive thoughts precede and result in depressed mood rather than the other way round.

Beck proposed that the 'cognitive triad', comprising the individual's view of himself, the world and the future, is central to an understanding of the individual's thinking, mood and behaviour. Depressed individuals are said to produce elaborate cognitive distortions or negative automatic thoughts which explain their pessimistic view of themselves, the world and the future. Negative automatic thoughts can take many forms (Table 17.8). For example, the following two statements illustrate dichotomous reasoning and selective abstraction respectively: 'As I am no good at tennis, this means that I am no good at any sport' and 'If the teacher does not ask me in class, this means that he does not like me'. Moreover, Beck argued that these negative automatic thoughts have a pervasively disabling effect on the individual's daily life, as they become his habitual, ingrained and automatic way of

**Table 17.8**   Examples of cognitive distortions

| Cognitive distortion | Example |
| --- | --- |
| Over-generalisation | A depressed person who makes one mistake concludes 'Everything I do goes wrong' |
| Selective abstraction | 'If the teacher does not ask me in class, this means he does not like me' |
| Dichotomous reasoning | 'If I am no good at tennis, I am no good at any other sport' |
| Personalisation | 'I am responsible for my parents' divorce'. 'If my mother does not watch me playing football, it means she does not love me' |
| Minimalisation | 'If I got good marks in my exams, anyone could do so' |
| Magnification | 'As I only got two good marks from my three exams, I should not carry on with my studying' |

thinking about himself, the world and the future, with disastrous results for the individual.

In order to modify these thoughts and to treat depressed mood, Beck devised a comprehensive treatment strategy employing many principles common to the behavioural approach. The main features are:

- a detailed preclinical assessment
- a clear definition of the aims and objectives of treatment
- the explanation of the rationale for treatment to the patient
- the accurate recording of changes during treatment
- the assignment of 'homework' tasks between therapy sessions in order to introduce beneficial change.

An extensive literature is now available on the application of these techniques for a wide variety of neurotic disorders (Hawton et al 1989).

## Cognitive therapy with children and adolescents

The extension of Beck's theories to child and adolescent disorders is more recent (Braswell & Kendall 1988). The techniques used with adults have been applied to a diverse range of childhood disorders such as depression, anxiety states, impulsivity and hyperactivity. The same principles of clear problem definition, accurate recording of thoughts and behaviour and the initiation of problem-solving strategies are used with appropriate modifications according to the age and the developmental skills of the child.

Particular problems include the ability of the child to verbalise his cognitions, the stability of his beliefs and the assignment of age-appropriate 'homework' tasks. In many children and adolescents, distorted cognitions are less important than the lack of effective strategies for controlling behaviour and a predominantly impulsive rather than reflective cognitive style. The emphasis is therefore on active co-operation between the child and therapist in developing strategies to alter cognitions and to modify behaviour. Common techniques include verbal self-instruction training, cognitive problem solving and self-management skills. The main aims of these techniques are:

- to train the child to monitor and to record accurately the maladaptive thoughts and behaviour
- to suggest alternative explanations for the present situation and to propose new more adaptive behaviour
- to evaluate the outcome.

The comparative effectiveness of these approaches has not been established, but it is likely that they will become more popular, as they have great flexibility and can be used by a variety of professionals after appropriate training.

**Table 17.9**   Functions of families for children

- Satisfaction of basis physical needs such as food and shelter
- Provision of love and security
- Promotion of psychosocial development
  - social relationships with peers and adults
  - cognitive and language skills
  - experience of appropriate role models and socialisation
  - acquisition of ethical and moral values

## FAMILY THERAPY (BARKER 1992)

Family therapy has become an extremely popular treatment approach for many problems referred to child psychiatry services. The literature is vast, with many books, articles and journals devoted to the theory and practice of family therapy. Rather than discussing in detail the various aspects of the subject, this section summarises the principles underlying the approach, with a recommendation to consult more specialist texts such as Barker (1992) for more information. This section is divided into four parts:

- normal family functioning
- the origins of family therapy
- the assessment of families
- the schools of family therapy.

### Normal family functioning

Families fulfil three main functions for children:

- the satisfaction of basic needs such as food and shelter
- the provision of love and security
- the promotion of psychosocial development (Table 17.9).

Children are clearly very likely to show signs of disturbance and maladaptive behaviour when the family is unable to discharge these tasks effectively.

Most family therapists also believe that two other concepts are of general importance in understanding how families function — first, the *developmental sequence* to family life and second, *systems thinking*.

### *The family life cycle*

Just as the individual undergoes an orderly sequences of development throughout childhood, so too does the family pass through a succession of developmental changes during its life cycle (Table 17.10). At the start of family life, the couple's main task is to establish their own relationship and to re-define their contact with their extended families and friends. The

**Table 17.10** Developmental cycle of family life

| Family life-cycle stage | Changes necessary for successful adaptation |
| --- | --- |
| Commitment as a couple | Formation of marital system<br>Re-alignment of relationships with extended families and friends |
| The family with young children | Assumption of parenting roles<br>Adjustment of marital system to allow for children<br>Introduction of children to outside institutions such as school |
| The family with adolescents | Fostering increased independence for adolescents<br>Mid-life re-assessment of marital and career roles for parents |
| Children leaving home | Adult relationship between children and parents<br>Regeneration of marital relationship for couple |
| Couple alone again | Acceptance of mortality as an individual and as a couple<br>Role as in-law and grandparent |

arrival of children requires that the couple assume parental roles as well as adapting their own relationship to accommodate the children. Couples and families vary widely in the ease or difficulty with which they make this adjustment. Stress within the parental roles is likely to affect adversely the marital system as well.

An important role for parents slightly later is to introduce the child to organisations outside the family, particularly nursery groups and schools. Children often take some time to adapt to the contrast in style between adult authority within the family and that outside. Later on, families have major roles in promoting the independence of their adolescent children, so that the latter are able to complete their other maturational tasks of career choice and assumption of adult sexual roles. Finally, the departure of the child from the family requires considerable adaptation from the parents in order for them to establish a more equal adult relationship with their children, as well as re-assessing their own relationship as a couple.

*Systems theory*

Systems theory is a general theory (von Bertalanffy 1968) to explain the interactions and relationships between the individual components comprising a larger or more complex unit or structure. The theory can be applied to mechanical systems such as feedback systems or clocks as well as to social systems such as families or schools.

The theory attracted the attention of family therapists as it provided a framework to understand the behaviour of the individual subsystems of the family — such as the children or the parents — as well as their relationships

**Table 17.11**   Systems thinking and families

| General features of systems | Applications to families |
| --- | --- |
| Systems have a purpose | Provision of love, security, etc |
| A system is composed of sub-systems and is part of wider systems | Subsystems – parents, children and grandparents |
| | Suprasystems – community, schools |
| Each system and subsystem has a boundary around it | Parents and children are separate units with different functions |
| Boundaries should be clear | The parental subsystem should not involve the grandparents or the children |
| Boundaries should be semi-permeable | Communication and expression of feelings between parents and children essential |
| Properties of each boundary change from time to time | Children require more autonomy and independence as they grow up |
| Systems are more than the sum of their parts | A family is more than a collection of individuals |
| There are general rules governing the behaviour of systems | A family regulates its behaviour according to its own values and beliefs |

to each other and to the outside world. Table 17.11 summarises the application of system theories to families and their functioning.

The attractiveness of the theory is that it appears not only to explain how families work and function but also to provide a method of analysing faults and flaws in the daily activities of family life. For instance, poor delineation of the boundaries between the parental and child subsystems can be responsible for problems of control and discipline with the children. As discussed later, Minuchin and colleagues (Minuchin 1974) have developed a school of family therapy based clearly on the application of systems theory to family functioning.

## Origins of family therapy

Contemporary family therapy practice is characterised by a plethora of techniques and schools. It is therefore helpful to look at the origins of family therapy in order to make some sense of the seemingly idiosyncratic and diverse developments that have occurred.

Ackerman, in his book *The Psychodynamics of Family Life* (1958), is regarded as the first person to provide a comprehensive account of family therapy. He applied psychodynamic concepts of individual and group processes to normal and abnormal family functioning. Contemporaneously with Ackerman, three other groups in North America were studying families with a psychiatrically disturbed member, usually someone with schizophrenia. Lidz and colleagues (Lidz & Lidz 1949) developed the notions of *schism* and *skew*. The former refers to the continual competing and undermining conflict between the parents for the loyalty of the children, while the latter occurs when the main emotional support is directed towards one of the parents rather than to the children. Wynne and colleagues (1958) coined the terms *pseudomutuality* and *pseudohostility* to describe the interactions of families with a schizophrenic member. Pseudomutuality refers to the expression of overt warmth but with an underlying sense of antagonism, while the latter is the reverse.

Bateson et al (1956) introduced the most influential concept of the *double-bind* interaction to explain how the thought processes of someone with schizophrenia become distorted. The double-bind interaction has three components:

- there is an overt demand or expectation to do something or to refrain from doing something
- simultaneously, there is a covert message, usually non-verbal, which contradicts the overt message
- finally, and most crucially, the recipient of the messages is prohibited or unable to expose the conflict in the situation, usually because of the mutually dependent relationship between the two people.

For example, a mother may tell her teenage son to go out and enjoy himself, while simultaneously communicating that she will be lonely when the adolescent is away from home. Bateson argued that it was the insoluble nature of the contradictory and conflictual interactions between the family members, shown by the double-bind, that was responsible for the development of the distorted thinking found in schizophrenia.

The central premise underlying the research by these three groups was that family interactions induced or caused schizophrenia in the individual, that is, they argued for a psychogenic or psychological explanation for the disorder. Subsequent research has largely discredited this hypothesis for two main reasons. First, the genetic predisposition to schizophrenia has been increasingly demonstrated (Kendell & Zealley 1993). Second, the fundamental methodological flaw with these studies is that the findings were based upon studies of families after the individual had developed schizophrenia. Consequently, the family's behaviour could be interpreted as a response to the individual's schizophrenia rather than its cause. Despite such criticisms, these research groups were influential in demonstrating to clinicians that family interactions could have widespread effects upon the behaviour of individual members. They provided the impetus to look at family behaviour in close detail.

Subsequently, two main schools of family therapy developed in the USA, the *structural approach* associated with Minuchin and colleagues (1974, 1981) and the *strategic approach* of Haley and colleagues (Haley 1976). The two schools acknowledge the importance of systems thinking to family functioning and its dysfunction, but they differ in their approach to assessment and in therapeutic techniques (see later section).

The third and most recent group to evolve a distinctive approach has been the Milan Systemic Group (Palazzoli et al 1978). The members of this group were trained originally as psychoanalysts and subsequently worked together as a therapeutic team. The team approach is one of the distinctive features of the group. In addition, they incorporated and developed ideas from the strategic school of family therapy in North America about the nature of and prerequisites for effective change in family functioning. The latter aspect of their work has attracted much interest and debate, resulting in considerable enhancement of their reputation among family therapists.

Finally, an unfortunate feature in the evolution of family therapy has been the tendency to overvalue the importance of the individual or group associated with one school or approach. Consequently, there has been little appreciation of the fact that non-specific factors such as the therapeutic alliance and empathy are just as important in producing beneficial change as the individual techniques or schools associated with one style of family therapy.

## Assessment procedures

Despite the numerous styles and schools of family therapy, most adopt similar methods of assessment. The important components of family assessment are summarised in Table 17.12.

Family therapists stress the importance of observed interaction between family members during the family interview as the basis for the formulation

**Table 17.12** Principles of family assessment

---

- Problem definition
- Observation of family interactions
    - Communication patterns
        - is it clear?
        - who controls communication?
        - are individuals allowed to speak for themselves?
        - main mode of communication – verbal or non-verbal
        - repertoire of affective response – range from indifference to over-involvement
    - Structural aspects
        - subsystem definition
        - relationship between subsystems
        - regulation of control between subsystems within and outside the family
        - role regulation
- Developmental stage of family life
- Sociocultural context of the family
- Problem solving abilities of the family

---

of the family's problems. This 'here and now' approach is the main focus for attention rather than a detailed description of problems obtained through the more traditional history-taking assessment procedures.

## Problem definition

Family therapists devote a large portion of the assessment interview to obtaining a clear definition of the problem(s). They are interested in knowing whether the problem is viewed by family members as a problem for the individual or a reflection of family interaction. Other important questions are:

- Do family members agree about the nature of the problem?
- What is each family member's explanation for the problem?
- What is each family member's response to the problem?
- Is the family's response appropriate?

## Observation of family interactions

Though family therapists ask some questions about the family's usual patterns of interaction and their response to problems, they attach much more significance to their own observations of the family's behaviour during the interview. The pattern of communication and the functioning of the family system is seen as crucial to assessment and understanding of the family's problems.

Important features of the family's communication patterns are the following:

- Is the communication between family members clear and unequivocal?
- Which family member dominates and controls communication?
- Are individuals allowed to speak for themselves?
- Is the main mode of communication verbal or non-verbal?
- What is the range of emotional or affective response from family members?

This last feature is central in deciding whether the family is capable of responding appropriately to the emotional needs of its members. Assessment of the systems functioning within the family involves determining whether there are clear boundaries between the subsystems — for instance, between the parents and the children — and the regulation and relationship of the subsystems with each other and the outside world.

## Developmental stage of the family cycle

Family therapists believe that the various stages of the family life-cycle impose different stresses on family members. For instance, problems of control and discipline feature frequently in families with young children, whereas independence and autonomy are more important in families with adolescent children. It is important for the family therapist to assess how well the family is coping with the tasks of their current developmental stage. For instance, some parents find younger children more difficult to bring up than adolescents, and others vice versa. Family therapists also believe that the transition from one developmental stage to the next is the time when problems are more likely to occur. These developmental transitions require the family to re-assess and possibly alter their roles and responsibilities.

## Sociocultural context of family life

The religious, sociocultural and ethnic values of the family are important variables determining the family's perception of problems and how they deal with them. The family therapist must not impose his own values on the family but rather utilise the strengths of the family's value system in order to introduce beneficial change.

## Problem solving abilities

As family therapists emphasise the present rather than the past, the family's competence at problem solving is a major determinant affecting treatment outcome. A distinction is often drawn between the practical needs of the family (e.g. for food and shelter) and their emotional needs (e.g. for security and support). Problem-solving abilities are assessed along the following dimensions: can the family

- identify the problem?
- communicate about the problem?
- consider options?
- decide upon options?
- initiate actions?
- monitor response?
- evaluate outcome?

## Schools of family therapy

Many styles or schools of family therapy have developed over the past 40 years, for instance, psychodynamic, behavioural, structural, strategic and systemic. Indeed, a cynic might argue that there are as many schools of family therapy as there are family therapists. Despite this unsatisfactory situation, a brief synopsis of the three most popular approaches is presented.

## Structural school of family therapy

This style of family therapy is particularly associated with Minuchin and his colleagues (Minuchin 1974, Minuchin & Fishman 1981). The approach applies systems theory thinking to families and their behaviour. It attaches particular importance as to whether there is effective working of the family's subsystems, for instance the parental and the child subsystems, and the delineation of the boundary between the family system and the outside world, the *suprasystem*.

The family's emotional responsiveness is described along a bipolar dimension with *enmeshment* at one extreme and *disengagement* at the other. Enmeshment refers to the over-involvement of the parents in the children's affairs, whereas disengagement is lack of interest in or concern for each other's welfare. Healthy family functioning operates between these two extremes.

The therapist should also be aware of the sociocultural context of the family: for instance, the ethos of a severely disadvantaged family is likely to be different from that of an economically affluent, aspiring family.

The therapist is particularly interested in determining the clarity of the boundaries between the parental and child subsystems and the distribution of power and decision-making within the family. Minuchin introduced the terms *alignment* and *coalition* to describe the situation when family members unite together, often in opposition to another member. This pattern of alliances is often seen in dysfunctional families, where it is accompanied by *triangulation* and *detouring*. Triangulation occurs when the child is allied with and used by one parent to criticise the other parent. Detouring arises when the parents, instead of arguing with each other about their own differences, transfer their combined aggression into disapproval of the child's behaviour.

The therapist adopts two main therapeutic strategies when working with the family. First, the therapist demonstrates or points out to the family dysfunctional patterns of interaction that occur during the session, for instance weak parental–child subsystem boundaries or the presence of triangulation. Second, the family or parts of the family subsystem are set tasks during and/or between sessions to remedy the distorted patterns of behaviour and to promote healthy family functioning.

Minuchin and colleagues studied two types of families extensively, those with severe psychosocial disadvantage and those with a member who had physical symptoms, the so-called *psychosomatic family*. He believed that the socially disadvantaged family had weak structural characteristics with unclear boundaries and poor parent–child subsystem functioning. Consequently, he thought the structural approach to be suitable as it provides a framework to enable the family to function more effectively.

Psychosomatic families are divided into *primary*, where there is a definite physical illness such as diabetes or epilepsy, and *secondary*, where the physical symptom is psychological, for instance abdominal pain or anorexia. All psychosomatic families share the same four characteristic patterns of interaction:

- enmeshment
- parental over-protectiveness
- rigidity or the inability to adapt to the developmental needs of the child
- conflict avoidance or the failure to resolve conflicts.

The parental enmeshment, over-protectiveness and rigidity produces an ill-defined parent–child subsystem which is further compounded by the inability to resolve conflicts. Rather than overtly express anger or hostility, the conflict is transferred into the development of physical symptoms.

Clearly, the goals with this type of family are:

- to promote the establishment of clear boundaries between the parents and the children
- to encourage the overt expression of anger
- to teach the family the skills necessary for conflict resolution.

### Strategic family therapy

Many therapies are included within this category, so that only the general principles and techniques will be mentioned. While recognising the importance of systems thinking and the developmental cycle to family life, this group of family therapies attaches particular importance to communication theory, theories of change and strategies or techniques to alter behaviour.

The main premise underlying this approach is that all forms of behaviour, whether between individuals or within families, are a form of communication. A well-known statement which typifies this philosophy advises: 'It is impossible NOT to communicate'. Communication is divided into two categories, *verbal* or *digital* and *non-verbal* or *analogue*. Families vary markedly in the relative balance between the two types of communication and also in the clarity with which they are expressed.

Another feature of the approach is the distinction drawn between first order and second order change in the family's behaviour. Strategic family therapists recognise the self-regulatory or homeostatic characteristics of the family system, so that as one member improves, another may become symptomatic, the so-called *first order change*. By contrast, *second order change* involves a reorganisation and realignment of the family's system functioning, so that no other symptomatology arises. Not surprisingly, second order change is more difficult to achieve.

Perhaps the most unique feature of the strategic family therapy school is its reliance upon strategies or techniques to produce change. The approach is entirely pragmatic, that is, any technique can be used providing it works. Insight or understanding are not necessary in order to produce beneficial change, a position radically different from the conventional psychodynamic viewpoint.

The most original and creative technique associated with this approach is the use of paradox or *paradoxical interventions*. Essentially this comprises instructing the family to continue with the symptomatic behaviour rather than attempt to stop the behaviour. For example, the mother and the child who argue incessantly are asked to have an argument each day at 4 p.m. for half an hour. If they comply with this request, it demonstrates that the arguments are under their own control, and hence modifiable. If they are unable to comply with the instructions, then the undesirable behaviour is eliminated. The therapist thereby demonstrates his control over the problem in the two outcome situations.

Other paradoxical techniques include restraining and positioning strategies. With the *restraining strategy*, the therapist advises against too rapid progress as this may be followed by a relapse. Similarly, *positioning strategies* involve adopting a pessimistic position about improvement, for example: 'Change is most unlikely to occur for the foreseeable future'. Again, these strategies increase the power of the therapist, as even the most gloomy outcome has been predicted beforehand.

### Milan System family therapy (Palazzoli et al 1978)

This group achieved prominence through their appearances at international meetings and conferences in the 1980s. Originally trained as psychoanalysts, they adopted strategic techniques to produce a distinctive approach combining elements from many sources. They maintain that it is essential for therapists to work together as a team, one member conducting the interview while the others observe it, often through a one-way screen. This is in order to prevent the interviewing therapist from becoming part of the family system. Prior to the interview, the therapy team meets to discuss the problem and produces an initial hypothesis to explain the basis for the problem behaviour. The purpose of the assessment interview is to confirm or refute this hypothesis.

This group developed a particular style of interviewing known as *circular questioning*. This involves asking each member of the family in turn to comment on the behaviour of other family members, so that a complete or circular view is obtained of the problem(s). This technique is designed to elicit the relative strength of relationships between family members. During the interview, the therapist actively seeks to maintain a position of neutrality in which every statement or communication from a family member is accepted at face value. A statement is neither better nor worse, good nor bad.

At the end of the interview, the therapist rejoins the other members of the team to review the hypothesis and to discuss their observations of the family's interactions. Subsequently, after an extensive and thorough discussion, the therapist returns to the family with an intervention or summary of the team's views of the problem(s).

A distinctive feature of the intervention is that the contribution and involvement of each family member is acknowledged and valued, hence the term 'systemic'. Frequently, the intervention contains a paradoxical injunction, for instance a statement containing a positive connotation. The latter is the attribution of good intention to the individual's symptomatic behaviour. For example, the adolescent girl with anorexia nervosa is making a sacrifice of her own needs in order to preserve the family's stability and to prevent even more disastrous change from happening. Restraining and positioning strategies are also commonly used .

The family is often asked to carry out a task, usually of the paradoxical variety, between therapy sessions. The time period between sessions is frequently long in order to 'allow therapeutic change to occur'. At the conclusion of the interview, the therapy team meets to review the family's response to the information and to amend their hypothesis accordingly.

## INDIVIDUAL PSYCHOTHERAPY (WOLFF 1986)

Historically, individual psychotherapy has been a major treatment method for disturbed children. The recent introduction of alternative treatment approaches, particularly family therapy and behaviour therapy, has meant that individual psychotherapy has become less popular. The time-consuming nature of the therapy and uncertainty over its usefulness have further eroded the importance of individual work with children. Despite these reservations, the therapeutic skills of individual assessment and treatment are still an important aspect of contemporary child psychiatric practice.

Most models of individual psychotherapy are derived from psychodynamic theories of psychopathology. Anna Freud (1946) and Melanie Klein (1932) made important contributions to the understanding and treatment of disturbed children, using insights derived from their clinical work. Winnicott (1970) developed his own imaginative techniques, particularly the *squiggle game*, to facilitate communication with the child. The squiggle game is a collaborative exercise involving the child and the therapist alternatively drawing, elaborating and commenting on the evolving drawing. For instance, the child draws a squiggle, the therapist says what he thinks it represents and

**Table 17.13**   Axline's principles of psychotherapy with children

- Warm and friendly relationship with child
- Total acceptance of child
- Freedom for child to express feelings openly with the therapist
- Therapist reflects child's feeling back to the child to promote increased awareness
- Child is responsible for own behaviour and for initiating change
- Child determines course of the session, not the therapist
- Treatment proceeds at own pace
- Limit setting is confined to the avoidance of danger and to acquaint the child with his role in the relationship with the therapist

then draws his/her own squiggle, which in turn is commented upon by the child, who then adds his/her own squiggle, followed by the therapist and so on. This process can be extremely useful, when used skilfully, in revealing the child's fantasies and worries. Considerable empathy with and understanding of the child are necessary for the successful use of this technique.

Axline (1969) has outlined the general principles underlying individual therapy with children. Table 17.13 summarises the key points which are elaborated in the next sections.

### Indications for individual psychotherapy

Despite its widespread use, the criteria for suitability for individual psychotherapy have not been clearly established. Two considerations are important, the problem and the capacities of the child. Generally speaking, children with reactive or neurotic disturbance are more likely to benefit than those with constitutionally determined disorders. Children who have had earlier traumatic experiences resulting in excessive use of defence mechanisms and the arrest of personality development often require the sustained and intensive nature of individual therapy to resolve their difficulties. Children with chronic illness or disability may also benefit from the prolonged support and contact provided by individual therapy.

The child also requires certain skills and abilities in order to benefit from individual work. He should possess the following abilities to some degree:

- sufficient trust and security to form and maintain a relationship with another individual
- the ability to distinguish fantasy from reality
- the ability to tolerate the anxiety and intense emotion aroused by treatment without losing control
- the ability to recognise and to verbalise thoughts and feelings
- the ability to be sufficiently self-reflective to be able to distinguish between thoughts, feelings and behaviour.

### General principles of individual psychotherapy

*Interview(s) with the child*

Three phases are discernible: the initial, middle and final stages. In most instances, the child is referred because of concerns expressed by parents, teachers or other adults rather than by his own choice or initiative. Consequently, a major task of the initial interview is to clarify the purpose of the meeting for the child. This also provides an ideal opportunity for the therapist to demonstrate his concern for and interest in the child as well as a willingness to help. Finally, the therapist negotiates with the parents and the child the contract for further individual assessment and treatment.

The middle section comprises the detailed assessment and treatment of the child's difficulties. An important role for the therapist is to explain to the child the purpose and format of the sessions. This includes telling the child about the frequency and duration of the sessions and that the sessions will provide the opportunity to use play materials. Most therapists set aside a tray or box containing the play materials that the child uses in the therapy sessions for the exclusive use of that child. Children commonly attend therapy sessions on a weekly basis.

Though the active expression of feelings is encouraged in the sessions, the therapist must also indicate the limits of acceptable behaviour, for instance, when the therapist will intervene to protect the child. Unrestrained expression of aggression or destruction is not helpful, as failure to control the situation induces more anxiety in the child. The skilful therapist is able to contain the explosive situation without making the child feel more guilty and responsible. Acknowledgement of the child's feelings, coupled with firm instructions, is the best tactic, for instance: 'I know you are very angry and upset at the moment, but I am not going to let you hurt yourself'.

The termination of treatment is an important aspect with individual psychotherapy cases. The timing and management of this process requires considerable skill and expertise. The child's altered understanding of himself inevitably affects the relationship with his parents, so that joint session(s) are often useful towards the end of therapy.

## Role of the therapist

Child psychotherapy is based on two principles, the relationship between the child and the therapist and the interpretation of the transactions occurring during the therapy sessions. The establishment of a therapeutic relationship with the child is dependent on the personal qualities and professional training of the therapist. Empathy, respect, non-possessive warmth and a desire to help are essential for the child psychotherapist, along with an intimate knowledge of children's cognitive and emotional development. The therapist must have the ability to understand and delineate the basis for the child's response to traumatic events such as loss or injury according to age and developmental stage. For instance, the inability of the preschool child to appreciate the permanence of death is in marked contrast to the adolescent with terminal illness who is only too aware of death's imminence and irreversibility.

The therapist has four tasks:

- to establish a therapeutic relationship with the child
- to facilitate the child's expression of feelings and thoughts
- to understand the basis for the child's conflicts
- to communicate this understanding to the child.

The personal qualities of the therapist are important in developing the relationship with the child. The provision of security and safety during the session enables the child to relax and to trust the therapist. The therapist must respond to the limited capacity of the child to tolerate anger and anxiety, so that intervention may be more necessary than with adult patients. Active interest and, when appropriate, participation in the child's play activities are a ready means by which the therapist's involvement is demonstrated to the child. Declarative statements such as 'You must have been upset by that' are often more necessary as well as more helpful than open-ended questions such as 'Did you feel upset when that happened?' Willingness to enter the child's world is the core ingredient necessary for developing a fruitful therapeutic relationship.

The most distinctive feature of child psychotherapy is the extensive use of play materials to facilitate the expression of feelings and conflicts. This applies particularly to the younger child, as older children do have the capacity to use verbal interchange to express their concerns. Preschool children enjoy and utilise sand/table play with sand, water and miniature people and animals. Make-belief play with the dolls' house is popular with school-age children who readily act out their conflicts via the family figures and materials provided by the dolls' house. Drawing, painting and modelling with Plasticine are other useful techniques with school-age children.

The purpose of these techniques is to establish the connections between conflicts enacted or depicted in the play activity and the real life concerns of the child. The child's conflicts more commonly centre on feelings of loss, insecurity and anger towards the parent(s) than the rivalrous oedipal conflicts of adult patients. Conflicts are also concerned with the present rather than the past, unlike adult patients. Once identified, the therapist's task is to convey or interpret this link to the child. The same themes are likely to recur throughout the sessions, so that interpretations are modified on the basis of further information.

The therapist must also ensure that the child has complete confidence in the privacy and confidentiality of the sessions. Honesty and openness are essential prerequisites to enable the child to disclose painful and distressing events. The exclusiveness of the child's therapy material and the exclusion of the parents from the therapy room are tangible signs to the child that the therapist is trustworthy and respects the child's integrity.

Finally, the therapist has two further tasks. First, the child inevitably regards the therapist as an important figure who provides him with a role model for adult behaviour. Second, the therapist should focus on strengthening the child's adaptive and coping skills through the acknowledgement and encouragement of the child's accomplishments during therapy.

*Relationships with parents*

Parents are usually responsible for initiating the referral and ensuring regular attendance, so that they must have regular contact with the therapist. They are also valuable sources of information about previous and current behaviour. In spite of these factors, the therapist must make clear to the parents the confidential nature of the child's disclosures during therapy. Separate meetings with the parents to discuss problems and to review progress are the best way to resolve these dilemmas. Finally, periodic joint meetings with the child and the parents are also useful.

## PARENTAL COUNSELLING AND SUPPORTIVE THERAPY

Parents are often involved in treatment programmes, for instance as co-therapists or supervisors in a behaviour modification programme or receiving advice about the management of specific problems. In both instances, the parental role is prescriptive, that is they are told what to do, or how to do something. By contrast, parental counselling is based on the premise that listening to and exploring the parents' feelings and attitudes will enable them to utilise their own resources to resolve difficulties. It is used most frequently in three situations:

- in response to an acutely stressful experience affecting the child, for instance the diagnosis of a serious malignant disease
- in parallel with other treatments that the child may be receiving, for instance individual or group psychotherapy
- when their child has a chronic illness or disability which is affecting the psychosocial adjustment of the parents.

Depending on the problem, two approaches are adopted: a brief, intensive but time-limited series of interviews or a more long-term but less frequent number of sessions.

Counselling involves using several techniques, including ventilation, clarification, encouragement and the promotion of insight.

*Ventilation*

This provides the parents with the opportunity to express their emotional response, commonly anger, guilt or sadness, to the situation. The acceptance of these responses by the therapist is emotionally cathartic for the parents, so that they find the discussion beneficial.

*Clarification*

This is the systematic examination of the parents' anxieties, so that the basis for their concerns can be identified, scrutinised and modified — for instance, the nature of the illness, treatment implications and long-term prognosis.

*Encouragement*

This strategy relies upon utilising the parents' resources and skills to find a more effective solution to the problem and also to help them overcome their doubts and lack of confidence.

*Promotion of insight*

While not attempting to explore in detail the predisposing factors for the parents' predicament, it is nevertheless beneficial to make them more aware of the links between their current attitudes and behaviour and their own childhood experience of family life. This increased understanding should enhance the parents' coping pattern and also promote a more adaptive response.

Finally, the 'common sense' nature of these various methods, allied with limited goals, means that they can be used in many situations and by the various professionals involved in the care of disturbed children and their families.

## SOCIAL SKILLS TRAINING (SPENCE 1983)

This approach rests on two major assumptions: that social skills are deficient in disturbed children and that social skills can be taught. There is indeed evidence to support both these propositions. Deficient social skills may be a primary feature of some conditions, such as pervasive developmental disorder, but are more commonly a secondary or accompanying feature of many conditions, for instance the aggressive behaviour of the conduct-disordered child or the socially withdrawn behaviour of the child with phobic disorder. Poor social skills can result in a deficit in prosocial behaviour and/or an excess of socially maladaptive behaviour. The acquisition of desirable social behaviour is dependent on:

- the accurate identification of the necessary social skills
- the design of a suitable training programme
- the application of the newly acquired skills to everyday situations.

The approach shares many similarities in style to cognitive–behavioural methods.

### Applications

Social skills training has been used to treat the following conditions:

- social deficits in children with pervasive developmental disorders
- aggressive antisocial behaviour
- the socially avoidant behaviour of children with anxiety and phobic states
- the poor language skills of children with learning and language disorders

- socially withdrawn behaviour
- poor peer group relationships.

A wide age range of children, from the preschool period to the adolescent period, can be involved in programmes, depending on the clinical problem. The programmes can be carried out on an individual or group basis, usually for an agreed number of sessions at weekly intervals.

## Techniques

Most programmes involve some or all of the following specialised techniques: modelling (watching a skilled trainer/peer demonstrate the desired behaviour); instructions (verbal or non-verbal directions to carry out the modelled behaviour); performance feedback (verbal or other rewards for participating in the session); role play (play-acting the desired behaviour in a social situation with rehearsal opportunities to practice the desired behaviour repeatedly). Finally, social reinforcement is used extensively for the performance of the new skills during the session(s).

## Outcome

Many programmes are successful in training the child to acquire new social skills, so that they become part of the individual's behavioural repertoire. Two major drawbacks are frequently found with these techniques: the failure to generalise the new skill into everyday life situations and the failure to persist with the new skills following the completion of the programme. Both these problems require careful attention in order to ensure that long-term benefits are obtained. 'Top up' meetings and regular post-treatment reviews go some way to resolving these difficulties.

## GROUP THERAPY

The treatment of children in a group setting is a common practice both in out-patient and in-patient work. Approaches vary widely, depending on the age of the child and the type of problem. Children can be usefully divided into three age bands: 4–7-year-olds, 8–12-year-olds and adolescents. With the two younger groups, parallel groups for parents are usually organised. The theoretical model underlying the group work can be psychodynamic, social skills or behavioural. The latter two types are more popular with the younger age groups where social or peer relationships are the major problems.

A psychodynamic approach is only possible with adolescents who are sufficiently mature to utilise the group dynamics to beneficial effect (Evans 1982). Essential features for successful group work are:

- a critical mass of group members

- shared expectations about the aims and methods used to resolve the difficulties
- the ability of the group to keep to task.

The group leader(s) should adopt an active leadership role to promote good relationships with individual group members. The leader(s) should also set clear limits about acceptable behaviour as well as encouraging members to assume the initiative and responsibility for group tasks. Group therapy as part of an in-patient treatment programme is clearly different in aims and structure from a 'closed' out-patient group. The latter would normally have between six and nine members and be run on a once-weekly basis by two group leaders. The group would have a definite life-span, usually 9–15 months, and an identified client group, for instance individuals with relationship difficulties or the victims of sexual abuse.

## OTHER TREATMENT APPROACHES

### HOSPITAL IN-PATIENT AND DAY PATIENT UNITS

Considerable changes have occurred recently in the provision of services for disturbed children by health services, social services and education departments. The remit of specialist psychiatric in-patient and day patient facilities is influenced by the availability of other residential resources provided by education and social services. Good provision of alternative care facilities for children from disturbed families by social services and a well-resourced education service for maladjusted children affects the role of specialist psychiatric services. Despite the recent changes, in-patient and day patient psychiatric facilities are likely to continue to have a small but important contribution to the provision of services for severely disturbed children. The continuation of these services at a local level may, however, often be a reflection of interest and commitment rather than absolute need.

In-patient and day patient units vary widely in treatment philosophy, age group of suitable children and type of problem treated. This section outlines the general characteristics of such units, while more detailed discussion is available elsewhere (Hersov & Bentovim 1985).

### In-patient units

There is a broad division into child (up to 13 years) and adolescent (13 years onwards) units. Within the children's unit there are also likely to be further subdivisions into preschool and school-age groups. The following list summarises the common reasons for admission:

- to manage acute seriously suicidal behaviour
- to manage acute psychotic illness

- to assess and manage the complex psychiatric problems associated with paediatric disorders, for instance the neuropsychiatric problems of childhood epilepsy
- to provide intensive management for disorders requiring strict medical and nursing supervision, for instance anorexia nervosa
- to manage chronic conditions that have failed to respond to extensive out-patient treatment, for instance encopresis
- to provide a comprehensive assessment of the child away from the family in order to obtain a more objective opinion and also to make plans for future needs
- to monitor the effectiveness of drug treatment for certain disorders, for instance stimulant drug treatment for hyperkinetic disorder
- occasionally, to provide respite for the family and/or the child or adolescent from mutually exhausting stress at home.

*Treatment methods*

Most units operate a therapeutic milieu policy which implies a collaborative effort involving nurses, teachers, psychologists, psychiatrists, social workers and occupational therapists. The nurses, who usually have a training in paediatrics and psychiatry, are the main front-line therapists and workers for the child on a daily basis. This multimodal approach relies upon utilising the different skills of the various professions to assess and to treat the various aspects of the child's disorder. Schooling, individual and group work are integral components of the child's daily activities combined with frequent family meetings. The latter are designed to treat the frequently co-existing family conflicts and also to review the child's progress within the unit. Regular case reviews and ward rounds are conducted by staff to assess progress and to formulate plans for the future. Careful planning is undertaken prior to the individual's discharge. Dependent on the problem and the unit's policy, admission is usually from 3 months to one year.

Some units, particularly those for adolescents, adopt a more explicitly therapeutic community model. The major emphasis with this model is the 'living learning' approach, in which the individual's daily interactions with staff and other patients are the main vehicle for therapeutic change. Daily community meetings where conflicts and disagreements are discussed openly and argued through assume major significance in the daily life of the unit.

**Day units**

These can have very similar benefits to in-patient treatment, with the advantage that the child is not removed from the home. Indeed, many units operate both in-patient and day patient programmes, so that the individual may graduate from the in-patient unit to day patient treatment. Usually the day units cater for well-defined age groups, preschool, middle childhood and adolescent. Preschool programmes usually require daily attendance and active participation from parents in the unit's activities. Preschool units often provide specialist assessment of the child's developmental needs as well as organising behaviourally based training programmes for parents in the management of behaviour problems. With older children and adolescents, the programmes centre on the school day, as most units have teachers attached to the unit.

The day patient resource provides a useful means to review the child's educational difficulties, for instance, specific learning disorders or behavioural problems in the school setting. Most units employ nurses, psychologists and occupational therapists, so that a comprehensive treatment programme can be organised. Admission to the day patient programme can last for several months, providing children with the opportunity to make substantial progress with their difficulties.

## LIAISON AND CONSULTATION

Child psychiatrists can make valuable contributions to the care of children through their collaborative work with the other professions more directly involved with children who are disturbed and/or in distressing circumstances. Two broad divisions can be made, paediatric liaison and consultation work.

### Paediatric liaison

This refers to the practice whereby the child psychiatrist, as a member of the paediatric team, attempts to provide an integrated approach to the medical and psychological needs of ill children. Charles West, the founder of the Hospital for Sick Children in London, noted that: 'If you are not fond of little children you cannot learn it, for they soon make up their minds as to who loves them, and when ill they will express their real feelings either by words or signs to no one else.'

Paediatric liaison is practised in diverse ways, ranging from the formal direct request about specific problems in individual children to active membership of the paediatric team in in-patient and out-patient work. Common reasons for consultation include:

- psychiatric disorder requiring collaborative care
- diagnostic dilemmas; paediatric illness with known psychiatric factors
- adverse reactions to hospitalisation
- psychological symptoms in physically ill children
- children with terminal illness.

The child psychiatrist has three roles in paediatric liaison: as an educator about the psychological aspects of illness in childhood, as a consultant for specific problems and as a research investigator into the causation and treatment of the psychiatric morbidity associated with paediatric illness. Paediatric staff, in their enthusiasm and eagerness to treat the medical aspects of illness, can be neglectful of the psychological impact of illness on the child and family. Advice about ward management, for instance admission practices, ward routines and the preparation for painful procedures, can alert staff to the stressful nature of illness and its treatment. The child psychiatrist has a role to inculcate a definite 'psychological mindedness' amongst staff, so that the child's reactions are placed in a developmental context, and responded to accordingly.

In many cases, the liaison psychiatrist acts as an advocate for the child, so that his needs are understood and appreciated. In order to discharge this task successfully, the child psychiatrist has to be accepted as a valued member of the paediatric team and not as an intrusive outsider. Specific meetings, such as the psychosocial ward rounds, are useful means to discuss the psychological aspects of the child's illness and its management. The success of these meetings is however totally dependent on the active support and participation of senior staff from all disciplines. Unless this occurs, they are doomed to failure, leading to further estrangement between paediatric and psychiatric staff.

Finally, among the more integrated paediatric teams, staff sensitivity groups run by the liaison psychiatrist can act as a forum to discuss the stressful nature of paediatric work. Again, in order to be successful, careful discussions of aims, objectives and membership has to be undertaken prior to the establishment of such groups.

The child psychiatrist is often asked about various aspects of illness, including:

- diagnostic dilemmas
- illnesses with physical and psychological components
- acute confusional or bizarre behaviour
- the psychological morbidity associated with chronic illness
- depressive or suicidal behaviour
- child protection work.

While these conditions have been mentioned in earlier chapters, some further brief comments will now be made.

## Diagnostic dilemmas

These arise most commonly with regard to the occurrence of physical symptoms without any known pathophysiological basis. The single most important contribution that the child psychiatrist can make is to stress that there should be positive psychological reasons for making a psychiatric diagnosis rather than merely the absence of physical explanations. If the psychiatrist is unconvinced about the psychological basis of the problem, this should be made clear. A verdict of 'not proven' is much preferable to assuming a psychological explanation to avoid uncertainty.

Useful indications of a psychological explanation are:

• the presence of identifiable stress at the onset of symptoms
• the previous use of physical symptoms as a psychological defence
• a reduction in stress following the onset of symptoms.

The child psychiatrist also has a useful role in assisting paediatric staff to implement the programme designed to minimise restrictions and promote rehabilitation in the child with physical symptoms without a pathological cause.

### Illness with physical and psychological components

Anorexia nervosa is the best example of a disorder in which a collaborative approach between the liaison psychiatrist and paediatric staff is essential. In addition to direct work with the child and family, the child psychiatrist should be involved in the design and implementation of the behaviourally based reward programme for weight gain. A busy paediatric ward is not the best place to manage anorexic patients, so that admission to the child psychiatric in-patient service is often necessary to manage the problem. When transfer has occurred, continued liaison with paediatric staff over medical management is still necessary.

### Acute confusional or bizarre behaviour

This arises commonly in four situations: the acute confusional state, post-traumatic head injury, the postepileptic seizure state and the psychotic reaction. The most important issue with acute confusional states is the detection and treatment of the underlying condition. Advice on managing the confused patient, for instance restricting nursing to a few well trained staff, avoiding excessive stimulation and the minimal use of psychotropic drugs, can give paediatric staff the confidence to look after the difficult patient. The rare occurrence of acutely disturbed behaviour due to a schizophrenic or hypomanic illness demands a much more active intervention from the child psychiatric service.

### Psychological morbidity associated with chronic illness

Chronic illness and disability form a major part of contemporary paediatric practice. Successful adaptation depends on collaborative and co-ordinated care from the paediatric team comprising the paediatrician and other professionals. Most hospital centres now run specific clinics dedicated to particular illnesses such as diabetes or cerebral palsy. This practice is designed to ensure that the various aspects of the condition such as diet or mobility restrictions are assessed and treated. The neurological impairments of some disorders such as epilepsy increase the risk of psychiatric disorder directly, while all disorders impose some additional risk of maladaptive behaviour because of their stressful nature.

The role of the liaison psychiatrist varies according to local circumstances. One model involves the child psychiatrist as an integral part of the clinical team with readily available consultation and advice, whereas in other situations specific referral to the child psychiatry service may be more appropriate. Irrespective of the local practice, the psychiatrist has two roles: as an educator for other members of the paediatric team and as a specialist therapy resource. The educational component involves familiarising team members with the following concepts:

- the impact of illness on the child and family
- the differing developmental crises that illness imposes on the child according to age
- ways of mobilising the coping resources of the child and family.

These tasks are most easily accomplished when the psychiatrist has regular and sustained contact with paediatric staff over individual children attending the clinic. Sometimes, the child and family benefit considerably from direct referral to the child psychiatric service for specific help with the problems associated with the illness and its treatment.

## Depressive and suicidal behaviour

Though paediatricians usually recognise when a child is sad or unhappy, they are less confident about whether this represents depressive disorder and whether it requires treatment. Similarly with children who have intentionally tried to harm themselves, the paediatrician often feels ill-equipped to assess the seriousness of the behaviour and the risk of recurrence. In both instances, the assessment and treatment skills of the liaison child psychiatrist can be extremely useful (see Ch. 8).

## Terminal illness and death

This situation is a major burden for the paediatric staff who feel that they have 'failed' to save the child. Similarly, the child and family are under tremendous strain during this period. The liaison child psychiatrist can be a therapeutic resource for both groups at this time. Considerable tact and sensitivity are necessary to undertake this work, so that careful negotiation with the staff, the child and the family is essential before any contact is made. Many units manage these problems extremely well without specific psychiatric input, so that local circumstances should determine the contribution of the child psychiatric liaison service.

*Child protection work*

This is now an important component of contemporary paediatric practice. It involves the assessment and treatment of the various aspects of physical, sexual and emotional abuse. Recently, many hospital units have established a multidisciplinary child protection team comprising a paediatric surgeon and physician, social workers and child psychiatry personnel. The main role of this team is to formulate and implement the agreed policies and practice related to child protection. The specialist skills of the child psychiatrist are used in two ways: individual disclosure work with children who have been sexually abused and individual and family therapy for the psychiatric problems found frequently in these families.

*Research into the psychiatric morbidity of paediatric illness*

The daily clinical work of liaison child psychiatrists demonstrates clearly the considerable morbidity in children with physical illness. Collaborative work between the child psychiatrist and the paediatrician shows that co-operation can be beneficial, one learning from the other. The academic and research skills of the liaison child psychiatrist can be used in two ways: to devise suitable instruments to measure the adjustment or otherwise of this group of children; and to evaluate the effectiveness of intervention strategies in reducing the psychiatric morbidity. The joint research endeavour could further strengthen the working relationship between the two professions, thereby enhancing mutual respect.

## Consultation

This approach shows some similarities to paediatric liaison psychiatry in that the child psychiatrist does not usually have direct contact with the particular child. Child psychiatrists provide consultation services to a variety of individuals and institutions working with disturbed children such as children's homes, residential schools and social services departments. Gallessich (1982) argues that consultative work has three components: one person, the consultee, asks another person, the consultant, about some aspect of their work, the consultation. The focus of the consultation may be client-centred, that is on the management of the clients or patients of the consultee; work-centred, that is focusing on the working relationships and structure of the consultee's organisation; or consultee-centred, that is to develop the professional skills of the consultee. Consultative work has several other distinctive features:

• There is an emphasis on helping the consultee utilise his own resources more effectively
• The consultee is not obliged to accept the opinion of the consultant
• The consultant has no formal responsibility over the consultee.

Before undertaking consultation work, it is important to establish some ground rules. Consultation shares with, but differs significantly from liaison work, supervision and counselling. Consequently, it is essential to confirm at the outset that consultative work is really required. At this time, the structure, format and membership of the consultative group should be clarified. Once these preliminaries have been agreed, the consultative work can begin.

Four components underlie consultative work:

- the personal qualities of the consultee
- the consultant–consultee relationship
- the consultee–client relationship
- the consultee's work setting.

An important initial task for the consultant is to get the consultee to acknowledge his skills as a professional and to value his own personal attributes. It is not lack of knowledge or of skills that cause the problem, but rather the close involvement of the consultee with the client's problem. The focus of the consultative work should be on the consultee's perception of the problem rather than that of the consultant. The consultant also needs to understand the structure and operation of the consultee's work setting. The consultee's status, role and relationships with colleagues as well as the process of decision making affect significantly the individual's ability to manage problems and to resolve conflicts. Understanding and clarification of these issues are central to successful consultative work.

## HYPNOSIS

Hypnosis involves the production of a state of altered awareness, perception and behaviour, enabling the subject to be more sensitive to persuasion and suggestion. It has many similarities to relaxation training. The main components are relaxation training, imagery and bio-feedback training.

Children from 5 years upwards can be taught the principles of self-hypnosis. The child is shown how to develop relaxation and imaginative skills. The latter involves the ability to visualise or imagine an unpleasant experience, for instance a painful procedure, and to contrast this image simultaneously with a pleasant experience, for instance lying on a beach in the sun. The major aim of treatment is to teach the child these skills, so that they can apply the techniques when an unpleasant experience is about to happen or does happen in everyday life.

Hypnosis has been used successfully in a wide variety of clinical situations including painful procedures, pain control and headaches (Olness & Gardiner 1988). It can be used as the main treatment approach or, more commonly, as part of an overall treatment plan. Training in hypnotherapy, essential for successful application of the techniques, is run by several organisations within the UK.

## DIETARY MEASURES

Apart from their obvious application for obesity and in the management of anorexia nervosa, dietary measures have become popular in the treatment of a variety of disorders, particularly the hyperkinetic syndromes. Essentially the approach involves the restriction and elimination of substances thought to be allergenic, for example tartrazine. The most convincing evidence for this approach has been the study conducted by Egger et al (1985), showing that rigorous restriction of substances produces a definite improvement. The unknown factor is, however, whether the findings would apply to the much larger group of children with overactive and disruptive behaviour. Application of dietary measures has also been extended to include other conditions with an allergenic component such as migraine or asthma, but their efficacy is not known.

## THE EFFICACY OF PSYCHOTHERAPEUTIC TREATMENTS

The empirical value of many psychotherapeutic treatments in child psychiatry is not clearly established. Many treatments were developed and became part of routine clinical practice without undergoing rigorous evaluation, so that it is difficult to persuade clinicians to stop using them. Several authors (Rutter 1982, Shaffer 1984) have provided reviews of the evidence, while others have looked at specific treatments in detail, for instance Wolff (1986) for individual therapy and Barker (1992) for family therapy.

Kolvin et al (1981) completed a large-scale intervention study of school-based therapies for children with behavioural difficulties. This study found that many treatments were effective, but some were more effective than others, depending on the problem. A major reservation with the study is that the children were identified from a school population rather than a clinic population, so that it is not known whether the findings would apply to children seen in clinical practice. The study did, however, highlight the problems associated with the evaluation of intervention studies as well as providing invaluable information about the future conduct of such studies in child psychiatry.

The consensus from the literature is that many treatments are effective, but that the comparative efficacy of treatments is unknown, an important gap given the expense and availability of contemporary child psychiatric services.

Rather than review individual studies or trials, this section looks at the principles underlying treatment evaluation. Table 17.14 lists the design characteristics of outcome studies that should be scrutinised when assessing the value of a particular study.

Many factors influence the referral of children with psychiatric disturbance. These include the type and severity of the problem(s), the availability of services and the attitude of parents to treatment. For instance, children

**Table 17.14**   Study design characteristics influencing the outcome of treatment interventions

- Type of children in the study
- Reliability and validity of measures of disturbance
- The allocation of children to different treatment groups
- Information about intervening variables that may influence outcome
- Distinction between specific and non-specific effects of treatment
- Therapist(s)' variables
- Follow-up period

referred to child psychiatric services with behavioural disturbance may well be different from those with similar problems seen in the community. Any treatment study should provide information about these factors as this will determine the value of the findings.

A major reason for the uncertainty of treatment effectiveness is that many studies have used outcome measures of unknown reliability or validity. It is clearly essential to ensure that the measures chosen are not only reliable and valid but also capable of repeated administration, so that they can detect changes during treatment. It is also useful, whenever possible, to evaluate outcome from different viewpoints, that is, from that of the child, the parents or the therapists, as well as an independent assessment.

The study should also include an adequate follow-up period, so that it is possible to determine whether the improvement persists in the post-trial period. Finally, the allocation of children to the different treatment arms of the study should be random, thereby reducing the risk of patient or treatment bias.

Several factors contribute to the improvement seen during treatment. These include the specific benefits associated with each treatment approach as well as other more general influences such as intervening variables, non-specific treatment effects and therapists' variables. *Intervening variables* are those factors not directly related to treatment that influence outcome, for instance changes in the marital relationship or the psychological adjustment of the parents may clearly influence the child's behaviour, even though these changes are not specifically related to the treatment of the child. *Non-specific treatment effects* influencing outcome include the successful engagement of the family, the adequate definition of the problem and the amount of therapeutic contact. Finally, therapists vary in their experience and expertise, so that it is important that these factors are considered when evaluating the outcome of the therapy.

Lastly, Table 17.15 lists the other factors that affect treatment evaluation and make decisions about correct choice of treatment more difficult in child psychiatry. Unlike adults, children are developing individuals, so that

**Table 17.15**   Constraints on treatment evaluation in child psychiatry

- Coincidental maturation
- Goals of treatment:
  - symptom reduction
  - independence
  - promotion of normal development
- Comparative efficacy of treatment
- Specificity of treatment
- Characteristics of responders
- Process of change
- Acceptability of treatment

changes in symptomatology should be seen against this background. For instance, the spontaneous cure rate for nocturnal enuresis is such that the problem is 10 times less frequent in 15-year-olds than in 5-year-olds. The goals of treatment with children may also be more general and non-specific than with adults. For instance, treatment involves not only symptom reduction but also promoting independence and normal healthy development. Again, the relative merits of different treatments and the specific indications for certain treatment are not clearly established in child psychiatry. Similar uncertainties exist about the factors underlying the process of beneficial change and the characteristics of children and families most likely to benefit from treatment. The final factor influencing the choice of treatment is its acceptability, that is, whether the child and family are likely to comply with the treatment regime and continue with therapy.

# 18. Legal and forensic aspects

Child psychiatrists are involved increasingly in legal and forensic aspects of child care. Additionally, recent changes in UK legislation have important implications for child psychiatric practice. This chapter has three sections:

- the child psychiatrist and the court
- common medicolegal problems
- child-care law.

## THE CHILD PSYCHIATRIST AND THE COURT

The court is likely to ask for the assistance of the child psychiatrist in two ways, to prepare a court report and/or to appear as a witness. Psychiatric opinion is asked in many situations, including child-care cases, child protection work and custody and access disputes. On many occasions, the preparation of the court report is the prelude to appearance as a witness, whereas in other situations the two functions are separate and distinct. Both these situations require considerable skill and expertise from the psychiatrist if he is to discharge his responsibilities successfully, that is, to assist the court in finding the best solution to meet the child's needs.

The guiding principle underlying work with children and the law is the notion of 'the least detrimental available alternative' (Goldstein et al 1980). This idea emphasises that, in many situations, it is not possible to find an ideal solution as each option has some disadvantages. Consequently, the adoption of the plan with the least likelihood of damage is the preferred solution.

Many child psychiatrists also find it useful to incorporate findings from research to substantiate their views about the problem. While knowledge of research findings can provide the basis for an opinion, they are usually only of a general nature, so that they cannot take account of the individual features of the particular case. For instance, although the prognosis for conduct disorder is often gloomy, many children survive and mature successfully despite their circumstances.

Finally, it is important to remember that it is the court, not the psychiatrist, that has the responsibility for making the decision about the

319

child's needs. The psychiatrist can play a valuable role in enabling the court to arrive at an informed decision about the best course of action. The child psychiatrist should avoid prevarication and state his opinion as definitively as possible.

## Preparation of the court report

Child psychiatrists vary widely in their approach to this task, depending on their theoretical orientation and the nature of the referral request. Irrespective of this variation, all reports should incorporate three principles:

- the language should be clear, concise and comprehensible
- the report should not use jargon
- it should be understandable to a lay person.

Generally speaking, the report should not be too long. Unless there are special reasons, it should be no more than 4–5 pages as otherwise the reader is likely to lose the impact of the information provided. Pithiness and precision are the essentials of a good report.

Table 18.1 lists a standard format. The report should begin with a statement of the name(s), age(s) and address(es) of the child(ren) in the report. This is followed by an outline of the sources of information, for instance the documents and papers supplied to the psychiatrist, as well as a description of the interviews that were undertaken in the preparation of the report. The main body of the report then describes the current problems, the family history and the personal history of the persons in the report. This is followed by a summary of the findings of the interview(s) with the child

**Table 18.1** Format of court report

| | |
|---|---|
| Child | Name, age, address |
| Sources of information | Documents and papers supplied |
| | Interview(s) with child, parents, social workers etc |
| History<br>• Current problems<br>• Family history<br>• Personal history | |
| Examination | |
| Opinion | |
| Recommendation | |
| Signature<br>Date<br>Qualifications<br>Position<br>Place of work | |

and other persons. Opinion about the presence or absence of psychiatric disorder in the child or other people is normally included here.

The opinion section shares many features of the formulation part of the standard child psychiatric diagnostic assessment. It contains a succinct summary of the facts, a statement about the presence or otherwise of psychiatric disorder, the factors contributing to the disorder and the likely outcome or prognosis.

The recommendation section is often regarded as the most important aspect of the report. A common practice is to review the available options, listing their advantages and disadvantages. This frequently arises in cases involving the long-term placement of the child or in cases of disputed custody and access. The preferred choice should be stated clearly. It is often useful to stipulate a defined time period to see whether implementation of the recommendation has been successful. This provides the court with the opportunity to review the situation. Another statement outlining the plan of action following an unsuccessful outcome is also helpful. Finally, the report should be signed and dated, followed by a statement of the author's qualifications and place of work. The Appendix at the end of this chapter contains a specimen report.

## Appearance in court

The child psychiatrist can appear in two capacities, as a professional witness and as an expert witness. When present as a professional witness, the child psychiatrist's role is to inform the court about his clinical contact with the child and family, for instance outlining the referral problem, the contact with the clinic and the progress with treatment.

By contrast, the expert witness is defined as someone with specialist knowledge about children's behaviour as well as the ability to comment competently on the particular child and family. The general areas of expertise include:

- normal child development
- the factors influencing child development
- childhood disturbance
- the likely outcome of treatment or intervention.

The expert witness can be used by the court in three roles:

- as an expert to comment on and speak on a previously prepared court report
- to provide a report based upon a review of the papers and documents supplied by the court, but without interviewing the child
- less commonly, to sit through the court proceedings and to be introduced as a witness at the end of the proceedings to comment on evidence heard in the court.

Successful presentation as an expert witness depends upon thorough preparation, the appropriate demeanour and respect for court proceedings, clear exposition of opinions and acknowledgement of the limitations of one's expertise. Court proceedings can be confrontational and adversarial, so that the expert witness must avoid becoming over-involved in the drama of the occasion. Sensitivity to the effects of testimony on the family should also be remembered. Finally, a debriefing session with a colleague or solicitor after the court appearance is often useful.

## COMMON MEDICOLEGAL PROBLEMS

The child psychiatrist may be asked for an opinion in many situations when doubt exists about the best way to meet the child's needs. Six common types of referral are now discussed:

- parenting capacity
- child abuse and neglect
- custody and access disputes
- child placement
- the child's educational needs
- delinquency.


### Parenting capacity

Questions about the ability of the parents to look adequately after the child arise in many situations, for instance child abuse, custody proceedings and parental psychiatric disorder. Parenting is a complex task requiring many skills. Adequate parenting is a relative term, so that the idea of 'good enough parents' (Winnicott 1965) is a useful way to conceptualise the minimum attributes necessary for successful parenting.

A key question in the assessment of parenting skills is the quality of the parent–child relationship. Bowlby's attachment theory (1969), with its concepts of secure and insecure attachment, provides a useful framework with which to evaluate this relationship. There is no doubt that children require committed care from one or more adult over a prolonged period of time in order to ensure healthy development. Parents are most likely to provide this commitment, so that there must be overwhelming evidence that the child's parents are not providing such care before alternative provisions are considered. It is also true that children can do well in uncommon or unusual family circumstances, for instance children looked after solely by their father, children brought up by a couple who are lesbian and the children of teenage mothers. It is the quality of the relationships and the nature of emotional expression within the family that determine the child's adjustment and well-being in such circumstances.

While much emphasis is placed on the mother–child relationship, the role of the father may be sometimes crucial in compensating for the relative lack of care and affection provided by the mother. In many circumstances, the extended family and community network have additional resources to support an otherwise precarious situation.

Parental psychiatric disorder can have a major impact on children's development and adjustment (Rutter 1985a). Although episodic disorders such as schizophrenia or manic-depressive illness can have a devastating effect during an acute relapse, more pernicious effects can be produced by conditions such as personality disorder where the persistent and pervasive nature of the disability has a more handicapping affect on the child's daily activities and development.

The age, sex and temperament of the child affect his ability to withstand less than ideal parenting. The parenting skills required with young children, for instance the provision of food and security, are different from those with older children, so that the parents' competence varies with the age of the child. Boys appear more adversely affected by stress than girls, so that the presence of distress in girls is a cause for more serious concern. Temperamental characteristics such as adaptability or response to new situations influence the child's ability to withstand adverse circumstances.

The assessment of parenting capacity involves a comprehensive review of the previous reports on the child and parents along with separate and combined interviews with the parent(s) and the child. Observation of the parent–child interaction during the interview can often provide vital information about the contemporary quality of the relationship, while previous reports enable the present situation to be placed within the context of the child's overall development. The over-riding consideration in the assessment must be the needs of the child, not those of the parents.

## Child abuse and neglect

Originally, child abuse referred solely to physical abuse, but it now includes sexual abuse, emotional abuse and neglect. Frequently, the various forms of abuse exist together. The child psychiatrist's views are often requested in three situations:

- to provide an opinion about whether emotional abuse has occurred
- to determine whether sexual abuse has happened
- to make recommendations about the child's needs following the disclosure of abuse.

### Emotional abuse and neglect

These two conditions have common features and are often associated with non-organic failure to thrive. Emotional abuse is difficult to define precisely, and even harder to quantify. It refers to the persistent verbal criticism, threat, ridicule and rejection of the child by the parent, accompanied by adverse effects on the child's behaviour and emotional development. It can take many forms, ranging from a lack of care for physical needs through a failure to provide consistent love and nurture to, finally, overt hostility and rejection.

The deleterious effects vary according to the child's age and the most marked changes are evident in the preschool period. In infancy, failure to thrive, developmental delay, anxious attachment and poor social responsiveness are common. The older preschool child has short stature, developmental delay and a disinhibited, overactive and over-friendly pattern of behaviour. The school-age child has usually an unkempt appearance and short stature with learning difficulties, low self-esteem and poor social relationships.

Clearly, these patterns of behaviour and development can occur in many circumstances, but it is the combination of three features that is diagnostic. These are:

- the long-standing nature of the problem
- disturbed behaviour and delayed development
- a persistent pattern of parental criticism and rejection.

Investigation of emotional abuse is dependent on two sources of information, the previous history and the current parent–child interaction. Documentation from the health visitor, general practitioner and paediatrician usually shows a consistent pattern of failure to thrive, poor growth and persistent feeding problems. A diagnostic feature is a rapid improvement in weight and growth following a change in environment, for instance admission to hospital, followed by a relapse on returning home. Interviews with the parents and child show poor relationship patterns characterised by parental criticism, rejection and hostility. For instance, the parents describe the child as 'stealing' food from the refrigerator or say that he 'could do it if he wants, but never does'. In many circumstances, it is not possible to be sure about the severity of the emotional abuse, particularly on initial contact. Regular review over a period of time provides a useful way to monitor progress.

Despite these uncertainties, the child psychiatrist should be able to provide the court with an opinion about the child's needs at the present and in the future.

## Sexual abuse

Child psychiatrists are frequently involved in various aspects of the management of the sexually abused child, including membership of the local child protection team, assessment of the child's needs and therapeutic work with the child and family. The diagnostic and interview skills of the child psychiatrist are sometimes requested to help with disclosure work in cases of suspected sexual abuse. Disclosure work usually employs specially developed interview techniques, often recorded on videotape, using anatomically correct dolls (Bentovim et al 1988). These techniques are not without their critics, as the legal status and validity of these interviews are open to question.

Despite widespread interest in the diagnostic and disclosure aspects of emotional and sexual abuse, the most common reason for psychiatric referral is to provide a recommendation about the best way to meet the child's needs. In these circumstances, the general principles underlying the preparation of a psychiatric report apply.

## Custody and access disputes

The child psychiatrist is not infrequently asked to provide an expert opinion about custody and access for children following the parents' divorce. The following general principles apply to the preparation of the report:

- Obtain agreement from both parties and/or the court to provide a report
- The report is made available to both parents
- See the parents both individually and with the children
- See the children alone where appropriate
- Custody is usually awarded to one parent
- Regular access should be granted to the non-custodial parent unless there are specific reasons to the contrary
- Advocate a conciliation service to resolve disputes and/or to assess parents' commitment to the children's needs.

The views of the children assume increasing importance as they grow older, hence the value of individual interviews. The non-custodial parent often complains that the custodial parent is obstructing regular contact with the children. Though joint custody may seem a preferable solution, continuing disagreements and disputes increase the risk of instability and insecurity, so that a clearer division of responsibilities may be desirable in many cases. There must be overwhelming reasons for denying access to the non-custodial parent, as most evidence suggests clearly that continued contact with both parents is beneficial. The establishment of conciliation services to assist couples to resolve the remaining disagreements over their marriage following their divorce has been useful. Referral to this service also provides the clinician with some indication about the individual motivation of the partners to arrive at an agreement.

In many cases, a major problem for the psychiatrist is the length of time that has elapsed between the time of separation and the request for a report. Often this is 2–3 years, so that any change in the current arrangements is likely to be extremely disruptive to the children, even though such a change might have had some advantages initially. This often affects the amount of contact between the children and the non-resident or non-custodial parent, usually the father. The latter is justifiably aggrieved that the passage of time has prejudiced his contact with the children.

The maxim of 'the least detrimental available alternative' is particularly applicable to recommendations about custody and access cases.

## Child placement

The current policies of social services departments demand that plans and decisions are made for children who are in the care of the local authority. This practice arose out of the previously unsatisfactory situation whereby children in care were often allowed to 'drift' in and out of care without the provision of an agreed strategy to meet their needs in the short or long term.

Frequent reception into care is often the lot of children from disorganised and disadvantaged families where abuse, neglect and deprivation are common. With some clear-cut exceptions, contemporary practice is based upon the premise that families should be given every assistance and support to enable the child to return home after a period of care. If this is unsuccessful and the problems persist, the social service department will eventually consider making alternative long-term arrangements involving the child living away from home permanently, the assumption of parental rights by the local authority and the placement of the child for adoption.

The child psychiatrist is often invited to participate at the various stages of the decision-making process. This may well be at the request of the local authority, the court or occasionally parents opposing the proposed plans. The child psychiatrist can make the most useful contribution when his independence and expertise are acknowledged and agreed upon by all parties. If this position is not accepted, it is sensible to seek clarification before proceeding with the preparation of the report.

The following list summarises the important factors determining recommendations about the future placement of the child:

- the strength of the attachment between the child and his parents
- the age and developmental level of the child
- the presence of psychiatric disorder in the child
- the type and severity of psychiatric disorder in the parents (if any)
- the quality of the interaction between parents and child
- the reasons for the failure of the rehabilitation programme
- alternative care options available.

While it is difficult to quantify the strength of the attachment between the parents and their child, it is useful to consider this aspect from two perspectives:

- Will the child be damaged by the severance of contact with the parents?

• Does the child have the capacity to form new relationships?

The child's attachment to other family members, particularly the siblings, is also important. The nature and severity of any psychiatric disorder in the child or parent(s) will have considerable influence on the decision about placement. The child's age and developmental level and the duration of the exposure to unsatisfactory circumstances affect the most suitable choice available.

The local authority has a statutory responsibility to assist families in their role as the main provider of care for the child. Consequently, the adequacy of the rehabilitation plan and the reasons underlying its failure have a major bearing on decisions about future care. Finally, in most circumstances, there is no guarantee that the proposed alternative care arrangements will succeed. A realistic appraisal of available options is an important element in the overall assessment of the best interests of the child.

## Non-attendance at school

Parents have a legal responsibility to ensure that their child attends school regularly. Apart from legitimate reasons for absence from school, non-attendance can arise through school refusal, truancy and parentally condoned absence from school. School refusal is unlikely to require the preparation of a psychiatric report, as the parents are usually only too eager to co-operate with the treatment plan. Truancy is often part of a more widespread disturbance in the child and family, so that the psychiatrist may be asked by the court to provide an overall assessment of the situation and to make a recommendation about future needs. Parentally condoned absence from school occurs most commonly among families who are deprived and disorganised. There is often a family tradition of such problems. A major reason for the psychiatric referral is to exclude a psychiatric disorder in the parents or the child as a basis for the problem.

## Delinquency

This is a legal term referring to an offence or crime committed by a child or adolescent. In many circumstances, there is little indication of psychiatric disturbance in other aspects of the individual's behaviour. For a minority, however, a psychiatric opinion is valuable, especially when there is other evidence of psychiatric disturbance and/or the offence is so serious that it warrants further investigation. The same principles involved in the preparation of a court report apply in this situation. An important consideration is whether specific psychiatric treatment is likely to be beneficial and also acceptable to the child and family.

## CHILD-CARE LAW

Child-care legislation varies widely between countries, so that only some general comments about UK law will be made with the additional proviso that the law in Scotland differs from that in the rest of the UK.

### The Children Act 1989

This Act, implemented in 1991, produced a fundamental revision of the law relating to children in England and Wales. The Act was designed to combine private and public law provisions for children, to define children's rights, to strike a better balance between protection of the child and the retention of parental responsibilities for the child and, finally, to encourage greater co-operation between the parents and the statutory authorities.

The Act clearly states that the interests of the child are the over-riding consideration determining decisions about the child's welfare. The notion of parental rights is replaced by that of parental responsibilities. The Act defines the latter as 'all the rights, duties, powers, responsibility and authority which by law the parent of the child has in relation to the child and his property'. Children are recognised as separate parties with their own rights of representation in legal proceedings. Local authorities are obliged to identify children in need, to protect them and also to provide services to meet their needs and that of their families.

The Act also establishes the principle that the court has to be convinced that it is in the child's interest to make an order rather than rely upon voluntary measures. When the court is considering making an order, it has to have regard for the following:

- the ascertainable wishes and feelings of the child (depending on age and understanding)
- the physical, emotional and educational needs of the child
- the likely effect on the child of any change in circumstances
- the age, sex, background and any characteristics of the child which the court considers relevant
- any harm which the child has suffered or is at risk from suffering
- the competence of the parents, and any other person in relation to whom the court considers the question to be relevant, to meet the child's needs
- the range of powers available to the court in the proceedings in question.

The main purpose of the above checklist is to ensure that the individual needs and current circumstances of the child are examined carefully before statutory measures are implemented. The Act also insists that these matters are resolved as expeditiously as possible as 'any delay is likely to prejudice the welfare of the child'.

Three new sections of the Act, family proceedings, care and supervision, and the protection of children, have introduced important changes in child-care practice that have implications for child psychiatrists. The concepts of custody and access, and care and control, have been replaced by four new orders, the Residence Order, the Contact Order, the Specific Issue Order and the Prohibited Steps Order. The guiding principle of the new orders is that the child should retain contact with both parents and that they are jointly responsible for meeting the child's physical, moral and emotional needs.

The Residence Order specifies with whom the child will live, while the Contact Order requires that the resident parent allows the child to visit or to stay with the other parent. The Specific Issue Order and the Prohibited Steps Order specify the actions that the parents can or cannot perform with their child respectively. Some examples of possible contentious decisions would include access to medical treatment, the type of education or the raising of the child in a specified religious denomination. If an act of omission or commission by the parent is likely to jeopardise the child's welfare, these two Orders can be taken out in order to prevent this situation from arising.

The Act introduces new Orders — the Care Order, the Interim Care Order and the Supervision Order — to cover compulsory measures of care and control for children. Before the court takes out an order, certain 'tests' or 'threshold' criteria have to be satisfied (Fig. 18.1). The first criterion is whether the child is suffering or likely to suffer harm through ill treatment or from impairment of health or development. The second stage involves a comparison between the child's situation and that of any other child in a similar position in order to determine whether the difference is significant. The final stage involves determining whether the significant harm, if

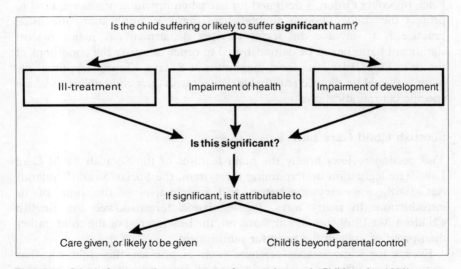

**Fig. 18.1**   Criteria for compulsory measures of care and control (Children Act 1989)

present, is attributable to the care given or likely to be given and/or whether the child is beyond parental control.

Providing the child meets one of the criteria, the court still has to decide whether making an Order would be better for the child than making no Order. The Care Order removes parental rights and places the social services department in charge of the child's welfare. Despite this position, the parents and the social services department are supposed to work together to meet the child's needs. The less drastic Supervision Order provides the social worker with the legal right to advise, assist and, where necessary, visit the child and the family. The Interim Care and Interim Supervision Orders are temporary arrangements to protect the child while definitive decisions about future care are made. Finally, the Act has a specific Education Supervision Order to ensure that the child receives a satisfactory education.

The Child Assessment Order and the Emergency Protection Order are the two orders designed to protect children. The main requirements of the Child Assessment Order are as follows:

- The child is suffering or likely to suffer from significant harm
- The assessment is necessary to enable the applicant to determine whether significant harm is present
- A satisfactory assessment cannot be completed unless an order is obtained.

The applicant is usually a local authority social worker or a specialist child protection social worker who has in addition a specific duty to keep the parents informed about the plan of action. The Order lasts for a maximum of 7 days.

The Emergency Protection Order, which replaces the previously existing Place of Safety Order, is designed for use when urgent action is required to protect the child. Though anybody can make an application, the usual practice is to involve the social services department. A major risk of significant harm has to be demonstrated in order to satisfy the conditions of the Act. The Order lasts for a maximum of 8 days. During this time, the parents should be allowed reasonable contact with their child unless there are specific contraindications.

## Scottish Child Care Law

This section reviews briefly the main features of the Scottish Child Care Law. The legislation underpinning the system, the Social Work (Scotland) Act 1968, was very innovative and imaginative at the time of its introduction. In many ways, the legislation foreshadowed the English Children Act 1989 with its emphasis on 'the best interest of the child' rather than proof of guilt or the need for punishment.

Except for some serious offences such as murder, the child who has committed an offence or who is in need of care and control goes before a

Children's Hearing rather than the Juvenile Court. The Hearing system comprises a Reporter, a Children's Panel and the social work department as well as regular contributions from child psychiatrists, teachers, educational and clinical psychologists, and the police.

The Reporter, who is the administrator of the system, has a background in law and/or social work, with considerable powers of discretion. Each Scottish Region employs a Regional Reporter along with a number of deputies and assistants. The Children's Panel comprises three specially trained lay persons who are advised and assisted by the Reporter.

Referral to a Children's Hearing can be made by any person or agency on the following grounds:

- The child is beyond parental control
- There is a lack of parental control leading to
  — exposure to moral danger
  — unnecessary suffering or serious impairment of health or development
- The child fails to attend school regularly without reasonable excuse
- The child has committed an offence.

Upon receipt of the referral, the Reporter then decides whether there are grounds for referral and whether to convene a Hearing. The parents can challenge the grounds for referral in which case 'proof' of the evidence is necessary at the Sheriff Court. If the child, usually because of age, is unable to understand the grounds for referral, the case also has to go to the Sheriff Court.

When the grounds are proved and/or accepted by the parents, the Reporter has three options:

- to take no further action
- to ask the social work department to advise and assist the family on a voluntary basis
- finally, to convene a Children's Hearing.

The Reporter is likely to take no further action if the parents and the child have recognised the seriousness of the problem and seem able to resolve the difficulties themselves. Similarly, the Reporter would endeavour to obtain the co-operation of the child and family, so that they can work together with the social work department on a voluntary basis to resolve the difficulties.

When the Reporter decides to convene a Hearing, this is usually because the voluntary and informal measures are not adequate to meet the child's needs, that is, compulsory measures of care and control are necessary. At the Hearing, the Panel members, one of whom is the chairperson, meet in private with the parents and the child to listen, question and discuss the concerns about the child. The social work department has the statutory obligation to provide the Hearing with a report about the child and family along with recommendations about their needs. The Reporter, who is also present at the Hearing, advises the Panel about points of law and the options available. The main aim of the Hearing is to decide upon the best course of action to meet the child's needs.

Three options are available to the Hearing:

● to discharge the referral
● to make a Supervision Order
● to make a Residential Supervision Order.

If the referral is discharged, the Hearing has concluded that the child's needs are being met on a voluntary basis with no need for further statutory involvement. If a Supervision Order is imposed, the child and the family have to meet regularly with the social worker to decide upon the child's needs and the best way to meet those needs. The most drastic measure, the Residential Supervision Order, removes the child from home and places him in a named residential provision, usually a children's home, foster home or school. This Order also requires that the social worker meets with the child and family regularly to devise and implement a care plan for the child. The Residential Supervision Order is rarely used at the first appearance before the Hearing, but more commonly when other measures such as a Supervision Order have been tried and have failed to improve the situation.

Finally, the legislation demands that further Hearings are called to review the requirement for the Supervision Order, usually on an annual basis. The child and family also have the right to request an earlier Hearing to review the position.

When the child is at immediate risk, an emergency order, the Place of Safety Order, can be obtained by application to the Sheriff or to a Justice of the Peace. The Order lasts for 7 days, during which a Hearing must be convened to review the child's need for compulsory measures of care and control.

## Mental Health Acts (UK)

This legislation provides for the compulsory detention, assessment and treatment of people who are suffering from a mental disorder that renders them liable to be a danger to themselves and/or likely to harm others. The legislation does not have an age limit, so that the Acts apply to children and adolescents. In practice, however, they are rarely invoked with children, as other measures such as the Children Act can be applied where necessary to ensure that the child receives treatment. For adolescents aged 16 and over, the Mental Health Acts provide the legal framework to ensure that the individual can be compulsorily detained when necessary.

### Consent to treatment

Usually, parental permission is sufficient for medical assessment and treatment to be undertaken. When the parents refuse treatment for the child and when the failure to provide treatment would impair significantly the child's health and development, this constitutes grounds for compulsory measures of care and control under the Children Act 1989.

The child also has a right to refuse treatment. In order to exercise this right, it has to be shown that the child has 'sufficient understanding and intelligence to be capable of making up their own mind'. Clearly, this ability is acquired in a gradual process, so that the judgement on competence is based on the assessment of the individual child rather than by fixed rules according to age. If the child's health is, however, likely to be adversely affected by the refusal to have treatment, this may again constitute grounds for compulsory measures of care and control.

Recently, English law has accepted that a child under 16 can receive treatment without parental consent under certain circumstances, for instance the prescription of the contraceptive pill. Despite this decision, the ethical stance of the doctor is that the parents and the child should be in agreement about treatment. For the adolescent of 16 years and over, the law adopts the principle that the young person is competent to make his own decision unless there is evidence to the contrary. Consequently, when there is serious concern that the young person is at risk or a danger to others, the Mental Health Act legislation is the most suitable way to obtain compulsory measures of treatment.

## APPENDIX

Department of Child and Family Psychiatry
Royal Hospital for Sick Children
3 Rillbank Terrace,
EDINBURGH EH9 1LL
Tel No: 031 668 2251
CONFIDENTIAL

### [Subject]

**Psychiatric Report on Brian Jones (01.10.81) 23 Home Drive, Edinburgh**

### [Sources of information]

This report is based upon papers supplied to me by the Court and also a review of the case notes of this boy at the Department of Child and Family Psychiatry, Royal Hospital for Sick Children. I have also interviewed Mrs Jones and Brian separately and also together on one occasion.

### [History]

There have been major problems with this boy's behaviour at home and in the community for some time. In December 1991 he was involved in an episode of vandalism at school. His behaviour at school has also been difficult in that he has been defiant and oppositional towards the teachers. He has subsequently been suspended and excluded from his primary school. I understand that he has recently been seen by Mr Simpson from the Education Department and it is likely that he will be recommended for special educational placement in the next academic session.

Brian has also been involved in other antisocial behaviour in the community. He has stolen several items from shops in the past and he has been cautioned by the police on account of this behaviour.

There have been two major stresses for the Jones household in the recent past. Mrs Jones had an ectopic pregnancy and also a miscarriage and I understand that she is likely to have a hysterectomy in the near future. Moreover, Mrs Jones's cohabitee left the family household at the end of 1991. He had previously been living in the household for 4 years.

*In the family history, Mrs Jones* is a 29-year-old lady who has been working on a part-time basis until recently. Mrs Jones has suffered with epilepsy since childhood and she has had a recurrence of her seizures in the last year. Mrs Jones was born and reared in Edinburgh and still has close contact with her own parents. The maternal grandparents supervise the children for Mrs Jones at the weekends. Mrs Jones was married when she was 16, but this marriage subsequently proved unsatisfactory. Mr Jones left the family household approximately 5 years ago. There has been infrequent contact with the father since that time. There are two other siblings, *George*, aged 12 and *Michelle*, aged 5. Michelle has also previously been investigated and received treatment for epilepsy.

*In the personal history,* the pregnancy with Brian was normal. There was some concern around the neonatal period but he was discharged from hospital at 6 days. His developmental milestones were delayed, particularly with speech. He also began to have seizures and nocturnal fits in 1987. He has been receiving treatment for epilepsy with sodium valproate since that time. He has had no seizures in the past 18 months. He was previously referred to our Department in 1990 by the paediatric neurologists for a psychometric assessment and also on account of his behaviour problems.

Psychometric assessment indicated that he was of low average ability and his attainments were commensurate with his overall ability. Consequently, his reading skills are behind those of his chronological age. He attended our Department for a series of meetings with our clinical psychologist to improve his behaviour. This contact was discontinued in 1991.

## [Examination]

*At interview* it was apparent that Mrs Jones had found Brian's behaviour difficult to manage for some time. Mrs Jones and Brian appeared to have a close relationship with evidence of mutual affection for each other. For his part, Brian acknowledged the seriousness of the present situation and that it would be necessary for him to change school. There was no evidence that Brian was suffering from a depressive illness.

**[Opinion]**

*Opinion:* This boy showed several features of conduct disturbance both at home and at school. Several factors are responsible for the situation: first, the boy's temperamental disposition, which makes him impulsive and also lacking in foresight; second, his low average intellectual ability and consequent educational retardation; third, his epilepsy, which further increases his vulnerability to behavioural disturbance; fourth, the family instability, particularly his mother's recent ill health, and also the departure of his mother's cohabitee. I think it is likely that Brian will remain a vulnerable boy throughout his childhood and will require close supervision to ensure that he does not have further behavioural difficulties, particularly as he approaches adolescence.

**[Recommendation]**

*Recommendation:* I think that Brian should be made the subject of a Supervision Order. This should provide the framework to enable Brian and his mother to work closely with the Social Work Department to help with the present difficulties. I think a community-based approach is likely to be most successful. Finally, I think it would be beneficial if Brian were transferred into a more specialised educational provision as this would provide him with more individual help with his educational and behavioural difficulties at school.

**[Signature]**


Dr P. Hoare

**[Date]**

**[Qualifications]**
DM, BM, BCh, MRCPsych

**[Position]**
Consultant Child and Adolescent Psychiatrist

**[Place of Work]**
Department of Child and Family Psychiatry, Royal Hospital for Sick Children, Edinburgh

# 19. Services for disturbed children

Services for disturbed children in the UK are provided by health, education, social services and voluntary agencies, often working collaboratively. The legal system is also indirectly involved as the court has the power to make and enforce recommendations about the care of disturbed children, for instance placement in specialised residential resources and attendance at child psychiatric services.

## HEALTH SERVICE PROVISION

Apart from child psychiatric services, three other groups of health care professionals have contact with disturbed children: family doctors, hospital and community paediatricians and school medical services.

In the UK, the family doctor, alternatively known as the general practitioner or primary care physician, has the central role in the health care of children and their families. Family doctors see on average about 90% of 0–4-year-olds and about 60% of 5–14-year-olds at least once a year for a consultation. Garralda & Bailey (1986) found that approximately 25% of children seen by family doctors showed signs of disturbance, at least twice the percentage of such children in the community. Although these disturbances do not fit readily into a formal psychiatric classification, they are nevertheless distressing to the child and the parents. Certain features categorise the contact between the family doctor and the mother/child:

- The child is usually accompanied by the mother
- Physical symptoms are often the presenting complaint
- Anxiety and bed wetting are the common psychiatric symptoms
- There are concurrent signs of stress within the family.

Family doctors vary markedly in their interest and expertise in the emotional and behavioural problems of children. The normal consultation time for the family doctor is approximately 10 minutes; this practice militates against a worthwhile discussion of the problem. Clearly the family doctor has to re-organise and/or set aside a specifically dedicated time or session to help with this type of problem.

Successful consultation depends upon the following features:

- Focus on current problem(s), taking note of their onset, frequency and severity
- Use open-ended questions to facilitate discussion about the presenting problem, usually a physical symptom with an underlying psychological basis
- Explain and advise in simple language
- Encourage further visits if the problems do not resolve.

Health visitors and other support staff within the family doctor's practice often provide invaluable long-term support for mothers, particularly with preschool behaviour problems. Special child health clinics, staffed jointly by family practitioners and health visitors, can be a useful way to help with this type of problem, though careful thought and planning are essential to ensure the clinic is successfully run. Support groups for mothers of preschool children with specific difficulties, for instance sleep problems, are another way to assist.

### Hospital and community paediatricians

In the UK, there is a definite move to integrate all aspects of child health provision (Hall 1989) though, in practice, hospital and community services are still organised separately. Community-based paediatric services are a potentially valuable way by which paediatric care can be made more available to socially disadvantaged or minority ethnic groups, who have traditionally had a low 'take-up' rate for services. In order to be successful, community-based programmes need to make themselves 'user-friendly' and 'consumer-conscious'. Attractive facilities, particularly the provision of toys and a suitable creche area, and a welcoming approach are essential for these ventures to succeed. Once the mothers begin to realise the benefits of contact, work can begin on a more long-term basis to look at the emotional and behavioural difficulties frequently present in this group of children.

Paediatricians working in hospital out-patient and in-patient services see a large number of children who show signs of disturbance. Garralda & Bailey (1989) found that approximately 25% of children referred to paediatric out-patients had symptoms of disturbance. In most cases, this is secondary to their physical illness, but in a minority it is the main reason for referral. The busy out-patient clinic is not the ideal setting to deal with these problems; a special dedicated clinic, often run jointly with the child psychiatrist or psychologist, is a better way to manage the service. In-patient admission is stressful for many children and the principles outlined in Chapter 16 for reducing distress should be incorporated into hospital practice.

*School medical service*

This service, staffed by school doctors, school nurses, occupational therapists and physiotherapists, is another avenue by which emotional and behavioural problems can be identified and hopefully helped. While the educational psychologists are mainly responsible for the management of psychological problems in school, the school medical service can be useful in providing advice and support to the teaching staff about the medical aspects of the illnesses that the children have as well as a more general health promotional role within the school.

## Child psychiatric services

In the UK, this service is organised into a hospital and community out-patient service, a hospital day patient service and an in-patient service. In many cases, staff members often divide their working week between the different facilities, though more recently there is an increasing specialisation into out-patient, day patient or in-patient work. As day patient and in-patient services were discussed in Chapter 17, they will not be mentioned any further.

The main child psychiatric service is a hospital or community out-patient service. The staffing usually comprises a consultant child psychiatrist and other child psychiatrists in training, educational and/or clinical psychologists, social workers and sometimes child psychotherapists and occupational therapists. The latter two groups tend to work in secondary or tertiary referral services where individual psychotherapeutic work with children is undertaken.

Child psychiatrists have an initial medical degree followed by specialised postgraduate training in psychiatry. This comprises general training in psychiatry followed by further subspeciality training in child and adolescent psychiatry. The consultant child psychiatrist has had approximately 7 years postgraduate training on first appointment as a consultant.

Educational and clinical psychologists have a first degree in psychology followed by specialised postgraduate training in teaching or clinical psychology respectively. Some educational psychologists work exclusively with schools, while others divide their work between the school and the clinic. The psychologist, educational or clinical, is particularly useful in providing an accurate psychometric assessment of the child's abilities and attainments as well as a more general contribution to the treatment of disturbed children, particularly through the application of behavioural programmes.

The social worker usually has a first degree, often in social sciences, followed by postgraduate training in social work or social policy. The child psychiatric social worker has specialist therapeutic skills in counselling and family therapy as well as expertise in the legal and statutory aspects of child care.

Child psychiatrists receive referrals from a wide range of sources including family practitioners, paediatricians, social services departments, schools and, less frequently, the court. The clinic is often organised to work as a multidisciplinary teams in which the different professions work jointly and collaboratively with the individual child and family. Very often the work will involve a family assessment and treatment model, so that two therapists, often from different professions, work together with the family. Indeed, the most striking feature of contemporary child psychiatry practice in the UK is the wide diversity of approach to clinical work.

## Educational services

In the UK, the local authority has a statutory responsibility to provide education for children. Historically, special education was first provided for children with physical handicap or mental handicap. Subsequently, further categories of special education, for instance for children with maladjustment, blindness or deafness, were identified, so that special education, often in a residential school, was provided according to the diagnostic category to which the child had been assigned.

More recently, widespread dissatisfaction with this approach has led to a major reform of the provisions for children with special educational needs with the implementation of the Education Act (1981). This Act recognised that about 15% of children have special educational needs at some point in their school career, and that this required accurate assessment and the formulation of an individually planned treatment programme.

The Act proposed that a formal 'statement' of the child's educational needs is drawn up and documented for each child for whom it is thought necessary. The statement has five sections: the teachers' report, the educational psychologist's report, the health professional's opinion, the parents' views on the child's educational needs and the education department's views of the child's requirements together with its ability to meet these needs. The philosophy of this approach is to tailor the educational resources for the individual child and to review regularly whether the child's needs are being adequately met. Another pillar of the Act is the principle of integration, whereby children with special educational needs should be educated within the ordinary school system whenever possible.

Critics of the Act argue that the 'statementing' procedures are bureaucratic and cumbersome with no good evidence that integration within the ordinary school system is the best strategy for many children with special needs. Indeed, many parents express a preference for their child to be placed in a special school rather than in a special unit in an ordinary school.

The range of special education options is wide, with the following resources available:

• additional help within the ordinary classroom

- specialist tuition in a remedial group on a part-time basis during the school week
- full-time placement in a special unit within the ordinary school
- placement at a special school devoted solely to children with special educational needs. Different categories of school, similar to the previous classification, exist, for instance for children with mild and severe learning disabilities, physical disability or emotional and behavioural problems
- placement at a residential school.

Residential school placement, particularly for psychiatrically disturbed children, is used much less frequently than previously, mainly because of concerns about the feasibility of maintaining the links between the child and family when the child is away from home and because of the precarious family situation created when the child returns home after leaving school. Despite these reservations, residential schools have considerable advantages for some groups of children, for instance children with childhood autism.

The education department employs two groups of professionals, educational psychologists and educational welfare officers or social workers, who make important contributions to the services for disturbed children. The educational psychologist has a pivotal role in the identification and formalisation of the requirements for children with special educational needs. Educational psychologists work closely with individual schools in a variety of ways:

- They provide individual assessment of children and their educational needs
- They advise staff about the management of behavioural difficulties within the classroom
- They provide teaching staff with information and support about educational policies and practice.

Additionally, many educational psychologists work closely with the child psychiatric service, providing a sessional commitment to a community-based child guidance service.

The education welfare officer has a variety of roles supporting children and their families over some aspect of the child's schooling. Often this involves practical assistance with arrangements for schooling or, more specifically, to helping the parents to ensure that the child goes to school regularly, usually when school non-attendance is the problem.

### Social services

To paraphrase Gilbert and Sullivan, 'a social worker's lot is not a happy one'. Social workers have a wide range of responsibilities, including important statutory responsibilities. These involve child protection work, the preparation of court reports, the provision of supervision for children on Statutory Care and Control Orders and the surveillance of care standards for children in residential establishments.

Social services departments usually organise their services into community-based offices serving a defined geographical area or 'patch'. Many departments further divide their responsibilities into work with particular client groups, for instance with children and families or with the elderly. Most departments also provide specialist units for work within the hospital service. This is the usual way in which social workers become members of the child psychiatry service, though in some regions some social workers are still seconded to work in the community-based child guidance service. Finally, social service departments are responsible for residential establishments for disturbed children such as children's homes or assessment units.

## Voluntary organisations

Large voluntary organisations such as the National Society for the Prevention of Cruelty to Children (NSPCC) and Dr Barnardo's have traditionally taken a major interest in particular aspects of child welfare such as child protection or the provision of substitute family care. Their current interests now concentrate on the development of specialist services that are not already provided by the statutory agencies. Examples of recent projects include the establishment of specialist treatment programmes for children subjected to non- accidental injury, the placement of 'hard to place' children for adoption and community-based specialist educational projects. Other agencies such as the British Association for Adoption and Fostering promote research and service initiatives for certain groups of children, while others such as the Society for Autistic Children cater for the needs of children with a specific disability or illness.

# 20. Multiple choice questions

Multiple Choice Questions (MCQs) have become an established part of undergraduate and postgraduate examinations in medicine over the past 20 years. In the UK, most medical schools include this format as a routine component of their assessment of undergraduate training, while the Royal Colleges have increasingly used this approach in the higher professional examinations. MCQs have several attractive features:

- they are objective
- they are easy to score, especially when computer marking facilities are available
- it is relatively simple to interpret the results.

The most common format is the multiple true/false style. This involves an introductory statement or *stem* followed by a series of options or *completions*. The stem and an option together are called an *item* and any of these may be true or false. False items are called *distractors*. The student has to decide whether the item is true or false together with a third category, don't know. Most marking systems score a correct response as a positive mark, an incorrect response as a negative mark and a don't know as zero. Generally, MCQs should be brief, understandable, relevant and discriminating. The most difficult aspect of question design is to compose suitable distractors, that is, questions that raise doubts in the candidate's mind.

Two useful objective measures of the MCQ examination are the facility index and the discrimination index. The value of these measures is not absolute and will vary with the requirements of the examination. The *facility index* is the proportion of candidates who answer an individual item correctly, for instance, two-thirds correct produces a facility index of 0.67. A high facility index is acceptable provided that other items have a lower index. The *discrimination index* is a measure of the ability of an item to distinguish between strong and weak candidates. This index is commonly derived in the following manner: the candidates' total scores are divided into quartile ranges; the top and the bottom quartiles are compared for each item. The number of correct answers given by the bottom group is subtracted from that of the top group and the result divided by 25%. In most cases, the results should be a positive number, so that a negative result requires scrutiny.

## MULTIPLE CHOICE QUESTIONS IN CHILD AND ADOLESCENT PSYCHIATRY

The following 30 questions are designed to test knowledge in child and adolescent psychiatry. The format is as described in the previous section, that is, a positive mark for a correct answer, a negative mark for an incorrect answer and a zero mark for don't know. The results are given at the end.

## QUESTIONS

Q 1   **Attachment and bonding:**
  A   is exclusively to the mother
  B   can only occur in the first year of life
  C   can be impaired if there is neonatal separation
  D   increases the risk of non-accidental injury
  E   was studied extensively by Bowlby

Q 2   **Piagetian theory states that:**
  A   stages in development are invariant
  B   the formal operational stage occurs before the concrete operational stage
  C   conservation of mass occurs before conservation of number
  D   object permanence occurs in the sensorimotor stage
  E   animistic thinking occurs in the preoperational period

Q 3   **The following people and concepts are associated together:**
  A   Sigmund Freud and identity crisis
  B   Melanie Klein and good enough mothering
  C   Anna Freud and projective identification
  D   Donald Winnicott and transitional object
  E   Erik Erikson and a basic sense of trust

Q 4   **Thomas & Chess's temperamental dimensions include:**
  A   approach versus withdrawal
  B   emotional versus impassive
  C   impulsive versus deliberate
  D   adaptable versus unadaptable
  E   gregarious versus detached

Q 5   **Non-accidental injury:**
  A   is less common in parents who were themselves abused
  B   is more common in children with low birthweight

C   usually affects the oldest child in the family
D   is initially admitted by the parents
E   was originally described by Melanie Klein

**Q 6   Schizophrenia in childhood and adolescence:**
A   has a general population prevalence of 3/1000
B   is more common in boys
C   is more common in higher socioeconomic groups
D   has a more acute onset in adolescence
E   usually has visual rather than auditory hallucinations

**Q 7   A 2½-year-old child should be able to:**
A   build a tower of seven or eight cubes
B   climb stairs one foot on each step
C   copy a circle with a pencil
D   remain dry at night
E   give his full name

**Q 8   Psychiatric disorder in childhood:**
A   occurs in 15% of 10-year-old children
B   is three times more common in adolescents than in 10-year-olds
C   is associated with learning problems
D   does not persist for longer than a year
E   usually requires hospital admission

**Q 9   The normal child of 4 years:**
A   can ride a tricycle
B   can eat skilfully with a spoon
C   can write his/her name
D   can give his/her age
E   soils his/her pants once per week

**Q10   Children with childhood autism:**
A   usually have symptoms before 30 months
B   often later develop schizophrenia
C   have brain damage in a high proportion of cases
D   use echolalic speech
E   prefer people to objects

**Q11   Encopresis (soiling):**
A   is more frequent in girls than boys
B   is always a sign of psychiatric disorder
C   may be preceded by fistula-in-ano
D   is often responsive to toilet training
E   persists into adult life

**Q12    Breath-holding attacks:**
  A    are commoner in children over $3\frac{1}{2}$ years
  B    are easily confused with a generalised seizure
  C    may be precipitated by minor injury
  D    should be treated with sedatives
  E    are an important cause of brain damage

**Q13    Nightmares:**
  A    are independent of daytime anxiety
  B    are a sign of severe emotional disturbance
  C    occur during non-REM sleep
  D    should be treated with psychotropic drugs
  E    cannot be remembered on waking up

**Q14    Children with nocturnal enuresis:**
  A    are less likely to have encopresis than other children
  B    commonly have a first-degree relative with nocturnal enuresis
  C    are usually dry by day
  D    are usually psychiatrically disturbed
  E    should be treated with drugs below the age of 5

**Q15    Tics:**
  A    are less common in girls than boys
  B    most commonly involve the hands
  C    are best treated with antidepressant drugs
  D    generally recur for at least 6 months
  E    are made worse by emotional stress

**Q16    Psychological reaction to hospitalisation:**
  A    is most common between 9 months and 4 years
  B    is least severe in children with unstable homes
  C    is prevented by daily parental visiting
  D    persists for several weeks after discharge
  E    is more severe when previous separations were happy

**Q17    Conduct disorder in childhood:**
  A    is more common in boys
  B    is associated with delinquency
  C    is not associated with learning difficulties
  D    may reflect parental disharmony
  E    does not persist into adult life

**Q18    Severe mental retardation (IQ less than 50):**
  A    occurs in 5% of the population
  B    is not associated with psychiatric disorder

C   is frequently caused by failure in mother–child bonding
D   is associated with epilepsy
E   always has a known cause

**Q19   Common features of anorexia nervosa in adolescents include:**
A   overactivity
B   hypersomnia
C   hypersexuality
D   distorted body image
E   bulimia

**Q20   Emotional disorders in childhood:**
A   are more common in boys
B   have a better prognosis than conduct disorders
C   are usually depressive in type
D   may be associated with school refusal
E   may persist into adult life

**Q21   Juvenile delinquency:**
A   is more common in boys
B   has a definite hereditary basis
C   is a common sequel of encephalitis
D   commonly leads to persistent criminal behaviour in adult life
E   is more common in children from low socioeconomic classes

**Q22   Hyperkinetic syndrome in childhood:**
A   is frequently associated with low intelligence
B   is more common in girls
C   is associated with aggressive behaviour
D   responds well to sedation
E   is characterised by long attention span

**Q23   School refusal:**
A   is usually associated with educational failure
B   can present as recurrent abdominal pain
C   characteristically occurs in children who steal and lie
D   is not improved by early return to school
E   may be treated with diazepam

**Q24   Children with recurrent abdominal pain:**
A   may suffer from school refusal
B   are best treated with drugs
C   are usually aggressive and extrovert
D   may have symptoms into adult life
E   are of high intelligence

**Q25   Psychiatric disorder in epileptic children:**
  A   is less common than in children with other physical illnesses
  B   is associated with learning difficulties
  C   is particularly responsive to treatment with psychotropic drugs
  D   is more common in children with temporal lobe epilepsy
  E   can be exacerbated by anticonvulsants

**Q26   Specific language disorder in childhood:**
  A   is more common in girls
  B   is often followed by later reading difficulties
  C   is caused by insufficient language stimulation in the preschool
      years
  D   occurs in children of all levels of intelligence
  E   is usually of an expressive type

**Q27   Pervasive refusal (adamant refusal to eat or drink) syndrome:**
  A   is more common among girls
  B   is associated with a previous history of sexual abuse
  C   responds well to out-patient psychotherapy
  D   is associated with a good long-term prognosis
  E   has diagnostic EEG findings

**Q28   The following are examples of operant techniques:**
  A   flooding
  B   punishment
  C   response prevention
  D   extinction
  E   negative reinforcement

**Q29   Suicide in adolescents:**
  A   is more common in females
  B   is usually accomplished by drug overdose
  C   is more likely among adolescents described as impulsive and
      volatile
  D   is more likely among adolescents described as withdrawn and
      uncommunicative
  E   is more likely among adolescents described as perfectionist and
      self-critical

**Q30   The following are examples of cognitive distortions or errors in
Beck's theory of depression:**
  A   intellectualisation
  B   repression
  C   minimalisation
  D   dichotomous reasoning
  E   personalisation

ANSWERS

**Q 1 Attachment and bonding:**
A False — infant capable of attachment to anyone in close contact, e.g. father
B False — begins in first year, but continues throughout infancy
C True — neonatal separation is disruptive
D False — common cause of NAI is poor parent–child attachment
E True — main person responsible for the concept

**Q 2 Piagetian theory states that**
A True — biological basis of theory means sequence is universal
B False — other way round
C False — conservation of number first
D True — main task of this stage
E True — characteristic of this stage

**Q 3 The following people and concepts are associated together:**
A False — identity crisis and Erikson
B False — good enough mothering and Winnicott
C False — projective identification and Klein
D True
E True

**Q 4 Thomas & Chess's temperamental dimensions include:**
A True
B False — dimension of Buss & Plomin
C False — dimension of Buss & Plomin
D True
E False — dimension of Buss & Plomin

**Q 5 Non-accidental injury:**
A False — poor childhood experiences increase risk of inadequate parenting
B True — major risk factor, as child may be more demanding
C False — no association with ordinal position
D False — parents extremely reluctant to admit responsibility at outset
E False — Kempe was pioneer with this topic

**Q 6 Schizophrenia in childhood and adolescence:**
A False — prevalence rate 3/10 000 or less
B True
C False — more common in lower socioeconomic groups
D True — insidious onset more likely in younger children
E False — though they occur, they are still less frequent than auditory

**Q 7    A 2½-year-old child should be able to:**

A    True — developmental fact
B    False — 3-year-old milestone
C    False — copy only vertical or horizontal line
D    True — most are dry, though stress may impede acquisition
E    True — can *only* give full name

**Q 8    Psychiatric disorder in childhood:**

A    False — nearer to 10%
B    False — only slight increase in adolescence
C    True — strong association with conduct disorder
D    False — 40% in IOW study persisted at least 4 years
E    False — only small percentage require in-patient admission

**Q 9    The normal child of 4 years:**

A    True
B    True, only skilfully by 4 years
C    False — give, but not write full name
D    True
E    False — children should be clean by fourth birthday

**Q10    Children with childhood autism:**

A    True — defining feature of disorder
B    False — no evidence to support this assertion
C    False — no abnormalities on investigation in most cases
D    True — common feature of deviant language
E    False — other way round

**Q11    Encopresis (soiling):**

A    False — other way round
B    False — as a group these children are disturbed, but not every one
C    True — preceding fissure makes defaecation painful, hence retention
D    True — effective treatment for the problem
E    False — symptoms resolve by adolescence, but others may replace them

**Q12    Breath-holding attacks:**

A    False — other way round
B    True — important consideration in differential diagnosis
C    True — common cause for attack
D    False — no indication, spontaneous recovery occurs
E    False — no indication whatsoever

**Q13    Nightmares:**
A    False — daytime anxiety a likely precipitant
B    True — no evidence
C    False — occurs during REM sleep
D    False — no indication per se
E    False — child able to describe event vividly

**Q14    Children with nocturnal enuresis:**
A    False — two problems often occur together
B    True — strong family history
C    True — daytime dryness usually precedes night-time dryness
D    False — only approximately 25% are disturbed occurs
E    False — high rate of spontaneous improvement

**Q15    Tics:**
A    True — more common in boys
B    False — most commonly affect face than hands
C    False — no indication, unless depression is also present
D    True — lasts at least for this period in many cases
E    True — tics are regarded as a means to reduce excessive anxiety

**Q16    Psychological reaction to hospitalisation:**
A    True — separation anxiety is very common during this age period
B    False — stress of hospitalisation exacerbates the instability
C    False — reduced, but not eliminated
D    True — stressful effects continue for some time
E    False — previously happy separation protects the child

**Q17    Conduct disorder in childhood:**
A    True — at least 3:1
B    True — strong association with older children and adolescents
C    False — strong association with learning difficulties
D    True — important aetiological factor
E    False — frequent persistence into adult life

**Q18    Severe mental retardation (IQ less than 50):**
A    False — 3–4/1000
B    False — approximately 50% show evidence of disorder
C    False — no evidence
D    True — epilepsy and brain damage commonly found
E    False — 10–20% cause unknown

**Q19    Common features of anorexia nervosa in adolescents include:**
A    True — increased activity undertaken to reduce weight

**B** False — no evidence
**C** False — opposite, if anything
**D** True — common finding
**E** True — frequently found in older adolescents

**Q20  Emotional disorders in childhood:**
**A** False — other way round
**B** True — often a response to identifiable stress which then disappears
**C** False — anxiety is most common
**D** True — school refusal is usually anxiety-based, hence association
**E** True — increased risk of neurosis in adult life

**Q21  Juvenile delinquency:**
**A** True — at least 8:1
**B** False — family dysfunction is most common cause
**C** False — no evidence
**D** False — most delinquency is transitory, not persistent
**E** True — epidemiological findings support this association

**Q22  Hyperkinetic syndrome in childhood:**
**A** True — frequent finding
**B** False — other way round
**C** True — common symptom
**D** False — stimulant drugs are most effective
**E** False — short attention span is the rule

**Q23  School refusal:**
**A** False — refusers have good academic attainments
**B** True — often symptom of anxiety
**C** False — no antisocial symptoms usually
**D** False — early return to school advisable to reduce secondary problems
**E** True — may reduce anxiety or phobic symptoms

**Q24  Children with recurrent abdominal pain:**
**A** True — sometimes a reason for non-attendance at school
**B** False — psychotherapeutic approach most useful
**C** False — antisocial symptoms uncommon
**D** True — increased risk of neurosis in adult life
**E** False — occurs in children of all abilities

**Q25  Psychiatric disorder in epileptic children:**
**A** False — at least twice more common
**B** True — definite association

C   False — no more than other types of psychiatric disorder
D   True — definite association
E   True — particularly older anticonvulsants

**Q26   Specific language disorder in childhood:**
A   False — other way round
B   True — definite association
C   False — maturational delay is most important cause
D   True — language delay is independent of cognitive ability
E   True — easily most common type, receptive type very rare

**Q27   Pervasive refusal (adamant refusal to eat or drink) syndrome:**
A   True — available evidence supports this association
B   True — available evidence supports this association
C   False — serious condition, unlikely to respond to out-patient contact
D   False — available evidence does not support this association
E   False — no diagnostic findings

**Q28   The following are examples of operant techniques:**
A   False — an exposure technique
B   True
C   False — an exposure technique
D   True
E   True

**Q29   Suicide in adolescents:**
A   False — other way round
B   False — more usually by violent means such as hanging or shooting
C   True — available evidence supports this association
D   True — available evidence supports this association
E   True — available evidence supports this association

**Q30   The following are examples of cognitive distortions or errors in Beck's theory of depression:**
A   False — a psychoanalytic defence mechanism
B   False — a psychoanalytic defence mechanism
C   True
D   True
E   True

# Glossary

This brief glossary is provided to assist the reader without a medical background with the definition of some common neurological, genetic and drug terms used in the text. The psychiatric terminology in the book is defined when it occurs first in the main text, so that it is not repeated again.

## NEUROLOGICAL

### Epilepsy
This is the recurrent tendency to have seizures. A seizure is defined as a series of paroxysmal motor movements along with a total or partial loss of consciousness which are thought to be due to an alteration of brain function or activity.

Epilepsy is categorised into *generalised* or *partial seizures*. Generalised seizures affect all parts of the body in a symmetrical manner, whereas partial seizures affect a focal or local part of the body. Common categories of generalised seizures are *grand mal* or *tonic–clonic epilepsy, absence seizures* or *petit mal*, and *myoclonic seizures* or *muscular jerking*. Partial seizures include *simple motor seizures* affecting one group of muscles or *complex partial seizures* involving motor and psychological symptoms. Complex partial seizures were previously often known as *psychomotor epilepsy* or *temporal lobe epilepsy*. Temporal lobe epilepsy refers to the site of origin of the seizure, whereas psychomotor epilepsy refers to the psychological and motor symptoms commonly present.

In addition to the common types of seizure such as tonic–clonic or psychomotor, children with epilepsy can often have a wide variety of other seizures including *atonic* or *loss of tone seizures, tonic* or *increased tone seizures* and *infantile spasms* or *drop attacks*.

Two severe forms of childhood epilepsy are *West's syndrome* and *Lennox–Gastaut syndrome*. These syndromes are characterised by frequent multiple seizures patterns with grossly disturbed EEG abnormalities and mental retardation.

355

## Cerebral palsy

This term is applied to a group of conditions whose main feature is a weakness affecting different muscle groups. It is usually present from early life and is not progressive. Examples include *hemiplegia* (loss of movement of the arm and leg on one side), *diplegia* (loss of movement of the lower limbs) and *quadriplegia*, affecting all four limbs.

## Extrapyramidal system

This neuronal network is involved in the control of motor movement. Abnormalities include *acute dystonic reactions* (sudden increase in muscular tone), *parkinsonian symptoms*, where there is muscular rigidity, tremor and difficulty starting movement, and *tardive dyskinesia*, in which there are rhythmic involuntary movements of the tongue, face, mouth or jaw. *Oculogyric crises* (upward movement of the eyes) and *acute torticollis* (abrupt turning of the neck muscles to one side into a fixed position) are common examples of acute dystonic reactions. Extrapyramidal movement disorders are often associated with long-standing treatment with phenothiazines. Antiparkinsonian drugs such as benzhexol or orphenadrine are used to control the parkinsonian side effects induced by phenothiazines.

## Other motor movements

*Chorea* is a group of conditions in which there are involuntary movements, commonly involving the face and limbs, which have some component of normal movement. The movements are not, however, under voluntary control and happen in an irregular and fragmented sequence. The movements are called *choreiform movements*.

*Athetosis/athetoid movements* are slow, sinuous writhing movements of the face and limbs, most marked with peripheral movements.

## Other neurological terms

*Ataxia*
Lack of muscular co-ordination

*Apraxia*
The inability to carry out purposeful movements correctly, so that a co-ordinated sequence of movements is not possible.

*Encephalitis*
Inflammation of the brain. It has many causes.

*Hydrocephalus*
Dilatation of the ventricles or fluid chambers in the inside of the brain with possible damage to brain function. Treatment can involve the insertion of a shunt to drain the excess fluid.

*Meningitis*
Inflammation of the linings surrounding the brain. Produces acute symptoms such as severe headache and vomiting. Potentially serious.

*Infections of the brain*
These include *rubella*, which can produce severe damage to the brain involving vision and hearing when the infection occurs during pregnancy.

*Toxoplasmosis* and *cytomegalovirus infections* also affect the developing fetus, with adverse effects on brain development.


GENETICS
The human genome or human genetic material consists of 23 pairs of *chromosomes*, threadlike structures present in each cell. The chromosomes are composed of several million *genes* or units of chromosome responsible for the production of enzymes and proteins. There are 22 pairs of *autosomal* or *non-sex chromosomes* and one pair of *sex chromosomes*. The male sex chromosomes comprise X and Y, the female X and X. Inheritance can involve either autosomal chromosomes or sex chromosomes. When it involves the latter it is called *sex-linked inheritance*. Inheritance can be *dominant* or *recessive* depending on whether one or both members of the chromosome pair have to be affected for the effect to be evident. Dominant inheritance requires only one member to be abnormal for the expression of the effect, while recessive inheritance requires both.

*Genotype* is the term for the total genetic material of the individual, whereas *phenotype* refers to the appearance or constitution of the individual which is the result of the interaction between the genotype and the environment.


DRUGS
Psychotropic drugs are divided into various categories:

**Anxiolytics**
Examples are *benzodiazepines* such as diazepam or chlordiazepoxide. Also known as *minor tranquillisers*.

**Major tranquillisers**
These include *phenothiazines* such as chlorpromazine and *butyrophenones* such as haloperidol. Used in treatment of acutely psychotic conditions such as schizophrenia and manic depressive psychosis. Sedative in large doses. Pronounced extrapyramidal side effects.

**Antidepressants**
*Tricyclics*, which have a chemical structure of three rings, are successful in the treatment of depression. Examples are imipramine and amitriptyline.

Newer antidepressants are drugs that affect serotonin (5-hydroxytryptamine) metabolism. Fluoxetine has been used in treatment of depression in children and adolescents.

## Stimulants

Examples are *methylphenidate* and *amphetamine*. The former is still used in the treatment of hyperkinetic disorders.

# References

Achenbach T, Edelbrock C 1983 Manual for child behaviour checklist and revised behaviour profile. Achenbach, Vermont

Ackerman N 1958 The psychodynamics of family life. Norton, New York

Ainsworth M 1982 Attachment: retrospect and prospect. In: Parkes C, Stevenson-Hinde J (eds) The place of attachment in human behaviour. Basic Books, New York

American Psychiatric Association 1987 Diagnostic and statistical manual of mental disorders (III). American Psychiatric Association Press, Washington, DC

Anthony E, Scott P 1960 Manic-depressive psychosis in childhood. Journal of Child Psychology and Psychiatry 4: 53–72

Apley J, MacKeith R 1968 The child and his symptoms. Blackwell, Oxford

Ashton C 1990 Solvent abuse: little progress after twenty years. British Medical Journal 300: 135–136

Asperger H 1944 Die 'autistischen Psychopathien' im Kindesalter. Archiv für Psychiatrie und Nervenkrankheiten 117: 76–136

August G , Stewart M 1983 Familial subtypes of childhood hyperactivity. Journal of Nervous and Mental Diseases 171: 362–368

Axline V 1969 Play therapy. Ballantine, New York

Bandura A 1969 Principles of behaviour modification. Rinehart & Winston, New York

Barker P 1992 Basic family therapy, 3rd edn. Blackwell Scientific Publications, Oxford

Bateson G, Jackson D, Haley J, Weakland J 1956 Towards a theory of schizophrenia. Behavioural Science 1: 251–264

Baumrind D 1972 Socialisation and instrumental competence in young children. In: Hartnup E (ed) Young child: reviews of research, vol 2. National Association for the Education of Young Children, Washington, DC

Bax M, MacKeith R (eds) 1963 Minimal cerebral dysfunction. Clinics in Developmental Medicine No. 10 SIMP/Heinemann, London

Bayley N 1969 Bayley scales of infant development: birth to two years. Psychological Corporation, New York

Beck A 1970 Cognitive therapy: nature in relation to behaviour therapy. Behaviour Therapy I: 184–200

Beck A 1976 Cognitive therapy and the emotional disorders. International Universities Press, New York

Beck A, Rush A, Shaw B, Emery G 1979 Cognitive therapy of depression. Wiley, New York

Bee H 1989 The developing child, 5th edn. Harper, New York

Belman M 1966 Studies in encopresis. Acta Paediatrica Scandinavica Suppl. 170

Bender L 1938 A visual motor gestalt test and its clinical use. American Orthopsychiatric Association, Albany, New York

Bender L, Schilder P 1940 Impulsions: A specific disorder of the behaviour of children. Archives of Neurology and Psychiatry 44: 990–1008

Bentovim A, Elton A, Hildebrand J, Tranter M, Vizard E 1988 Child sexual abuse within the family: assessment and treatment. Wright, Bristol

Berg I 1970 Follow-up study of school phobic adolescents admitted to an in-patient unit. Journal of Child Psychology and Psychiatry 11: 37–47

Berg I 1982 When truants and school refusers grow up. British Journal of Psychiatry 141: 208–210

Berg I 1985 The management of truancy. Journal of Child Psychology and Psychiatry 26: 325–331

Berger M, Yule W, Rutter M 1975 Attainment and adjustment in two geographical areas II. Prevalence of specific reading retardation. British Journal of Psychiatry 126: 510–519

Bishop D 1987 The causes of specific developmental language disorder ('developmental dysphasia'). Journal of Child Psychology and Psychiatry 28: 1–8

Black D 1986 Schoolgirl mothers. British Medical Journal 293: 1047

Bleuler E 1911 Dementia praecox or the group of schizophrenias (trans Z Zinkin 1950). Vienna International Universities Press, New York

Bloomfield S, Calder J, Chisholm V, Kelnar, C, Steel J, Farquhar J, Elton R 1990 A project in diabetes education for children. Diabetic Medicine 7: 137–142

Bolton D, Colins S, Steinberg D 1983 The treatment of obsessive-compulsive disorder in adolescents. British Journal of Psychiatry 142: 456–464

Bourne S, Lewis, E 1991 Perinatal bereavement. British Medical Journal 302: 1167–1168

Bowlby J 1969 Attachment and loss, vol 1: Attachment. Hogarth Press, London

Bradley C 1937 Behaviour of children receiving Benzedrine. American Journal of Psychiatry 94: 577–585

Braswell L, Kendall P 1988 Cognitive-behavioral methods with children. In: Dobson K (ed) Handbook of cognitive-behavioural therapies. Guilford Press, New York

Brown G, Harris T 1978 Social origins of depression: a study of psychiatric disorder in women. Tavistock, London

Brown G, Chadwick O, Shaffter D, Rutter M, Traub N 1981 A prospective study of children with head injuries: III. Psychiatric sequelae. Psychological Medicine 11: 63–78

Bruch H 1973 Eating disorders: obesity and anorexia. Basic Books, New York

Bruinincks R 1978 Bruinincks–Oseretsky test of motor proficiency. American Guidance Service, Minnesota, USA

Bryant P 1974 Perception and understanding in young children. Methuen, London

Buss A, Plomin R 1975 A temperament theory of personality. Wiley, New York

Byrne E, Cunningham C 1985 The effects of mentally handicapped children on families – a conceptual review. Journal of Child Psychology and Psychiatry 26: 847–864

Campbell A, McIntosh N (eds) 1992 Forfar & Arneil's textbook of paediatrics, 4th edn. Churchill Livingstone, Edinburgh

Campbell M, Spencer E 1988 Psychopharmacology in child and adolescent psychiatry: a review of the past five years. Journal of the American Academy of Child and Adolescent Psychiatry 27: 269–279

Cantwell D, Baker L 1985 Psychiatric and learning disorders in children with speech and language disorders: A descriptive analysis. Advances in Learning and Behaviour Disabilities 4: 29–47

Caplan H L 1970 Hysterical 'conversion' symptoms in childhood. MPhil Dissertation, University of London

Carlson G, Davenport Y, Jamison K 1977 A comparison of outcome in adolescent and late-onset bipolar manic depressive illness. American Journal of Psychiatry 134: 919–922

Carroll B 1982 Dexamethasone of suppression test: a review of contemporary confusion. Journal of Clinical Psychiatry 46, 13–24

Chadwick O, Rutter R, Brown G, Shaffer D, Traub M 1981 A prospective study of children with head injuries: II. Cognitive sequelae. Psychological Medicine 11: 49–61

Chambers W, Puig-Antich J, Hirsch M, Paez P, Ambrosini P, Tabrizi M, Davies N 1985 The assessment of affective disorders in children and adolescents by semi-structured interview. Archives of General Psychiatry 42: 696–702

Chomsky N 1965 Aspects of theory of syntax. MIT Press, Cambridge, MA

Clements S, Peters J 1962 Minimal brain dysfunction in school-age children. Archives of General Psychiatry 6: 185–197

Corbett J 1979 Psychiatric morbidity and mental retardation: In: James F, Snaith R (eds) Psychiatric illness and mental handicap. Gaskell Press, London

Corbett J, Mathews A, Connell P, Shapiro D 1969 Tics and Gilles de la Tourette's syndrome: a follow-up study and critical review. British Journal of Psychiatry 115: 229–241

Corbett J , Harris R, Taylor E, Trimble M 1977 Progressive disintegrative psychosis of childhood. Journal of Child Psychology and Psychiatry 18: 211–219

Cousens P, Waters B, Said J, Stevens M 1988 Cognitive effects of cranial irradiation in leukaemia: a survey and meta analysis. Journal of Child Psychology and Psychiatry 29: 839–852

Craigen G, Kennedy S, Garfinkel P, Jeejeebhoy K 1987 Drugs that facilitate gastric emptying. In: Garfinkel P, Garner D (eds) The role of drug treatments for eating disorders. Brunner/Mazel, New York

Crisp A, Palmer R, Kalucy R 1976 How common is anorexia? A prevalence study. British Journal of Psychiatry 128: 549–554

Crome L 1960 The brain and mental retardation. British Medical Journal i: 897–904

Department of Health and Social Security 1988 Report of inquiry into child abuse in Cleveland 1987. Cm 413. HMSO, London

De Sanctis S 1906 Sopra alcune varieta della demenzi precoce. Rivista Sperimentale de Freniatria e di Medicina Legale 32: 141–165

Deykin E, McMahon B 1979 The incidence of seizures among children with autistic symptoms. American Journal of Psychiatry 136: 1310–1312

Donaldson M 1978 Children's minds. Fontana/Collins, Glasgow

Dorner S 1976 Adolescents with spina bifida: how they see their situation. Archives of Diseases in Childhood 51: 439–444

Douglas J, Richman M 1984 My child won't sleep. Penguin, Harmondsworth

Dreifuss F 1989 Childhood epilepsies. In: Hermann B, Seidenberg N (eds) Childhood epilepsies: neuropsychological, psychosocial and intervention aspects. Wiley, Chichester

Dubovitz V, Hersov L 1976 Management of children with non-organic (hysterical) disorders of motor function. Developmental Medicine and Child Neurology 18: 358–368

Dunnell K 1990 Monitoring children's health. Population Trends No 60, HMSO, London

Eaton-Evans J, Dugdale A 1988 Sleep patterns of infants in the first year of life. Archives of Disease in Childhood 63: 647–649

Egger J, Carter C, Graham P, Gumley D, Soothil J 1985 A controlled trial of oligoantigenic treatment in the hyperkinetic syndrome. Lancet i: 540–545

Eggers C 1978 Course and prognosis of childhood schizophrenia. Journal of Autism and Childhood Schizophrenia 7: 21–36

Elliott C, Murray D J, Pearson L 1983 The British abilities scales (new edn). National Foundation for Educational Research/Nelson, Windsor

Erikson E 1965 Childhood and society. Penguin, London

Evans J 1982 Adolescent and pre-adolescent psychiatry. Academic Press, London

Farrington D 1978 The family backgrounds of aggressive youths. In: Hersov, L, Berger M, Shaffer D (eds) Aggression and antisocial behaviour in childhood and adolescence. Pergamon, Oxford

Farrington D 1990 Long-term criminal outcomes of hyperactivity-impulsivity-attention deficit (HIA) and conduct problems in childhood. In: Robins L, Rutter M (eds) Straight and devious pathways from childhood to adult life. Cambridge University Press, Cambridge

Faull C, Nicol R 1986 Abdominal pain in six-year-olds: an epidemiological study in a new town. Journal of Child Psychology and Psychiatry 27: 251–261

Feingold B 1975 Hyperkinesis and learning difficulties linked to artificial food flavors and colors. American Journal of Nursing 75: 797–803

Flament M, Rapoport J, Berg C, Sceery W, Kitts C, Mellstromm B, Linnolia M 1985 Clomipramine treatment of childhood obsessive-compulsive disorder. Archives of General Psychiatry 42: 977–983

Flament M, Coby E, Rapoport J, Berg C, Zahn T, Cox C, Denckla M, Lemane M 1990 Childhood obsessive-compulsive disorder: A prospective follow-up study. Journal of Child Psychology and Psychiatry 31: 363–380

Fogelman D, Tibbenham A, Lambert L 1980 Attendance in school: findings from the national child development study. In: Hersov L, Berg I (eds) Out of School. Wiley, Chichester

Fordham K, Meadow R 1988 Control trial of standard pad and bell alarm against mini-alarm for nocturnal enuresis. Archives of Disease in Childhood 64: 651–656

Forrest G, Claridge R S, Baum D 1981 Practical management of perinatal death. British Medical Journal 281: 31–32

Forrest G, Standish E, Baum D 1982 Support after perinatal death: a study of support and counselling after perinatal death. British Medical Journal 285: 1475–1478

Frankenberg W, Dodds J, Fandal A, Kazuk E, Cohrs M 1975 Denver screening test. Ladoca Project and Publishing Foundation, Denver, CO

Fraser A, Taylor D 1986 Childhood encopresis extended into adult life. British Journal of Psychiatry 149: 370–371

Freeman R 1977 Psychiatric aspects of sensory disorders and intervention. In: Graham P (ed) Epidemiological approaches in child psychiatry. Academic Press, London

Freeman R, Malkin S, Hastings J 1975 Psychological problems of deaf children and their families: a comparative study. American Annals of the Deaf 120: 391–405

Freud A 1936 The ego and the mechanisms of defence. Hogarth Press, London

Freud A 1946 The psychological treatment of children. Imago, London

Freud S 1953 Three essays on the theory of sexuality (1905). In: Collected papers, vol 7, standard edn. Hogarth, London

Fritz G, William J, Amylan M 1988 After treatment ends: psychosocial sequelae in pediatric cancer survivors. American Journal of Orthopsychiatry 58: 552–561

Gadow K 1992 Paediatric psychopharmacotherapy: a review of recent research. Journal of Child Psychology and Psychiatry 33: 153–196

Gallessich J 1982 The profession and practice of consultation: a handbook for consultants, trainers of consultants and consumers of consultation services. Jossey-Bass, London

Garralda M, Bailey D 1986 Children with psychiatric disorders in primary care. Journal of Child Psychology and Psychiatry 27: 611–624

Garralda M, Bailey D 1989 Psychiatric disorders in general paediatric referrals. Archives of Disease in Childhood 64: 727–733

Gaynor J, Hatcher C 1987 The psychology of child firesetting. Detection and intervention. Brunner/Mazel, New York

Gilles de la Tourette G 1885 Étude sur une affection nerveuse caractérisé par de l'incoordination motrice accompagné d'echolalie et de copralalie. Reprinted in: Archives of Neurology 9: 158–200

Gittelmain-Klein R 1987 Pharmacology in childhood hyperactivity: an update. In: Meltzer H (ed) Psychopharmacology: the third generation of progress. Raven Press, New York

Goldman A, Beardsmore S, Hunt J 1990 Palliative care for children with cancer — home, hospital or hospice. Archives of Disease in Childhood 65: 641–644.

Goldstein J, Freud A, Solnit A 1980 Beyond the best interest of the child. Burnett Books, London

Goodman R, Stevenson J 1989 A twin study of hyperactivity: II. The aetiological role of genes, family relationships and perinatal adversity. Journal of Child Psychology and Psychiatry 30: 691–709

Goodyer I 1981 Hysterical conversion reactions in childhood. Journal of Child Psychology and Psychiatry 22: 179–188

Goodyer I 1990 Life experiences, development and childhood psychopathology. Wiley, Chichester

Goodyer I, Kolvin I, Gatzanis S 1985 Recent undesirable life events and psychiatric disorder in childhood. British Journal of Psychiatry 147: 517–523

Gordon N, MacKinlay I 1986 Motor learning difficulties: 'clumsy' children. In: Gordon N, MacKinlay I (eds) Children with neurodevelopmental disorders, vol 1. Neurologically handicapped children: treatment and management. Blackwell, Oxford

Graham P 1974 Depression in pre-pubertal children. Developmental Medicine and Child Neurology 16: 340–349

Graham P, Rutter M 1973 Psychiatric disorder in the young adolescent: a follow-up study. Proceedings of the Royal Society of Medicine 66: 1226–1229

Green W, Campbell M, Hardesty A, Grega D, Pradron-Gylon M, Shell J, Erlenmeyer-Kimling L 1984 A comparison of schizophrenic and autistic children. Journal of the American Academy of Child Psychiatry 23: 399–409

Griffiths R 1954 The abilities of babies. McGraw Hill, New York

Gurman A, Kniskern D, Pinsof W 1986 Research on the process and outcome of marital and family therapy. In: Garfield S, Bergin A (eds) Handbook of psychotherapy and behavior change. Wiley, New York

Hagberg B, Aicardi J, Dias K, Ramos O 1983 A progressive syndrome of autism, dementia, ataxia and loss of purposeful hand use in girls: Rett's syndrome. Archives of Neurology 14: 471–479

Haley J 1976 Problem solving therapy. Jossey-Bass, San Francisco

Hall D (ed) 1989 Health for all children. Oxford Medical Publications, Oxford

Hall R, Tice L, Beresford T, Wooley B, Klassen A 1989 Sexual abuse in patients with anorexia nervosa and bulimia. Psychosomatics 30: 73–79

Hamilton M 1960 A rating scale for depression. Journal of Neurology and Neurosurgery 23: 56–61

Harlow H, Harlow M 1969 Effects of various mother–infant relationships on rhesus monkey behaviours. In: Foss B M (ed) Determinants of infant behaviour, vol 4. Methuen, London

Harris, P 1989 Children and emotion: the development of psychological understanding. Basil Blackwell, Oxford

Harter S 1983 Developmental perspectives on the self esteem. In: Mussen P (ed) Handbook of child psychology, vol 4: Socialisation, personality and social development, 4th edn. Wiley, New York

Harter S 1985 Manual for the self perception profile for children. University of Denver, Denver, CO

Hawton K, Salkovskis P, Kirk J, Clark D 1989 Cognitive behaviour therapy for psychiatric problems: a practical guide. Oxford University Press, Oxford

Heller T 1930 About dementia infantilis. Reprinted in: Howells JG (ed) 1969 Modern perspectives in international child psychiatry. Oliver & Boyd, Edinburgh

Henderson S 1987 The assessment of 'clumsy' children: old and new approaches. Journal of Child Psychology and Psychiatry 28: 511–527

Herbert M 1981 Behavioural assessment and treatment of problem children: a practice manual. Academic Press, London

Hersov L, Bentovim A 1985 In-patient and day hospital units. In: Rutter M, Hersov L (eds) Child and adolescent psychiatry: modern approaches. Blackwell Scientific Publications, Oxford

Hersov L, Berg I (eds) 1980 Out of school. Wiley, Chichester

Hewitt L, Jenkins R, 1946 Fundamental patterns of maladjustment: the dynamics of their origin. CC Thomas, Springfield, IL

Higgs J, Goodyer I, Birch J 1989 Anorexia nervosa and food avoidance emotional disorder. Archives of Disease in Childhood 64: 346–351

Hinde R, Spencer-Booth Y 1970 Individual differences in the responses of rhesus monkeys to a period of separation from their mothers. Journal of Child Psychology and Psychiatry 11: 159–176

Hoare P 1984a Development of psychiatric disorder among school children with epilepsy. Developmental Medicine and Child Neurology 26: 3–13

Hoare P 1984b Psychiatric disturbance in the families of epileptic children. Developmental Medicine and Child Neurology 26: 14–19

Hoare P, Kerley S 1991 Psychological adjustment of children with chronic epilepsy and their families. Developmental Medicine and Child Neurology 33: 201–215

Hoare P, Elton R, Greer A, Kerley S 1993 The modification and standardisation of the Harter self-esteem questionnaire with Scottish school children. European Child and Adolescent Psychiatry 2: 19–33

Hobson P 1986 The autistic child's appraisal of expressions of emotions: an experimental investigation. Journal of Child Psychology and Psychiatry 27: 321–342

Holland J, Roland J (eds) 1989 Handbook of psycho-oncology: psychological care of the patient with cancer. Oxford University Press, New York

Horne J 1992 Sleep and its disorders in children. Journal of Child Psychology and Child Psychiatry 33: 473–487

Jacobson R 1985a Fire-setters: a clinical investigation. Journal of Child Psychology and Psychiatry 26: 759–768

Jacobson R 1985b The sub-classification of fire-setters. Journal of Child Psychology and Psychiatry 26: 769–775

James W 1890 The principles of psychology. Holt, New York

Jenkins R 1969 Classification of behaviour problems in children. American Journal of Psychiatry 125: 1032–1039

Johnson S 1988 Psychological aspects of juvenile diabetes. Journal of Child Psychology and Psychiatry 29: 729–738

Jones D (ed) 1982 Understanding child abuse. Hodder & Stoughton Educational, Sevenoaks

Kanner L 1942 Child psychiatry. CC Thomas, Springfield, IL

Kanner L 1943 Autistic disturbances of affective contact. The Nervous Child 2: 217–250

Kazdin A 1990 Childhood depression. Journal of Child Psychology and Psychiatry 31: 121–160

Kempe R, Kempe C 1978 Child abuse. Fontana, London

Kendell R, Zealley A 1993 Companion to psychiatric studies, 5th edn, Churchill Livingstone, Edinburgh

Kerr A, Stephenson J 1985 Rett's syndrome in the west of Scotland. British Medical Journal 291: 579–582

Klein M 1932 The psycho-analysis of children. Hogarth Press, London

Klein M 1948 Contributions to psycho-analysis 1921–45. Hogarth Press, London

Knobloch H, Pasamanick B 1966 Prospective studies on the epidemiology of reproductive casualty: methods, findings and some implications. Merrill Palmer Quarterly 12: 27–43.

Kohlberg L 1964 Development of moral character and moral ideology. In: Hoffman M, Hoffman L (eds) Review of child development research, vol 1. Russel Sage Foundation, New York.

Kohlberg L 1966 A cognitive-developmental analysis of children's sex-role concepts and attitudes. In: Maccoby E (ed) The development of sex differences. Stanford University Press, Stanford, CA

Kolvin I 1971 Studies in childhood psychoses I. Diagnostic criteria and classification. British Journal of Psychiatry 118: 381–384

Kolvin I, Fundudis T 1981 Elective mute children: psychological development and background factors. Journal of Child Psychology and Psychiatry 22: 219–232

Kolvin I, Garside R, Nicol A, MacMillan A, Wolfstenhome F, Leitch I 1981 Help starts here: the maladjusted child in the ordinary school. Tavistock Publications, London

Kolvin I, Bernie T, Bhate S 1984 Classification and diagnosis of depression in school phobia. British Journal of Psychiatry 145: 347–357

Koocher G, O'Malley J 1981 The Damocles syndrome. McGraw-Hill, New York

Kraepelin E 1919 Dementia praecox and paraphrenia (trans Barclay R M). Livingstone, Edinburgh

Kramer H, Awiszus D, Sterzel U, Van Haltern A, Classen R 1989 Development of personality and intelligence in children with congenital heart disease. Journal of Child Psychology and Psychiatry 30: 299–308

Krenner P, Millar F 1989 Psychiatric response to HIV spectrum disease in children and adolescents. Journal of the American Academy of Child and Adolescent Psychiatry 28: 596–605

Kun L, Mulhern R, Chrisco J 1983 Quality of life in children treated with brain tumours: intellectual, emotional and academic function. Journal of Neurosurgery 58: 1–6

Lannering B, Markey I, Lundberg A, Olsson E 1990 Long-term sequelae after paediatric brain tumours: their effect on disability and quality of life. Medical Paediatric Oncology 18: 304–310

Lask B 1988 Novel and non-toxic treatment for night terrors. British Medical Journal 297: 592

Lask B, Bryant-Waugh R 1992 Early onset anorexia and related eating disorders. Journal of Child Psychology and Psychiatry 33: 281–300

Lask B, Fosson A. 1989 Childhood illness: the psychosomatic approach. John Wiley, Chichester

Lask B, Matthew D 1979 Childhood asthma — a controlled trial of family psychotherapy. Archives of Diseases in Childhood 54: 116–119

Lask B, Britten C, Kroll L, Magana J, Tranter N 1991 Children with pervasive refusal. Archives of Disease in Childhood 66: 866–869

Last C, Francis G, Hersen M, Kazdin A, Strauss C 1987 Separation anxiety in school phobia: a comparison using DSM-III criteria. American Journal of Psychiatry 144: 653–657

Leff J, Cuipers L, Berkowitz R, Erberlein-Vries R, Sturgeon D 1982 A Controlled trial of social intervention in the families of schizophrenic patients. British Journal of Psychiatry 141: 121–134

Lidz R, Lidz T 1949 A family environment of schizophrenic patients. American Journal of Psychiatry 106: 332–345

Lockyer L, Rutter M 1969 A five to fifteen year follow-up study of infantile psychosis III psychological aspects. British Journal of Psychiatry 115: 865–882

Lotter V 1966 Epidemiology of autistic conditions in young children: I. Prevalence. Social Psychiatry 1: 1241–1247

McAdam E, Gilbert P 1985 Cognitive behavioural therapy as a psychotherapy for mood disturbance in child, adolescent and family psychiatry. Newsletter, Association for Child Psychology and Psychiatry 7: 19–27

McAuley R, McAuley P 1977 Child behavioural problems. An empirical approach to management. Macmillan, London

McClure G 1984 Recent trends in suicide amongst the young. British Journal of Psychiatry 144: 134–138

McConville B, Boag L, Purohit A 1973 Three types of childhood depression. Canadian Psychiatric Association Journal 18: 133–138

McEvedy C, Griffiths A, Hall T 1966 Two school epidemics. British Medical Journal 2: 1300–1302

McGoldrick M, Carter E 1982 The family life style. In: Walsh F (ed) Normal family processes. Guilford, New York

McGuffin P 1987 The new genetics and childhood psychiatric disorder. Journal of Child Psychology and Psychiatry 28: 215–222

MacKeith R, Rutter M 1972 A note on the prevalence of speech and language disorders. In: Rutter M, Martin J (eds) The child with delayed speech. Clinics in Developmental Medicine 43. SIMP, Heinemann Medical, London

Maguire P 1982 Psychological and social consequences of cancer. In: William C, Whitehouse J (eds) Recent advances on clinical oncology. Churchill Livingstone, Edinburgh

Maguire P, Rutter D 1976 History taking for medical students: I. Deficiencies in performance. Lancet ii: 556–558

Mannuzza S, Gittelman-Klein R, Horowitz-Konig P, Giampino T 1989 Hyperactive boys almost grown up: IV. Criminality and its relationship to psychiatric status. Archives of General Psychiatry 46: 1073–1079

Meadow R 1982 Munchausen syndrome by proxy. Archives of Disease in Childhood 57: 92–98

Minuchin S 1974 Families and family therapy. Harvard University Press, Cambridge, USA

Minuchin S, Fishman H 1981 Family therapy techniques. Harvard University Press, Cambridge, MA

Minuchin S, Baker L, Rosman B, Liebman R, Millman M, Todd G 1975 A conceptual model of psychosomatic illness in children. Archives of General Psychiatry 32: 1031–1038

Minuchin S, Rosman B, Baker L 1978 Psychosomatic families: anorexia in context. Harvard University Press, Cambridge, Massachusetts

Mischel W 1970 Sex typing and socialisation. In: Mussen P (ed) Carmichael's manual of child psychology, 3rd edn, vol 2. Wiley, New York

Mrazek D 1985 Child psychiatric consultation and liaison to paediatrics. In: Rutter M, Hersov L (eds) Child and adolescent psychiatry: modern approaches, 2nd edn. Blackwell, Oxford

Mrazek D, Mrazek P 1985 Child maltreatment In: Rutter M, Hersov L (eds) Child and adolescent psychiatry: modern approaches, 2nd edn. Blackwell, Oxford

Mulhearn R, Horowitz M, Ochs J, Friedman A, Armstrong D, Copeland D 1989 Assessment of quality of life among paediatric patients with cancer. Psychological assessment: A Journal of Consulting and Clinical Psychology 1: 130–138

Mullen P, Romans-Clarkson S, Walton V, Herbison G 1988 Impact of sexual and physical abuse on women's mental health. Lancet i 841–845

Murphy G 1985 Update — self-injuring behaviour in the mentally handicapped. Newsletter, Association for Child Psychology and Psychiatry 7: 2–11

Neale M 1958 Neale analysis of reading ability manual. Macmillan, London

Needleman H, Gunnoe C, Leviton A, Reed R, Peresie H, Maher C, Barnett P 1979 Deficits in psychological and classroom performance of children with elevated dentine lead levels. New England Journal of Medicine 300: 689–695

Nolan T, Zvagulia I, Pless I 1987 Controlled trial of social work in childhood chronic illness. Lancet ii : 411–415

Offord D, Boyle M, Szatmari P, Rae-Grant N, Links P, Cadman D, Byles J, Crawford J, Blum H, Byrne C, Thomas H, Woodward C 1987 Ontario child health study: prevalence of disorder and rates of service utilisation. Archives of General Psychiatry 44: 832–836

Oglethorpe R 1989 Parenting after perinatal bereavement — a review of the literature. Journal of Reproductive and Infant Psychology 7: 227–244

Olness K, Gardiner G 1988 Hypnosis and hypnotherapy with children. Grune & Stratton, Philadelphia

Ounsted C, Lindsey J, Richards P 1986 Temporal lobe epilepsy 1948–1986. A biographical study. Clinics in Developmental Medicine 103. Blackwell Scientific Publications, Oxford

Ousten J (ed) 1990 Occasional papers 3. The consequences of child sexual abuse. Association of Child Psychology and Psychiatry, London

Palazzoli M, Boscolo L, Cecchin G, Prata G 1978 Paradox and counter paradox. Jason Aronson, New York

Palmer R, Oppenheimer R, Dignon A, Chaloner D, Howells K 1990 Childhood sexual experience with adults reported by women with eating disorders: an extended series. British Journal of Psychiatry 156: 699–703

Parsons T 1951 The social system. Free Press, New York

Patterson G 1982 Coercive family processes. Castalia, Oregon

Patterson G, Chamberlain P, Reed J 1982 A comparative evaluation of a parent-training programme. Behaviour Therapy 13: 638–650

Pauls D, Leckman J 1988 The genetics of Tourette's syndrome. In: Cohen D, Brunn R, Leckman J (eds) Tourette's syndrome and tic disorders. Wiley, New York

Pearce J 1978 The recognition of depressive disorder in children. Journal of the Royal Society of Medicine 71: 494–500

Petersen L 1989 Coping by children undergoing stressful medical procedures: some conceptual, methodological and therapeutic issues. Journal of Consulting and Clinical Psychology 57: 380–387

Piaget J 1929 The child's conception of the world. Kegan Paul, London

Pilowsky I 1969 Abnormal illness behaviour. British Journal of Medical Psychology 42: 347–351

Plant M, Peck D, Stuart T 1982 Self-reported drinking habits and alcohol related consequences among a cohort of Scottish teenagers. British Journal of Addiction 77: 75–90

Pomeroy J, Sprafkin J, Gaddow F 1988 Minor physical anomalies as a biological marker for behavior disorders. Journal of the American Academy of Child and Adolescent Psychiatry 27: 466–473.

Porter R (ed) 1984 Child sexual abuse within the family. Tavistock, London

Potter H 1933 Schizophrenia in children. American Journal of Psychiatry 89: 1253–1270

Powell G, Brazel J, Blizzard R 1967 Emotional deprivation and growth retardation simulating idiopathic hypopituitarism: I. Clinical evaluation of the syndrome. New England Journal of Medicine 276: 1271–1278

Poznanski E, Grossman J, Buchsbaum Y, Banegas M, Freeman L, Gibbons R 1984 Preliminary study of the reliability and validity of the children's depression rating scale. Journal of the American Academy of Child Psychiatry 23: 191–197

Quinton D, Rutter M 1976 Early hospital admission and later disturbances of behaviour: an attempted replication of Douglas's findings. Developmental Medicine and Child Neurology 18: 447–459

Redd W, Jacobson P, Die-Trill M, Dermatis H, McEvoy M, Holland J 1987 Cognitive-attentional distraction in the control of conditioned nausea in paediatric cancer patients receiving chemotherapy. Journal of Consulting and Clinical Psychology 55: 391–395

Reitan R, Woolfson D 1985 The Halstead–Reitan neuropsychological test battery. Neuropsychological Press, Tucson, AZ

Rett A 1966 Über ein eigenartiges hiratrophisches Syndrom bei Hyperammonamie im Kinderalter. Wiener Medizinishe Wochenschrift 116: 723–726

Reynell J 1969 Reynell developmental language scales. NFER, Windsor

Rich J 1956 Types of stealing. Lancet 1: 496–498

Richman N 1977 Behavioural problems in pre-school children. Family and social factors. British Journal of Psychiatry 131: 523–527

Richman N 1981 A community survey of characteristics of one-to-two-year-olds with sleep disruptions. Journal of the American Academy of Child Psychiatry 20: 281–291

Richman N, Lansdown R 1988 Problems of pre-school children. Wiley, Chichester

Richman N, Stevenson J, Graham P 1975 Prevalence of behaviour problems in three-year-old children: an epidemiological study in a London borough. Journal of Child Psychology and Psychiatry 16: 277–287

Richman N, Stevenson J, Graham P 1982 Pre-school to school: a behavioural study. Academic Press, London

Rivinus T, Jamison D, Graham P 1975 Childhood organic neurological disease presenting as psychiatric disorder. Archives of Disease in Childhood 50: 115–119

Robins L 1966 Deviant children grown up. Williams & Wilkins, Baltimore, MD

Robins L 1991 Conduct disorder. Journal of Child Psychology and Psychiatry 32: 193–212

Rosenberg D 1987 Web of deceit: a literature review of Munchausen's syndrome by proxy. Child Abuse and Neglect 11: 547–563

Rosenberg K, McEwan H 1991 Teenage pregnancy in Scotland: trends and risks. Scottish Medical Journal 36: 172–174

Russel A, Bott L, Sammons C 1989 The phenomenology of schizophrenia occurring in childhood. Journal of the Academy of Adolescent Psychiatry 28: 399–407

Russell G, Szmulker G, Dare C, Eisler I 1987 An evaluation of family therapy in anorexia nervosa and bulimia nervosa. Archives of General Psychiatry 44: 1047–1056

Rutter M 1981 Stress, coping and development: some issues and some questions. Journal of Child Psychology and Psychiatry 22: 323–356

Rutter M 1982 Psychological therapies in child psychiatry: issues and prospects. Psychological Medicine 12: 723–740

Rutter M 1985a The role of the family. In: Rutter M, Hersov L (eds) Child and adolescent psychiatry: modern approaches, 2nd edn. Blackwell, Oxford

Rutter M 1985b Infantile autism and other pervasive developmental disorders. In: Rutter M, Hersov L (eds) Child and adolescent psychiatry: modern approaches, 2nd edn. Blackwell, Oxford

Rutter M 1988 Depressive disorders. In: Rutter M, Tuma A, Lann I (eds) Assessment and diagnosis in child psychopathology. Fulton, London

Rutter M, Lord C 1987 Language disorders associated with psychiatric disturbance. In: Yule W, Rutter M (eds) Language development and disorders. Clinics in Developmental Medicine 101/102. Blackwell Scientific Publications, Oxford.

Rutter M, Schopler E (eds) 1978 Autism: a reappraisal of concepts and treatment. Plenum Press, New York

Rutter M, Graham P, Yule W 1970a A neuropsychiatric study of childhood. Clinics in Developmental Medicine 35/36. SMIP/Heinemann, London

Rutter M, Tizard J, Whitmore K 1970b Education, health and behaviour. Longman, London

Rutter M, Cox A, Tupling C, Berger M, Yule W 1975a Attainment and adjustment in two geographical areas: I. Prevalence of Psychiatric Disorders. British Journal of Psychiatry 126: 493–509

Rutter M, Yule B, Quinton D, Rowlands O, Yule W, Berger M 1975b Attainment and adjustment in two geographical areas: III. Some factors accounting for area differences. British Journal of Psychiatry 126: 520–533

Rutter M, Graham P, Chadwick O, Yule W 1976 Adolescent turmoil: fact or fiction? Journal of Child Psychology and Psychiatry 17: 35–56

Rutter M, Maughan B, Mortimore P, Ouston J 1979 Fifteen thousand hours. Open Books, London

Rutter M, Macdonald H, Le Couteur A, Harrington R, Bolton P, Bailey A 1990 The genetic factors in child psychiatric disorder: II. Empirical findings. Journal of Child Psychology and Psychiatry 31: 39–84

Salter A 1988 Treating child sex offenders and victims: a practical guide. Sage, Beverley Hills, CA

Satterfield J, Satterfield B, Schell A 1987 Therapeutic interventions to prevent delinquency in hyperactive boys. Journal of the American Academy of Child Psychiatry 26: 56–64

Sawyer M, Minde K, Zuker R 1983 The burnt child — scarred for life? A study of the psychosocial impact of a burn injury at different developmental stages. Burns Including Thermal Injury 9: 205–214

Schacher R 1991 Childhood hyperactivity. Journal of Child Psychology and Psychiatry 32 : 155–212

Schonell F, Schonell F 1950 Diagnostic and attainment testing. Oliver & Boyd, Edinburgh

Schultz J 1983 Timing of elective hypospadias repair in children. Paediatrics 71: 242–351

Seligman M 1975 Helplessness: on depression development and death. W Freeman, San Francisco, CA

Shaffer D 1974 Suicide in childhood and early adolescence. Journal of Child Psychology and Child Psychiatry 45: 406–451

Shaffer D 1984 Notes on psychotherapy research among children and adolescents. Journal of the American Academy of Child Psychiatry 23: 522–561

Shaffer D 1985 Brain damage. In: Rutter M, Hersov L (eds) Child and adolescent psychiatry: modern approaches, 2nd edn. Blackwell, Oxford

Shapiro A, Shapiro E 1988 Treatment of tic disorders with haloperidol. In: Cohen D, Brunn R, Leckman J (eds) Tourette's syndrome and tic disorders. Wiley, New York

Shapiro S, Garfinkel B 1986 The occurrence of behaviour disorders in children: the interdependence of attention deficit disorder and conduct disorder. Journal of the American Academy of Child Psychiatry 25: 809–819

Shepherd M, Oppenheim A, Mitchell S 1971 Childhood behaviour and mental health. University of London Press, London

Silver J, Yudofsky S, Hales R 1987 Neuropsychiatric aspects of traumatic brain injury. In: Hales R, Yudofsky S (eds) The American Psychiatric Press text book of neuropsychiatry. American Psychiatric Press, Washington, DC

Skuse D 1985 Non-organic failure to thrive: a reappraisal. Archives of Disease in Childhood 60: 173–178

Skuse D 1988 Psychosocial adversity and impaired growth in children: in search of causal mechanisms. In: Williams P, G, K (eds) The scope of epidemiological psychiatry: essays in honour of Michael Shepherd, Routledge, London

Snowling M 1991 Developmental reading disorders. Journal of Child Psychology and Child Psychiatry 32: 49–77.

Sparrow S, Balla D, Cicchetti D 1984 The Vineland adaptive behavior scales. American Guidance Service, Minnesota

Spence S 1983 Teaching social skills to children. Journal of Child Psychology and Psychiatry 24: 621–627

Spitz R 1946 Anaclitic depression. Journal of Psychoanalytic Study of the Child II; 313–342

Spitzer R, Endicott J 1978 Schedule for affective disorders in schizophrenia. New York State Psychiatric Institute, New York

Stein R, Jessop D 1984 Does paediatric home care make a difference for children with chronic illness? Findings from the paediatric ambulatory care treatment study. Paediatrics 73: 845–853

Stoddard F, Norma D, Murphy J, Beardslee W 1989 Psychiatric outcome of burnt children and adolescents. Journal of the American Academy of Child and Adolescent Psychiatry 28: 589–595

Stores G 1978 School children with epilepsy at risk for learning and behaviour problems. Developmental Medicine and Child Neurology 20: 502–508

Strauss A, Lehtinen, L 1947 Psychopathology and education of the brain injured child, vol I. Grune & Stratton, New York.

Szatmari P, Offord D, Boyle, M 1989a Correlates, associated impairments and patterns of service utilisation of children with attention deficit disorder: Finding from the Ontario child health study. Journal of Child Psychology and Psychiatry 30: 205–218

Szatmari P, Offord D, Boyle, M 1989b Ontario child health study: prevalence of attention deficit disorder with hyperactivity. Journal of Child Psychology and Psychiatry 30: 219–230.

Taylor E 1985 Attention deficit and conduct disorder syndromes In: Rutter M, Hersov L (eds) Child and adolescent psychiatry: modern approaches, 2nd edn. Blackwell, Oxford

Taylor E (ed) 1986 The overactive child. SIMP/Blackwell, Oxford

Thomas A, Chess S 1982 Temperament and development. Brunner/Mazel, New York

Thomas A, Chess S, Birch H 1968 Temperament and behaviour disorders in childhood. New York University Press, New York

Thomson G, Raals G, Hepburn W, Hunter R, Fulton M, Laxen D 1989 Blood-lead levels and children's behaviour-results from the Edinburgh Lead Study. Journal of Child Psychology and Psychiatry 30: 515–528

Thorndike R 1973 Stanford Binet intelligence scale, form L–M, 1972 norms tables. Houghton Mifflin, Boston

Vandenberg S, Singer S, Pauls D 1986 The hereditary of behaviour disorders in children and adults. Plenum, New York

Volkmar F, Cohen D, Hoshimoy 1988 Phenomenology and classification of childhood psychoses. Psychological Medicine 18: 191–201

von Bertalanffy 1968 General systems theory. Brazillier, New York

Waller D, Eisenberg L 1980 School refusal in childhood — a psychiatric–paediatric perspective. In: Hersov L, Berg I (eds) Out of school. Wiley, Chichester

Wechsler D 1974 Manual for the Wechsler intelligence scale for children — revised Psychological Corporation, New York

Weller R, Weller E, Tucker S 1986 Mania in prepubertal children: has it been underdiagnosed? Journal of Affective Disorders 11: 151–154

White S, Strom G, Santilli G, Halpin B 1986 Interviewing young sexually abused victims with anatomically correct dolls. Child Abuse and Neglect 10: 519–529

Wing L 1981 Asperger's syndrome: a clinical account. Psychological Medicine 11: 115–129

Wing L, Gould J 1979 Severe impairments of social interaction and associated abnormalities in children: epidemiology and classification. Journal of Autism and Developmental Disorders 9: 11–30

Winnicott D 1957 The child and the family. Tavistock Publications, London

Winnicott D 1958 Collective papers: through paediatrics to psycho-analysis. Tavistock Publications, London

Winnicott D 1965 The maturational processes and the facilitating environment. Hogarth Press, London

Winnicott D 1970 Therapeutic consultations in child psychiatry. Hogarth Press 1970

Wolff S 1985 Non-delinquent disturbances of conduct. In: Rutter M, Hersov L (eds) Child and adolescent psychiatry: modern approaches. Blackwell Oxford

Wolff S 1986 Child psychotherapy. In: Bloch S (ed) Introduction to the psychotherapies, 2nd edn. Oxford University Press, Oxford

Wolff S 1991 Schizoid personality in childhood and adult life: III. The childhood picture. British Journal of Psychiatry 159: 629–635

Wolff S, Chick J 1980 Schizoid personality in childhood: a controlled follow-up study. Psychological Medicine 10: 85–100

Wooley H, Stein A, Forrest G, Baum D 1989 Imparting the diagnosis of life threatening illness in children. British Medical Journal 298: 1623–1626

Wooley H, Stein A, Forrest G, Baum D 1991 Cornerstone care for families of children with life-threatening illnesses. Developmental Medicine and Child Neurology 33: 216–224

World Health Organization 1980 International classification of impairments, disabilities and handicaps. World Health Organization, Geneva

World Health Organization 1992 The ICD-10 classification of mental and behaviour disorders: clinical descriptions and diagnostic guidelines. World Health Organization, Geneva

Wynne L, Ryckoff I, Day J, Hirsch S 1958 Pseudomutuality in the family relations of schizophrenics. Psychiatry 21: 205–220

Yule W 1991 Work with children following disasters. In: Herbert M (ed) Clinical child psychology. Wiley, Chichester

Yule W, Udwin O, Murdoch K 1990 The 'Jupiter' sinking: effects on children's fears, depression and anxiety. Journal of Child Psychology and Psychiatry 71: 1051–1062

Zeitlin H 1986 Natural history of psychiatric disorder in childhood. Maudsley Monograph 29. Oxford University Press, Oxford

Zeltzer L, Jay S, Fisher D 1989 The management of pain associated with pediatric procedures. Pediatric Clinics of North America 36: 941–964

Zuker K, Green R 1991 Gender identity disorders. In: Lewis M (ed) Child and adolescent psychiatry: a comprehensive text book. Williams & Wilkins, Baltimore, MD

# Index